F.V.

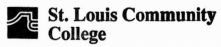

Springer Series

FOCUS ON MEN

Daniel Jay Sonkin, Ph.D., Series Editor
James H. Hennessy, Ph.D., Founding Editor

*Focus on Men provides a wide range of books on the major
psychological, medical, and social issues confronting men today.*

JORDAN I. KOSBERG, PhD, ACSW, is Professor and Coordinator of the Ph.D. Program in the School of Social Work at Florida International University (North Miami) and Faculty Associate in the University's Southeast Florida Center on Aging. Previously, he had been the Philip S. Fisher Professor, and Director of The Centre for Applied Family Studies, in the School of Social Work at McGill University (Montreal, Quebec) and Professor of Gerontology at the University of South Florida. His BS and MSW degrees are from the University of Wisconsin-Milwaukee and his Ph.D. is from the School of Social Service Administration at the University of Chicago. He is a member of the Editorial Board of the *Journal of Gerontological Social Work* and a Fellow of the Gerontological Society of America, and has been elected to the Board of Directors for the National Committee for Gerontology in Social Work Education. He has authored over 75 articles and book chapters and has edited *Working With and For the Aged* (1979), *Abuse and Maltreatment of the Elderly* (1984), *Family Care of the Elderly: Social and Cultural Changes* (1992), *International Handbook of Services for the Elderly* (1994), and *Elder Abuse in World-Wide Perspective* (1995).

LENARD W. KAYE, DSW, received his MSW from the New York University School of Social Work and his DSW from the Columbia University School of Social Work. He is Professor of Social Work and Social Research at the Graduate School of Social Work and Social Research at Bryn Mawr College. He has written widely in the field of social gerontology, and his recent books include: *Self-Help Support Groups for Older Women* (1997), *Part-Time Employment for the Lower-Income Elderly* (1997), *Controversial Issues in Aging* (1997), *New Developments in Home Care Services for the Elderly* (1995), *Home Health Care* (1992), *Congregate Housing for the Elderly* (1991), and *Men as Caregivers to the Elderly* (1991). He is currently writing a text on human services planning and administration. Dr. Kaye sits on the editorial boards of the *Journal of Gerontological Social Work* and *Geriatric Care Management Journal*, reviews manuscripts for a variety of professional journals, and is a Fellow of the Gerontological Society of America. His research interests focus on assessments of the effectiveness of innovative services for older adults.

Elderly Men

Special Problems and
Professional Challenges

Jordan I. Kosberg, PhD
Lenard W. Kaye, DSW

Editors

Springer Publishing Company

Springer Publishing Company, Inc.
536 Broadway
New York, NY 10012-3955

Cover design by: Margaret Dunin
Acquisitions Editor: Bill Tucker
Production Editor: Kathleen Kelly

Library of Congress Cataloging-in-Publication Data

Elderly men: special problems and professional challenges/edited by
    Jordan I. Kosberg and Lenard W. Kaye.
        p.   cm. — (Springer series, focus on men)
    Includes bibliographical references and index.
    ISBN 0-8261-9670-5
    1. Aged men—United States—Social conditions.   2. Aged
men—United States—Economic conditions.   3. Aged men—
United States—Psychology.   4. Social work with the aged—
United States.
    I. Kosberg, Jordan I., 1939–   .   II. Kaye, Lenard W.   III. Series.
HQ1064.U5E425   1997
305.26—DC21   97-6653
                                                                      CIP

Printed in the United States of America

I am dedicating this book to my brother, Larry, who has consistently and stoically challenged popular conventions to lead a life on his own terms, true to his values and dreams. He is the most honest person I know—to others and with himself. Age well, my brother; may the best be yet to come for you.

J. I. K.

This book is dedicated to my late father, Jerome Kaye, whose unfaltering professional energy, curiosity, and commitment to hard work served to defy stereotypes of a sedentary old age.

L. W. K.

Contents

C. SPECIAL POPULATIONS

D. SPECIAL PROBLEMS

E. FORMAL AND INFORMAL ASSISTANCE

F. CONCLUSION

Contributors

Christopher F. Abel, M.A.
Research Assistant
Department of Criminal Justice
University of Alabama
Tuscaloosa, AL

Jeffrey S. Applegate, D.S.W.
Associate Professor
Graduate School of Social Work and Social Research
Bryn Mawr College
Bryn Mawr, PA

Amanda S. Barusch, D.S.W.
Professor
Graduate School of Social Work
University of Utah
Salt Lake City, UT

Stan L. Bowie, Ph.D.
Assistant Professor
School of Social Work
Florida International University
North Miami, FL

Burton D. Dunlop, Ph.D.
Associate Director of Research
Southeast Florida Center on Aging
Florida International University
North Miami, FL

J. Kevin Eckert, Ph.D.
Professor
Department of Sociology and Anthropology
University of Maryland—Baltimore County
Baltimore, MD

Kathleen J. Farkas, Ph.D.
Associate Professor
Mandel School of Applied Social Sciences
Case Western Reserve University
Cleveland, OH

William A. Formby, Ph.D.
Associate Professor
Department of Criminal Justice
University of Alabama
Tuscaloosa, AL

George Getzel, D.S.W.
Professor
School of Social Work
Hunter College of the City
University of New York
New York, NY

Lenard W. Kaye, D.S.W.
Professor
Graduate School of Social Work and Social Research
Bryn Mawr College
Bryn Mawr, PA

Vira R. Kivett, Ph.D.
Excellence Professor
Department of Human Development and Family Studies
School of Human Environment Sciences
University of North Carolina at Greensboro
Greensboro, NC

Theodore H. Koff, Ed.D.
Director, Arizona Center on Aging
Professor, School of Public Administration and Policy

University of Arizona
Tucson, AZ

Lenore A. Kola, Ph.D.
Associate Professor
Mandel School of Applied Social Sciences
Case Western Reserve University
Cleveland, OH

Jordan I. Kosberg, Ph.D.
Professor
School of Social Work
Florida International University
North Miami, FL

John A. Krout, Ph.D.
Director
Gerontology Institute
Ithaca College
Ithaca, NY

Barry D. Lebowitz, Ph.D.
Chief
Mental Disorders of the Aging Research Branch
National Institute of Mental Health
Rockville, MD

Wiley P. Mangum, Ph.D.
Associate Professor
Department of Gerontology
University of South Florida
Tampa, FL

B. Jan McCulloch, Ph.D.
Assistant Professor
Department of Family Studies and
Sanders-Brown Center on Aging
University of Kentucky
Lexington, KY

John L. McIntosh, Ph.D.
Professor
Department of Psychology
Indiana University at South Bend
South Bend, IN

Abraham Monk, Ph.D.
Professor
School of Social Work
Columbia University
New York, NY

Terry Peak, Ph.D.
Assistant Professor
Department of Sociology, Social Work, and Anthropology
Utah State University
Logan, UT

Jane L. Pearson, Ph.D.
Chief
Clinical and Developmental Psychopathology Program
Mental Disorders of the Aging Research Branch
National Institute of Mental Health
Rockville, MD

Chandra Rambali, M.H.S.A.
Area Supervisor
American Red Cross
Miami, FL

Lucy Geissler Repaci, M.A.
Research Assistant
Center for Health Program Development and Management
University of Maryland—Baltimore County
Baltimore, MD

Max Rothman, J.D.
Executive Director
Southeast Florida Center on Aging

Florida International University
North Miami, FL

William A. Satariano, Ph.D., M.P.H.
Professor of Epidemiology and Director
Center on Aging
University of California at Berkeley
Berkeley, CA

Sheldon S. Tobin, Ph.D.
Professor
School of Social Welfare
State University of New York at Albany
Albany, NY

Donna L. Wagner, Ph.D.
Vice President for Research and Development
National Council on the Aging, Inc.
Washington, DC

Foreword

Robert L. Rubinstein, Ph.D.

Elderly Men: Special Problems and Professional Challenges represents an important landmark in understanding the lives of older men. It is one of the very few scholarly efforts aimed at synthesizing materials in a subject matter that has, for far too long, been neglected.

It is certainly the case that, in American society, elders as a group are socially devalued, As a class of persons within this larger category, older men are often shunned or unnoticed. They are truly hidden and forgotten people.

The chapters in this book are diverse, treating demography, the workplace, life in the inner city, retirement communities and prisons, rural residents, gay men, and retirement from work. Key problems of older men are also directly addressed, including health, substance abuse, and suicide, which is especially prevalent among older men. Finally, a variety of formal and informal interventions and means of assistance are described in a concluding series of chapters.

The strengths of this work, I believe, can be found in three areas, First, *Elderly Men: Special Problems and Professional Challenges* is a work that is topically comprehensive, regarding men from the perspectives of theory, social settings, social categories, special problems, and interventions. Most literature on older men rarely covers such a broad spectrum of concerns and interests. This focus makes the book truly unique. Second, this work emphasizes variation and diversity among older males. While older men represent an important and neglected social category, within this category, there can be considerable variation on the basis of key demographic variables, lifestyle, and in how social problems are experienced. For example, in terms of longevity, African-American older men may be the most disadvantaged of all groups, although men as a group have significantly less longevity than do older women.

Third, *Elderly Men: Special Problems and Professional Challenges* takes us to the point of encountering the social construction of gender as a central issue in social theory and in life as experienced individually. As with other social categories, older men are not a fixed or given entity, but emerge through socially constituting processes that involve cohort, generation, chronological and social age, gender, and the culturally constructed life course. Older men are the product of the 20th century and its political and economic, as well as social and cultural, forces.

In a sense, then, this book is the story of these forces at work in the aggregate lives of individuals. The editors and authors are to be congratulated for their efforts to shed light on these lives. There is little doubt that this book will inspire continued research on older men and issues that concern them.

Preface

Elderly men in the United States (and, indeed, around the world) have tended to be a forgotten minority who are often misunderstood and underserved. Because of their status as a numerical and proportional minority group in comparison to elderly women, the needs of older men may not receive sufficient attention by those in the health and social sciences, engaged in research activities, and practicing in the helping professions. Elderly men (themselves), their wives or partners, and children, and the general public tend not to be aware of the unique and diverse characteristics of elderly men in contemporary society.

There has been a great deal of attention directed toward elderly women in the literature and in program planning. Certainly this, in part, can be explained by the greater proportional representation of women among all elderly persons. Books have been written about them (e.g., Barusch, 1994; Lopata, 1995; Thone, 1992); periodicals are published for them (e.g., *The Women and Aging Letter*, published by the National Policy and Resource Center on Women and Aging of the American Society on Aging, and the *Journal of Women and Aging*, published by The Haworth Press, Inc.); and organizations have been formed with their specific needs in mind (e.g., the Older Women's League [OWL] and The Women's Initiative of the American Association of Retired Persons). Equivalent organizations and publications do not exist currently for elderly men. Further, book chapters on elderly minority groups often include sections on women, and subject indexes within books on aging and old age generally list many references to women's issues, but seldom are there references to elderly men.

THE CO-EDITORS

Our interest in the topic has developed independently over the years.

Jordan I. Kosberg, while a professor at Florida State University, was President of the Senior Society Planning Council in Tallahassee, Florida and, upon visiting one of the Council's three multiservice senior citizens' centers, noticed that the few men present were sitting alone and were not involved in any activities. Upon inquiring, it was learned that the programs catered to the female participants and were female-oriented and that center staff was all female.

In the 1980s, along with a colleague, Kosberg co-chaired a roundtable on elderly men as caregivers at the annual meeting of the Gerontological Society of America, which drew only a handful of participants. In 1986, Kosberg (along with Drs. Tom Rich and Wiley Mangum) presented the paper "The Older Male: A Forgotten Minority?" at the annual meeting of the Association of Gerontology in Higher Education.

And, while director of the Centre for Applied Family Studies at Montreal's McGill University, Kosberg's interest in the topic was "reignited" as result of the influence of his research associate, Dr. Germain Dulac, who was a leading writer on masculine issues in Canada. Kosberg and Dulac presented papers on elderly men at national gerontological conferences in Canada and in the United States.

Finally, for almost a decade, Kosberg has taught courses on ethical issues in aging and old age (at the University of South Florida and at McGill University) and in social work practice (at Florida International University). An important part of such a course pertains to sensitizing students to the need for gender equity, whether for younger or older women or men.

Lenard W. Kaye has been interested in the experience of men's old age for the past 20 years. His research and publications have emphasized gender comparisons in the consumption patterns of a wide range of gerontological services, including nursing home ombudsman programs, both traditional and high-technology home health care, adult day care, retirement planning programs, senior citizen centers, and congregate housing.

Interest in the differences in older men's and women's use of social and health services, and their perspectives on the aging process, came to fruition in 1988. At that time, Kaye and Dr. Jeffrey Applegate, his colleague at Bryn Mawr College's Graduate School of Social Work and Social Research, embarked on formal research aimed at presenting an in-depth analysis of older men who assume the role of caregiver for incapacitated relatives and friends. During the course of that research, Kaye and Applegate investigated men's attitudes, tasks, sources of support, and use of caregiver support groups during their engagement in the caregiving enterprise.

As a result of this work, Kaye was able to provide new insight into the impact of changing family structures and gender roles in caregiving. More than anything else, though, his work was able to promote an increased understanding of, and appreciation for, a heretofore unrecognized source of family support: the older man.

Through his continuing research, teaching, presentations, and publications, Kaye has continued to promote attention to gender in analyses of the impact of diversity in old age. His prominence in the field led Kosberg to invite him to appear on the symposium on "Elderly Men: Research Findings and Applied Ramifications" during the 1994 annual scientific meetings of the Gerontological Society of America. It was at this time that Kosberg and Kaye first began to consider the possibility of a book of readings on elderly men.

ORGANIZATION OF THE BOOK

The book provides an overview of elderly men and the problems they face which affect the quality of their lives from social, cultural, psychological, physical, and economic perspectives. It supplies the reader with helpful insights on common and unique features of elderly men, relative to elderly women, in the aging process and in old age. The heterogeneity of elderly men is discussed in relation to race, ethnicity, religion, social class, and other important sociodemographic variables. Readers should be aware that discussions of elderly men, as a group, are always in danger of over-generalization, and that there is a need for specificity regarding any reference to an elderly man and to groups of elderly men.

As the co-editors are social workers, the book has an applied, rather than a theoretical, perspective. Accordingly, a portion of each chapter focuses upon appropriate interventive efforts (whether clinical, pro-grammatic, or policy-formulation) which attempt to meet the specific needs of elderly male populations. The chapters address the needs of elderly men through alternative interventions including community-based programs, institutionally based care, and therapeutic and support group efforts.

Research has found that elderly men face a greater likelihood of experiencing certain types of problems and challenges which result from their masculine socialization, lifestyles, and health conditions. The organization of chapters emanates out of such considerations, and the list of chapters included is meant to be more indicative of various issues facing elderly persons than to be all-inclusive. Admittedly, there are important areas which are not addressed in this book. Rather than having specific chapters on elderly men from particular ethnic, racial, religious, and social class groups, *each chapter* pays attention to such important considerations.

A final chapter summarizes and integrates the material covered in the chapters of the book. This chapter makes projections about likely social changes in elderly men in the future which affects their relationships with spouses and significant others, lifestyles, family responsibilities, and work histories. Such changes, in turn, are discussed with regard to the needs of future cohorts of elderly men, and the steps that must be taken to meet their needs.

THE AUTHORS

Having established the general parameters and objectives for the book, we sought to identify experts to write the specific chapters. In most instances, we were familiar with individuals who had developed reputa-tions for research and/or writing on the elderly, as a group, with regard to particular topics. Yet, in the majority of cases, these experts—when contacted and asked to write a chapter for a book on elderly men— indicated that they had not focused their work specifically upon such a subgroup of the elderly. To their credit, all who were asked were undaunted and agreed to undertake the challenge. Those who were initially contacted were free to involve others as co-authors. It is expected that for many of the authors or co-authors, this initial effort focusing upon elderly men might result in further work by them specifically on elderly men or on gender-related comparative analyses.

Without many exceptions, the authors produced their chapters in a timely fashion and were sympathetic to our task of ensuring that each chapter be written with clarity, and in a format and language somewhat comparable across chapters. Authors generally adhered to the maximum length of pages set for chapters. It should be noted that Chapter Twelve, "Mental Disorders of Elderly Men," is lengthier than the others. This anomaly is based upon the request made by the original authors of two separate chapters on mental health and on suicide to combine their efforts, given the overlap of material and its implications within the two chapters. It should be noted, also, that authors were asked to limit the number of references utilized in a chapter. The purpose was to have authors write in a more definitive than a scholarly fashion, and to permit the use of more pages for substantive text and less for bibliography. Most (including the editors themselves!) were not able to exorcise their usual writing style and limit the references to the requested number.

JIK and LWK
January, 1997

REFERENCES

Barusch, A. S. (1994). *Older women in poverty: Private lives in public places.* New York: Springer.

Lopata, H. Z. (1995). *Current widowhood: Myths and realities.* Thousand Oaks, CA: Sage Publications.

Thone, R. R. (1992). *Women and aging: Celebrating ourselves.* New York: The Haworth Press.

A. Introduction

CHAPTER 1

Theorizing Older Men

Jeffrey S. Applegate, D.S.W.

In a popular mid-1990s television advertisement, a convivial quartet of white men, dressed in farm clothes and appearing to be in their 60s or 70s, gathers in a country diner for a breakfast of Rice Krispies cereal. On a cue, they lift their bowls in unison in order to better hear the cereal's trademark "snap, crackle and pop," provoking a bemused, indulgent smirk from a nearby waitress. In another ad for this product, the same group assembles on a rural front porch where they share Rice Krispies squares prepared by a female acquaintance. When one of the men expresses surprise at another's delight at the low-fat content of this confection, the latter man exclaims, to chuckles all around, "How do you think I keep my girlish figure!"

What is the viewing public to make of this humorous, seemingly benign ad campaign? At first, we might be heartened by the inclusion of older men in television advertising, a medium so dominated by images of youth. Moreover, in a medium that typically depicts older people as preoccupied with chronic ailments, the apparent health and well-being of these men strike a positive chord. But a second glance reveals more troubling messages. These men appear in bucolic settings, suggesting that they have been put out to pasture. Their basic needs apparently met, they have so much idle time on their hands that they must find entertainment in listening to their cereal. They are depicted as childlike and, especially in the second scenario, feminized. Their lives appear to be organized around quotidian trivia.

Such public images both reflect and shape the contemporary discourse on older men—a discourse characterized by lack of attention to their diversity and the nuanced complexity of their lives. This chapter examines some of the theories and assumptions that have influenced this discourse and considers the utility of a contemporary process-focused conceptual model that may be helpful in informing 21st-century research, service, and social policy related to older men.

THE DISCOVERY OF OLDER MEN

Among the unanticipated consequences of the Women's Movement was the opening of a conceptual space for critical inquiry about men. Prior to the societal push for women's liberation and the simultaneous development of women's studies in the academy, men were assumed and implicit in social and behavioral theory. The assumption of men and men's experience as the human norm kept women and women's experience in the background, thus obscuring them. Paradoxically, men's position in the foreground had the effect of obscuring the differences among them as well (Brod, 1987). But in the last 20 years, scholars have drawn attention to men's diversity through inquiry about the costs and benefits of male privilege, as well as about differences in men associated with their race, ethnicity, social class, bodily ability, religion, and sexual orientation. Gay studies in particular have contributed to an expanded appreciation of the rich array of masculinities among men. Such inquiry has begun to erode the traditional monolithic view of men by capturing the pluralism of their lives.

There remains, however, a blind spot in this widening perspective. Older men have been strikingly absent from mainstream men's studies. As Thompson (1994) points out in the lead chapter of the only recent book on the topic, they have been largely ignored by gerontology as well. Thompson suggests several factors that converge to explain this oversight. Until very recently, elderly men as well as women were grouped by the Bureau of the Census into the age band "65 and over," a catchall category that had the effect of glossing over their diversity and reducing them to a demographic afterthought. Now that life expectancies are increasing and the numbers of older people are burgeoning, distinct age groups, ranging from the "young elderly" (65–69) to the "very elderly" (85 and over), are explicated.

Earlier categories, while homogenizing older people of both sexes, were particularly obscuring of men, who were and continue to be in the minority due to the well-documented sex ratio in a longevity that overwhelmingly favors women. Because fewer older men than women reach old age, inquiry about them has seemed irrelevant. And those men reaching old age have often been perceived as physically impaired or sick, a stereotype reinforced by a booming medical industry that thrives on such procedures as angioplasty, cardiac bypass surgery, and the installation of pacemakers. This medicalization of older men not only focuses attention away from prevention, but further conceals their diversity by keeping their nonmedical needs in the shadows, ignoring the concerns of the majority who enjoy good health.

Indeed, more men are living longer and healthier lives. The sex difference in life expectancy is likely to narrow as more women experience the rise in mortality associated with full-time paid employment. Demographers predict that a swelling army of male baby boomers, privileged by advances in health care and increased longevity, can expect to march, as Thompson (1994) puts it, "deep into the Third Age" (p. 6).

Defining older men by comparing their life expectancy to that of women has had the effect of conflating sex and gender in ways that have concealed older men's experience as gendered social beings. In gerontological scholarship, gender is often used as a synonym for sex, a practice that keeps the focus on sex differences rather than on the range of masculinities among older men. By differentiating gender, a social construction, from sex, a biological distinction, newer scholars can look more carefully at the plurality of older men's lives and experiences.

Focusing on older men, however, has been controversial in some sectors of the academy. Socially, older men have fared better than their female counterparts. As a group, they tend to have more assets, fewer debts, and are much more likely than older women to live with a spouse and benefit from the enhanced morale and social support afforded by this arrangement. Their resulting advantages in life satisfaction and well-being render them less interesting to researchers than older women, whose stresses and burdens are amplified by reduced financial security, social disadvantage, and domestic isolation. Older men's smaller numbers and apparently privileged status mean that they are also less apt to attract research funds than are their disenfranchised female counterparts.

But the idealized view of older men as a privileged gerontocracy fades when we look beyond the confines of the white, middle-class, traditionally structured nuclear family. Thompson (1994) reminds us, for example, that older African-American and Hispanic men are far less likely than white men to live with a spouse. Moreover, heterosexual men who are widowed, those who never married, and gay men have been largely overlooked in inquiry about older men's lives. Thompson concludes that "the diversity among young and middle-aged men does not disappear at age 65, 70, or 75, when older men leave the workplace to take up more assiduously their semipublic and private social worlds. Their gendered lives continue" (p. 15). But research and theory-building have not reflected this diversity. It is as though once men meet and presumably resolve the midlife crisis, they drift into a never-never land of degendered homogeneity. This perception constitutes a subtle yet insidious form of sexism and ageism whose origins can be traced to the psychologizing of aging so prevalent in our most treasured behavioral and social theories.

OLDER MEN IN LIFE-STAGE THEORY

The idea of specific age ranges and concomitant age-driven concerns and behavior is relatively new, appearing in the late 19th century and laying the groundwork for a "categorized age consciousness" (Brok, 1992, p. 173) that we have come to take for granted. Motivated by the modernist penchant for classification and building on Freud's division of early life into specific psychosexual states, a number of well-known theorists began to conceptualize adult development as a series of recognizable periods with predictable characteristic markers. Most influential on gerontological inquiry has been the work of Erikson (1959), whose well-known eight-stage model is still widely employed in thinking about older people's lives. As Erikson conceived it, successful development through successive life stages requires the mastery of key developmental tasks and the resolution of associated developmental crises. Most pertinent to elderly men is Stage Eight, called Older Adulthood, whose defining developmental polarity is Ego Integrity versus Despair and Disgust. In this stage, healthy resolution presumably results in wisdom born of a serene acceptance of the fundamental integrity of one's life as it was lived. Failure to achieve this acceptance results in a fear of death, despair that time is running out, and a general misanthropy that may be projected onto other people or institutions. Based on the principle of epigenesis, this deterministic conceptual model assumes that failures in earlier life stages will haunt the "final" stage, compromising the older man's capacity to transcend previous difficulties in order to forge new perspectives.

A stage model applied explicitly to adult male development was introduced by Levinson and his associates (Levinson, Darrow, Klein, Levinson, & McKee, 1978), whose book, *The Seasons of a Man's Life*, reported findings from a sample of 40 men drawn from four occupational groups: hourly workers in industry, business executives, university biologists, and novelists. From biographical interviews, Levinson et al. concluded that men's lives evolve in an orderly sequence of stable "eras" punctuated by 4- to 5-year unsettled "transitional periods." Devoting only seven pages of a lengthy book to late adulthood, the authors suggest that, in response to bodily decline, death, or serious illness of loved ones, medical wake-up calls, and increasingly peripheral social status, older men turn inward to become preoccupied with "immediate bodily needs and personal comforts" (p. 38) as well as with the specter of their mortality and its philosophical implications. Such interiority is believed to promote reflective integration of the positive and negative aspects of one's life. Failure to achieve this integration may result in depression and anxiety related to an exaggerated fear of death and a sense of incompletion.

These and other popular stage theories posit a kind of either-or outcome, suggesting that those older men who fail to come to grips with previous developmental vulnerabilities and consolidate a coherent personal meaning system end life unhappily. Such a polarized view fails to capture the intricate complexity and variability of older men's lives, either idealizing or catastrophizing them. More realistically, older men will have lived lives characterized by ambiguity, uncertainty, struggles, triumphs, good days and bad. Similarly, their later years are likely to be composed of periods of relative serenity and well-being, bouts of depression and anxiety, and the range of affective experiences in between. The timing and intensity of these subjective experiences will vary widely according to health status, finances, levels of social support, and other variables.

Moreover, stage models are tethered to an Anglo-Western conception of the nuclear family and a family life cycle which evolves through heterosexual marriage, child-rearing, the empty nest, and, for men, retirement from a fulfilling career. As late 20th-century culture wreaks havoc on the traditional life cycle, stage models of adult development become increasingly obsolete in understanding aging. Predictable crises and transitions seem doomed to extinction, upended by an economy requiring two incomes per family, increasing life expectancy, soaring divorce and remarriage rates, the growing incidence of nonmarital cohabitation, and the gay liberation movement. The family of the 1950s, comprised of a man who provides economically for a wife who stays home to raise the children, now represents only about 12% of American society (Skolnick & Skolnick, 1989).

Nevertheless, one of the most influential and enduring psychological theories informing contemporary gerontology depends on a model of traditional family structure organized around childbearing. First proposed in the 1950s and kept in the spotlight by a recent book by Gutmann (1987), this theory suggests that, as people reach their middle and later years and move beyond parenthood, they naturally become more androgynous. Middle-aged and older men are believed to "reclaim" the feminine aspects of their identity that they have had to repress earlier in order to fulfill their roles as providers and protectors of the dependent mother-child dyad. According to this idea, once the "parental emergency" is past, there is a natural relaxation of the previously necessary gender role rigidity, and postparental men can enjoy the nurturant, affiliative aspects of their personalities that have been put on hold.

While this theory has the benefit of a strengths perspective that makes it possible to view aging as a period of developmental integration, it remains tied to the essentialist idea that men's life course is based on the biological reproductive imperative and its associated cultural conventions. Although Gutmann's (1987) cross-cultural findings offer some support for such an idea, other research fails to find support either for universally appearing gendered distinctions associated with the child-rearing cycle or for a masculine-to-feminine shift in older men (Solomon, 1982; Thompson, 1994). In contexts where such a shift is observed, it may be that the perception of older men as more feminine has more to do with their moving from rigidly institutionalized roles to more informal and tenuous ones than it does with postparental sex role flexibility. To grow old in the patriarchy, for example, may mean that men increasingly share the marginalized status of women and are, therefore, perceived as more womanlike. Further, this theory fails to account for men who do not become parents or who in other ways depart from the mainstream heterosexual norm.

SOCIAL THEORY AND THE OLDER MAN

We might assume that social theory captures the diversity of older men's lives more comprehensively; yet few social theories have looked at older men specifically. Among the most pertinent to the inquiry are role theory, activity theory, disengagement theory, continuity theory, and socioenvironmental theory, comprehensively reviewed and summarized by Fry (1992).

Role theory holds that aging brings a potentially traumatic loss of familiar roles, especially occupational and other institutionalized roles wherein behaviors and experiences are clearly defined. Looking at older men specifically, traditional socialization to clearly defined sex roles plays a crucial part in this scenario. In a culture that rewards men for their occupational success, their positions in male-dominated hierarchies of influence, their financial achievement, and their physical vigor, such life events as retirement, widowerhood, and physical illness or disability can, according to this theory, erode familiar role attachments and their accompanying sense of personal and social power.

Similarly, activity theory suggests that a decline in customary activity levels contributes to decreased well-being among older people. From this perspective, services and policies which promote continuation of familiar activities into old age can have preventive as well as salutary effects. Disengagement theory hypothesizes that, as people age, they naturally and inevitably become less involved with institutional structures of society, have less energy for social intercourse, and invest less in relationships with others. For aging men, this view implies disengagement from careers, withdrawal from previously meaningful social organizations and activities, and the loss of status associated with male privilege in these institutional structures. If things go well, men reach a gradual acceptance of this disengagement and place increasing value on introspection.

Continuity theory asserts that, despite role loss, activity decline and social disengagement, people's unique patterns of traits and behaviors persist across the life span into old age and retain their predictability. Although earlier versions of this theory betray a deterministic bent, more contemporary versions suggest that, while basic personality traits may persist over time, there is room for considerable variability in relation to varying life contexts of older men.

An emphasis on changing contexts for aging is highlighted in socioenvironmental theories of aging which focus on the dynamic inter-action between people's individual resources and the social resources available to them. In contrast to the linear perspective undergirding most social theories, socioenvironmental theory takes an ecosystemic person-in-environment approach. But, like other psychological and social theories informing the study of aging, most socioenvironmental inquiry fails to treat gender and other politically charged aspects of diversity as contextual factors in older men's lives. To learn more about the influence of these factors as they shape the experience of aging for men, we must turn to the growing body of scholarship that emerges primarily from profeminist men's studies and takes a political economy perspective.

POLITICAL ECONOMY THEORY
AND OLDER MEN'S LIVES

In contrast to prevalent biopsychosocial models for examining aging, a political economy perspective concentrates on the way in which the status and resources of elderly people are connected to their class position in the social structure and to other variables in the overall socio-economic, political, and cultural environment. According to this view, the age at which pivotal life events like retirement and loss of a partner occur is socially structured and carries social and political meaning in relation to gender, class, race, religion, and sexual orientation.

In this framework, gender is explicitly distinguished from biological sex assignment and is viewed as a primary category for understanding the personal and social world. Here, gender is regarded as a set of power relations that are both socially structured and individually embodied. From this perspective patriarchy is seen, not just as a system of men's power over women, but as a complex of hierarchies of power among different groups of men and among various masculinities (Kaufman, 1994). For example, degendered or feminized images of older men in the media keep in the forefront a masculinity that sustains the economic primacy of younger men.

Such social messages contribute to a defining paradox in many older men's lives—their contradictory experiences of power. As men, they are likely to have reaped the benefits of the aggregate mantle of privilege bestowed on them by the patriarchy; but, as older people, they are subject to ageist stereotypes that erode their sense of personal power and self-efficacy. Furthermore, the implicit privilege enjoyed by some groups of older men does not extend across racial, ethnic, and class lines. The broad economic expansion of the last 40 years that has profited white, well-educated, middle-class, employed men has eluded many working-class or unemployed men of color, groups for whom such goals as a planned-for comfortable retirement may be no more than an elusive dream. Even the class of men who have traditionally benefited from steady and lucrative employment faces an uncertain future in today's climate of fiscal austerity, company downsizing, declining unionization, and a shrinking manufacturing sector.

A political economy perspective also opens the door of inquiry to the variety of alternative life choices and life styles of older men. Older gay men, for example, have been stereotyped and stigmatized as marginal and lonely, sexually obsessed but unfulfilled. Recent research sketches a strikingly different, more affirmative picture. As reported in a book edited by Lee (1991), most older gay men report being neither unhappy, isolated, nor sexually inactive. Many take pride in having helped lay the social groundwork for the gay liberation movement, are in stable, loving partnerships, and enjoy valued positions in the gay community. Those stresses they experience appear to come less from personal dysphoria than from instances of institutional, legal, social service, and medical discrimination or oversight associated with homophobia.

In summary, the political economy perspective encourages a holistic, sociostructural approach to understanding the diversity that character-izes contemporary aging in general and older men's and women's lives in particular. Some critics worry that, in emphasizing this diversity, inquiry can lapse into individualized pluralism that risks detracting attention from the overarching structures of power and oppression that infiltrate whole groups and classes of older people. The challenge to theorists interested in older men is to preserve a degree of creative tension between the recognition of gender, race, class, and other politically meaningful factors, and an appreciation of the uniqueness of their individual perceptions and subjective experiences.

CONSTRUCTIVISM AND OLDER MEN

One effort to embrace this tension takes the form of a constructivist view of aging as lived experience. From this standpoint, a focus on instrumental, social, and politically structured meanings must be balanced by an equal emphasis on personally constructed meanings. As postmodernism raises questions about the suitability of the logical positivist paradigm for social science inquiry, constructivist theory suggests that subjective perceptions of experience constitute the only meaningful individual reality. Using this perspective, aging is seen as "a process of change in personal constructions over time, resulting from the reciprocal interplay between the biological and psychological processes of the organism and the social, cultural and historical contexts in which the individual is embedded" (Reker & Wong, 1988, p. 217).

Proponents of this interpretive paradigm suggest that we cannot make generalized statements about older people of either gender or about people of different races, classes, or sexual orientations. They propose instead taking a "personal existence" view of growing older—one that moves inquiry from a deficit framework of irretrievable decline and deterioration to a competence approach that focuses on self-creative potentials in the aging process. Kenyon (1988), for example, suggests that cognitive development in older people moves beyond Piagetian formal operational thought, traditionally seen as the pinnacle of cognitive development from which older people gradually retreat, to achieve more complex "dialectical operations" wherein contradictions are welcomed rather than avoided and an expanded capacity for knowledge synthesis appears. Here a life-events perspective becomes important, so that deterministic theories of aging are replaced by context-specific examinations of concrete actions and perceptions of individual persons in their unique social worlds. In relation to older men, inquiry moves from viewing them in terms of biological, psychological, or social-structural generalizations to considering the lived experiences of individual men as subjectively constructed. How do specific older men, in other words, make meaning of their changing biopsychosocial circumstances?

A PROCESS MODEL FOR CONCEPTUALIZING OLDER MEN'S LIVES

A contemporary process-focused model for looking at adult development, developed by Settlage and his associates (1988), offers a promising additional conceptual tool for thinking about older men. These researchers proceed from a definition of development that, while making room for temporary decline and regression, emphasizes outcomes that are forward and new. Even in late adulthood, when decline or losses of physical function, relationships, and resources may occur, changes are viewed as catalysts for new development and revised conceptions of the self.

According to this conceptualization, the primary stimulus for development at any age is disturbance of previously adequate self-regulatory and adaptive functioning. Different kinds of stimuli can set the developmental process in motion: (1) biological maturation or physical change; (2) environmental change, expectation, or demand; (3) losses or traumatic experiences; and/or (4) the perception of possibilities of achieving improved adaptation. Any of these stimuli singularly or in combination may create an unsettled state accompanied by varying degrees of mental and emotional stress. If not overwhelming, this stress serves to initiate a sequence of development.

First the individual perceives and accepts a *developmental challenge*, examples of which can be a need for new skills, new ways of regulating feelings, or new attitudes and values. Acceptance of the challenge sets the developmental process in motion and transforms the unsettled state into a more organized and goal-oriented state. With the need for change more apparent, the gap between where the individual is and where he or she wants or needs to be creates *developmental tension*. Unlike the negatively experienced disequilibrium of the previously unsettled state, this tension is positive and motivational. *Developmental conflict* results as the desire for change typically evokes fears of loss of the security experienced in the previous adaptation; fears of failure; or anxieties about unknown or imagined negative consequences of change. Typically, this period of conflict is transitory and abates with *resolution of developmental conflict* through mastery of new skills and the gradual integration of new ways of coping and adapting. Finally, this integration of alternative modes of functioning results in a *change in self-representation* and a revised view of the meaning ascribed to the original challenge. The results of successfully traversing this developmental process can include formation of a new function, refinement or expansion of a preexisting function, more flexible application of an existing function, and/or reorganization of cognitive and emotional structures toward a higher level of functioning.

This nonstage process model provides a way of individualizing older men's concerns and experiences in ways that can include consideration of their race, ethnicity, social class, physical ability, sexual orientation, religion and other aspects of their diversity. It permits consideration of the wide variety of situations that may challenge different older men in different ways. While recognizing their vulnerabilities, the model proceeds from a strengths perspective that searches out and builds on people's competencies.

In a study of older men who were called on to act as primary caregivers to an elderly relative (Kaye & Applegate, 1990), for example, it became clear that the prospect of caregiving confronted them with a developmental challenge for which many felt unprepared and ill-equipped. For some, the need to provide personal care and emotional sustenance challenged previous sex-role socialization that had prepared them for instrumental rather than for expressive functioning. Once the disequilibrium created by the challenge began to settle, most men experienced a positively motivating tension that led them to find out what they needed to learn in order to become capable caregivers. For some, the gap between their felt competencies and what they felt they needed to know created considerable conflict. Such conflict typically began to resolve, however, when they transferred to caregiving the organizational and time-management skills that had been effective in their work environments. With the creative integration of previously functional roles into a new context, many experienced a shift in their sense of themselves and felt pride and satisfaction in their new capabilities. It is not that these men had become more androgynous or feminized; rather, the developmental challenge posed by the need for them to become caregivers enabled them to change in flexible ways that were not so rigidly sex-role defined. They transposed and modified skills that were once effective in formal, rigidly institutionalized roles to the "softer," informal roles associated with caregiving.

A process model of late life development makes it possible to reframe such pivotal life events as retirement, physical decline, death or disability of a partner, or a change in economic status as challenges which, while distressing, are also potentially motivational of new development. Since developmental challenges can be viewed as arising from the environment as well, such oppressive social conditions as poverty, racial discrimination, ageism, and homophobia can also be considered potential targets for change.

In assessing the need for person-environment intervention, examination of the various points in the developmental sequence may be useful. Where in the sequence is the individual in need of service? Is he still experiencing the disequilibrium of a traumatic life event? In a post-crisis period of tension, with greater readiness to consider new coping strategies? In need of assistance, with conflicts aroused by the necessity for change? Or on the way to resolution of conflict and needing to work reflectively on modifications in self-concept already in progress? From this perspective, those planning interventions can consider where in the developmental sequence particular strengths and vulnerabilities lie— not just in terms of personality or other individual variables, but in relation to the socioeconomic and political forces that may be impeding the developmental process. Intervention at these macrosystem levels might include social activism, advocacy, and social policy reform.

IMPLICATIONS AND CONCLUSION

Process-focused models like the one described here have the advantages of cohering and synthesizing insights from a wide variety of ways of knowing and thinking about older men's lives and experiences. Such models permit scholars to consider the variations in older men's lives and the wide range of masculinities they express. This expanded perspective helps service planners and providers keep in check the tendency to homogenize older men while preserving their awareness of larger social-structural, institutional, and cultural forces that silently shape the lives of various constituencies.

Many of the life-stage and other theoretical frameworks reviewed in this chapter promote a tendency to idealize older men's lives, as though smooth and successful development in previous periods can lead to an old age of serenity, acceptance of limitations, and satisfaction from a life well lived. Those working in the human services know that the picture is much more complex and that a comfortable, financially secure old age eludes many. Similarly, developmental process models can foster looking for hopeful potentials in situations where few exist. While a minority, for example, many older men develop illnesses and disabilities that lead to their institutionalization in nursing homes or other continuing care facilities. As their longevity increases, many will face chronic conditions that virtually assure some level of dependency. Services to the most severely impaired will likely involve more intensive levels of costly care at a time in history when such previously dependable benefits as Social Security, Medicare, and Medicaid can no longer be taken for granted. A primary focus on such concerns, however, tends to perpetuate a discourse that compares older men to "productive" younger men and is dominated by the question, "What are we going to do with all these burdensome, impaired old men?" A more balanced, affirmative, and prevention-oriented posture will result only by studying older men *qua* older men, thus uncoupling their identities and concerns from invidious comparisons to the cultures of youth and work.

Indeed, impending changes in the ecology of elder care pose a developmental challenge to the field of aging and aging studies. The complexities of planning services for and studying older people are numerous and formidable. In this period of unprecedented social change, occurring in tandem with a paradigm shift in the academy toward a postmodern climate for inquiry, the growing interest in narrative and other interpretive qualitative research methods may prove especially pertinent to gerontology. Along with traditional methods that help track large group phenomena, these and other research innovations can facilitate creative engagement of the inevitable tension and conflict aroused by the changing face of aging and can lead to new and more effective ways of understanding and assisting 21st-century older men.

REFERENCES

Brod, H. (Ed.). (1987). *The making of masculinities: The new men's studies.* Boston: Allen & Bacon.

Brok, A. J. (1992). Some thoughts on gender role issues for men later in life. In B. R. Wainrib (Ed.), *Gender issues across the life cycle* (pp. 172–183). New York: Springer.

Erikson, E. H. (1959). *Identity and the life cycle.* New York: International Universities Press.

Fry, P. S. (1992). Major social theories of aging and their implications for counseling concepts and practice: A critical review. *The Counseling Psychologist, 20,* 246–329.

Gutmann, D. (1987). *Reclaimed powers: Toward a new psychology of men and women in later life.* New York: Basic Books.

Kaufman, M. (1994). Men, feminism, and men's contradictory experiences of power. In H. Brod & M. Kaufman (Eds.), *Theorizing masculinities* (pp. 142–163). Thousand Oaks, CA: Sage.

Kaye, L. W., & Applegate, J. S. (1990). *Men as caregivers to the elderly: Understanding and aiding unrecognized family support.* Lexington, MA: Lexington Books.

Kenyon, G. M. (1988). Basic assumptions in theories of human aging. In J. E. Birren & V. L. Bengtson (Eds.), *Emergent theories of aging* (pp. 3–18). New York: Springer.

Lee, J. A. (Ed.). (1991). *Gay midlife and maturity.* New York: Haworth.

Levinson, D. J., Darrow, C. N., Klein, E. B., Levinson, M. H., & McKee, B. (1978). *The seasons of a man's life.* New York: Ballantine Books.

Reker, G. L., & Wong, P. T. P. (1988). Aging as an individual process: Toward a theory of personal meaning. In J. E. Birren & V. L. Bengston (Eds.), *Emergent theories of aging* (pp. 214–246). New York: Springer.

Settlage, C. F., Curtis, J., Lozoff, M., Lozoff, M., Silberschatz, G., & Simburg, E. J. (1988). Conceptualizing adult development. *Journal of the American Psychoanalytic Association, 36,* 347–369.

Skolnick, A. S., & Skolnick, J. H. (1989). *Family in transition: Rethinking marriage, sexuality and children* (6th ed.). Glenview, IL: Scott Foresman.

Solomon, K. (1982). The older man. In K. Solomon & N. B. Levy (Eds.), *Men in transition: Theory and therapy* (pp. 205–240). New York: Plenum.

Thompson, E. H., Jr. (1994). Older men as invisible men in contemporary society. In E. H. Thompson, Jr., (Ed.), *Older men's lives* (pp. 1–21). Thousand Oaks, CA: Sage.

CHAPTER 2

A Demographic Overview of Elderly Men

Wiley P. Mangum, Ph.D.

The intent of this chapter is to locate elderly men in demographic space. Demographic space, similar in conception to social space and an aspect of it, refers to the set of demographic characteristics found among the inhabitants of a particular social environment, ranging from a cocktail party to a national society. The focus here is on elderly men in the United States, each of whom has various ascribed and achieved demographic characteristics such as age, racial/ethnic identity, marital status, educational level, and occupational status that, along with personality characteristics and environmental experiences, define the individual to himself and others through self-reflection and social interaction. In addition to their defining function, or perhaps because of it, demographic characteristics exert a powerful influence on the life chances of an individual. A 65-year-old man with a degree from a major university, a prestigious job, and who is happily married is likelier to have had a better quality of life and better prospects for the future than another 65-year-old man who is a never-married high school dropout with a modest job.

Before considering some major demographic characteristics of elderly men, however, it is necessary to ponder the question: Who, chronologically, are elderly men? Are they men 65 years of age and over, the administrative threshold established by the Social Security Act for eligible persons to receive standard retirement benefits and, thus, one traditional benchmark for the beginning of old age in our society? Are they men 62 years of age and over, another administrative threshold for receiving early and reduced Social Security retirement benefits or for eligibility for federally assisted housing for the elderly? Are they men 60 years of age and over, the age of eligibility for receiving services under the Older Americans Act? Are they men 55 years of age and over, eligible for treatment in community mental health centers as older clients? Are they, even, men 40 years of age and over, defined as older workers by the Age Discrimination in Employment Act? Each of these ages is used to define older age groups in American society for administrative purposes, and each is largely arbitrary. Nevertheless, an administratively defining age can have major practical and psychosocial consequences for the individuals involved and, for a particular analytic/descriptive purpose, it is necessary to select and use one or more of them. Because available summary demographic data for older age groups are usually presented for persons 65 years of age and over, this age group will generally provide the chronological point of reference for this discussion. Unless otherwise noted, all demographic data presented in this chapter are from the *Statistical Abstract of the United States, 1994* (U.S. Bureau of the Census, 1995a).

The concept of demographic space refers not only to a set of demographic characteristics held by the inhabitants of a social environment; as an aspect of social space, it also implies social relationships among them. Thus, although the focus of this chapter is on elderly men, these men will generally be viewed in relation to elderly women and, occasionally, in relation to younger persons. This will permit conventionally meaningful comparisons to be made, as with income and marital status where there are major gender differences, or in labor force participation, where there are major age group differences. In addition, this will make it possible to view particular characteristics of elderly men, vis-à-vis elderly women, as being either arguably advantageous or disadvantageous for elderly men in socially or physically significant ways. This chapter will begin, however, with some simple demographic facts about elderly men and women: their numbers and percentages in the U.S. population and the associated sex ratios.

NUMBERS, PERCENTAGES, AND SEX RATIOS
OF ELDERLY MALES AND FEMALES
IN THE UNITED STATES

As of November 22, 1995, the U.S. Bureau of the Census projected, via its online PopClock Projection, the resident population of the United States to be 26,378,984 (U.S. Bureau of the Census, 1995b). Of these, approximately 49% were males and 51% were females. Using 65 years of age and over as the threshold of "elderly," and numbers from a census estimate as of September 1, 1995, there were approximately 33,609,000 elderly persons in the United States, representing 12.8% of the total population. Of these, 40.8% were elderly males and 59.2% were elderly females, an appreciable percentage point decrease for the former and an increase for the latter relative to the earlier percentages of males and females without regard to age.

It is well known that older females outnumber older males in the United States and other industrialized societies, but a downward shift in the sex ratio, or number of men per 100 women, occurs long before old age. As Treas (1995, p. 3) has noted, "Although about 105 boys are born for every 100 girls, women outnumber men by age 30 because of . . . higher male mortality rates." By age 65 and older, the sex ratio has become highly skewed, and varies considerably among racial/ethnic groups. It is 69 for older whites (i.e., 69 older white males per 100 older white females); 63 among older African-Americans, and 76 among older Asians. While demographers and gerontologists have long been aware of and concerned about low sex ratios among older persons, with more females than males in all racial/ethnic groups, Treas (1995, p. 3) makes the socially significant point:

> The long downward slide in the sex ratio for older adults came to a surprising halt during the 1980s, probably because deaths from heart disease declined significantly for men but not for women. If the sex differential in mortality continues to narrow, it may help equalize the number of men and women in the older population and ease some of the loneliness, poverty, and other ill effects of an extremely low sex ratio.

Whether this will actually happen, only time will tell but, as Table 2.1 shows, increasing sex ratios among older persons from 1992 onward will provide numerical support for this possibility.

TABLE 2.1   Ratio of Males to Females, by Age Group, 1950 to 1992, and Projections, 2000 and 2025

Age	1950	1960	1970	1980	1990	1992	Projections 2000	2025
All ages	**98.6**	**97.1**	**94.8**	**94.5**	**95.1**	**95.3**	**95.7**	**96.3**
Under 14 years	103.7	103.4	103.9	104.6	104.9	104.9	105.2	105.4
14 to 24 years	98.2	98.7	98.7	101.9	104.6	104.6	104.4	104.7
25 to 44 years	96.4	95.7	95.5	97.4	98.9	99.2	99.1	98.6
45 to 64 years	100.1	95.7	91.6	90.7	92.5	93.1	94.1	94.2
65 years and over	89.6	82.8	72.1	67.6	67.2	67.8	70.5	82.0

Note: From *Statistical Abstract of the United States, 1994* (Table 14, p. 15), by the U.S. Bureau of the Census, 1995. Washington, DC: U.S. Government Printing Office.

Note first, in Table 2.1, that for persons less than 25 years of age, the sex ratio is either close to 100—indicating equal numbers of males and females—or over 100—indicating more males than females. When "All ages" are considered, the sex ratio is in the mid- to high 90s for the years shown, indicating rough numerical parity between males and females in American society. When persons 65 years of age and over are singled out, considerable variability emerges, but there are always more women than men in the population. For the years shown, numerical parity between men and women was at its highest in 1950, with a sex ratio of 89.6 and declined from decade to decade after that until 1990, where it reached a low point of 67.2. In 1992, however, the sex ratio increased slightly to 67.8, and is projected to reach 82.0 in the year 2025. It will still be below its 1950 level of 89.6, but it may be high enough to support Treas' (1995) earlier sanguine prediction about a possible decrease in the loneliness and poverty of older women because of the greater availability of older men. Numerical disparities between older males and females may interact with their major vital and sociodemographic characteristics to produce differences in quality of life and life satisfaction.

SOCIODEMOGRAPHIC CHARACTERISTICS OF OLDER MEN AND WOMEN

Life Expectancy

Next to the number and percentage of older persons in a population, life expectancy is, perhaps, the most frequently cited statistic in discussions of aging. As a social indicator, it immediately reflects something about the conditions of life in the social entity being described. Generally, the more favorable the conditions of life, the higher the life expectancy. More developed regions of the world have higher life expectancies than do less developed regions (Brown, 1996). Life expectancy is also a matter of gender. The imbalanced sex ratio between older males and females is, as noted earlier, a result of mortality differences between them. Such differences are reflected in life expectancy, which varies considerably between older males and females. In 1900, life expectancy in the United States for white males was 48.2 years, meaning that a white male born in 1900 could expect, on the average, to live to be 48.2 years old. For white females born in 1900, life expectancy was 51.1 years, an advantage of 2.9 years over white males. By contrast, males and females who were of "Other racial categories" had life expectancies of 32.5 and 35.0, respectively. Such racial/ethnic differences in expectation of life at birth have persisted throughout this century, although they are less marked at the present time than in the past. By 1992, life expectancy had increased to 72.3 years for males and to 79.0 years for females, a considerable widening of the longevity gap between males and females from what existed in 1900.

Less well known than general life expectancy figures, which are used as a rough gauge of longevity, is the fact that, at any age, people of that age still have some years of life remaining, up to the limits of the human life span which is 115–120 years. That is, while a person born in a certain year has, on the average, the life expectancy associated with that year; for example, 75.2 years, a person who is already 80 years old in that year, say 1991, has 7.1 years of expected life remaining, if male, and 9.0 years of life remaining, if female. More generally, for males who were 65 years of age in 1991, there were, on the average, 15.3 years of life remaining while for 65-year-old females, the corresponding figure was 19.1 years. Because of gender-based mortality differentials, such comparisons always favor females over males. Such figures certainly indicate an advantage in longevity for older women, although (as Treas, 1995, has suggested) the additional years for many of them may involve considerable loneliness and poverty. For some older women, to invert a gerontological "mantra," it seems that years may be added to life rather than life being added to years.

Mortality

In view of the centrality of mortality rates in determining life expectancy, it is well to consider differences between older males and females in death rates associated with leading causes of death. These are shown in Table 2.2.

As would be expected from the differences in life expectancy between older males and females discussed earlier, there are major differences in mortality rates between them. Elderly men, predictably, have a much higher overall death rate than elderly women: 5,719.9 deaths per 100,000 men 65 years of age or over in 1991 vs. 4,387.0 deaths per 100,000 women 65 years of age or over. Older men also have much higher death rates from the first two leading causes of death: heart disease and, especially, cancer. The rates are not, however, uniformly higher for men. Older

TABLE 2.2   Death Rates for Males and Females 65 Years of Age and Over by Leading Causes of Death, 1991

Causes of Death	Death Rate per 100,000 Population	
	Male	Female
All causes	**5,719.9**	**4,387.0**
Leading causes of death:		
Heart disease	2,131.3	1,712.0
Malignant neoplasms (cancer)	1,469.3	879.7
Cerebrovascular (stroke)	366.6	412.7
Chronic obstructive pulmonary disease	334.7	177.2
Pneumonia and influenza	240.1	201.7
Diabetes	114.1	115.7
Accidents	102.9	70.0
Motor vehicle	30.9	16.3

Note: From *Statistical Abstract of the United States, 1994* (Table 127, p. 95) by the U.S. Department of the Census, 1995. Washington, DC: U.S. Government Printing Office.

women are considerably more likely to die from strokes and somewhat more likely to die from diabetes than are older men. On the evidence, however, the grim reaper generally prefers older men to older women. Why?

There are hormonal, physiological, and (perhaps) genetic differences between men and women that account for some of the variance in death rates. In addition, however, there are lifestyle and workplace differences that must account for another large portion. Women are generally more health-conscious than men and differ in their health behaviors, such as seeking necessary medical care in a timelier fashion. They are also more likely to act on current advice on proper nutrition and exercise. While it is changing, the workplace tends to be more hazardous for men than for women because of the traditional male/female occupational structure. For instance, men have higher rates of chronic obstructive pulmonary disease because more of them work in coal mines, foundries, automobile paint shops, and other environments where they inhale noxious, lung-damaging particulates and fumes. Such exposure may not catch up with them until old age but, when it does, it often exacts a heavy toll not only on them but on society. Consider that in the Black Lung Division of the Department of Labor in Washington, about 30 young and middle-aged attorneys, male and female, labor mightily to resolve the legal claims of citizens, mainly widows of older male coal miners, for compensatory black lung benefits from coal mine operators or the federal government.

Health

Among older persons, the two major concerns are health and financial security, usually in that order. Health status is assessed in various ways, one of which is perceived health status. Among men and women between 65 and 74 years of age, the National Health Interview Survey of 1984 found that over two-thirds perceived their health to be good to excellent, with a slightly higher percentage of men saying their health was excellent (16.3% vs. 14.8%) as well as saying their health was poor (12.5% vs. 9.2%). Among persons 75 years of age and over, almost two-thirds say their health is good to excellent, with similar percentages saying their health is excellent and somewhat higher percentages of men and women saying their health is poor (Duensing, 1988).

Based on the 1991 National Health Interview Survey, 70.8% of males 65 and over reported their health to be good to excellent, while 10.9%

said it was poor. Among comparable older women, 71.2% reported their health as good to excellent while 8.9% said it was poor (National Center for Health Statistics, 1992).

Another way of assessing health status among age groups is in terms of their susceptibility to acute and chronic medical conditions. Older persons generally have lower rates of acute conditions and higher rates of chronic conditions than do younger persons. For chronic conditions, however, there is considerable variability by gender. For selected chronic conditions, women 65 years of age and over generally have higher rates than men of arthritis, cataracts, deformities or orthopedic impairments; trouble with ingrown toenails and corns and calluses; frequent constipation; diabetes; migraine; high blood pressure; varicose veins; hemorrhoids; chronic bronchitis; hay fever; and chronic sinusitis. Older men, by contrast, have higher rates than women of visual impairments; hearing impairments; ulcer; and heart conditions. Given the mortality differentials between older men and women, it seems fair to say that older women tend to be plagued by chronic conditions that gnaw away at their quality of life, while older men tend to be plagued by chronic conditions that gnaw away their lives; i.e, their chronic conditions tend to be more serious.

Another measure of health status among older persons is hospitalization utilization rates. In terms of days of care per 1,000 persons, both older males and females had much higher utilization rates than did all younger age and gender groups in 1992. For males 65 to 74 years of age, the rate was 2,240 while the comparable figure for females was 1,885. For persons 75 and over, the figures were 3,929 and 3,648 for males and females, respectively. At the same time, the average hospital stay was slightly longer for females 75 and over than for comparable males: 8.9 vs. 8.4 days.

Considering these findings, it would appear that older men have poorer health than older women. More recently, however, George (1996) concludes that for most health indicators other than mortality, older women exhibit poorer health than their male peers.

Suicide

Although suicide does not appear among the seven leading causes of death among older men and women shown in Table 2.2, there are large differences in suicide rates between older men and women and, espe-

TABLE 2.3   Suicide Rates for Persons 65 Years of Age and Over by Sex and Race, 1991 (per 100,000 population)

	Male		Female	
Age	White	Black	White	Black
All ages	**21.7**	**12.1**	**5.2**	**1.9**
65 to 74 years	32.6	13.8	6.4	2.4
75 to 84 years	56.1	21.6	6.0	(B)
85 years and over	75.1	(B)	6.6	(B)

Note: B Base figure too small to meet statistical standards for reliability of a derived figure. Adapted from *Statistical Abstract of the United States, 1994* (Table 136, p. 101), by the U.S. Bureau of the Census, 1995. Washington, DC: U.S. Government Printing Office.

cially, between older white males and other gender/racial categories. These differences are shown in Table 2.3.

Just as there are large differences between older males and females in overall mortality rates and in rates for most causes of death, Table 2.3 indicates that there also are large differences in suicide rates. When race is considered, it can be seen that white males have higher suicide rates than African-American males, who have higher rates than white females, who, in turn, have higher rates than African-American females. Indeed, for African-American females 75 years of age and over (and African-American males 85 and over), there are so few suicides that reliable rates cannot be calculated. Suicide is not, as indicated in Table 2.3, unheard of among women but the figures clearly indicate that it is primarily a male phenomenon and much more common among white males than among African-American males, particularly white males 85 years of age and over. Compared to white females of the same age group, white males 85 and over had a suicide rate in 1991 that was over 11 times higher.

Deaths from Accidents and Violence

Death rates from accidents and violence among older persons in 1991 followed a pattern similar to that for suicide: white males 85 and over had the highest rate (of all age groups) followed by African-American males who, in turn, were followed by white females and African-American females.

Being murdered, as often reported in the media, is mainly something that happens to young males, but it is not unknown among older persons. Predictably, based on a now-familiar gender pattern, older males are generally more likely to be murdered than are older females. In 1992, however, 245 females 75 years of age and over were murdered in comparison to 229 males in this age group. While this is a difference of only 16 persons, and the number pales in relation to the 22,540 overall murders in 1992, the reversal in the usual gender pattern may be significant. Some older women are murdered by strangers but, probably, more of them are murdered by their husbands, either as a means of euthanasia or out of anger. Interestingly, in a current, ongoing study of occasionally reported "suicide pacts" between older couples, in which the husband kills his wife and then kills himself, it is beginning to appear that most wives have no desire to be part of the pact; rather, they are murdered by their husbands as part of his fatal episode (D. Cohen, personal communication, March 17, 1995).

Although older women appear to suffer more from troublesome, as opposed to life-threatening, conditions than do older men, it appears that their health is generally better than that of older men. In this regard, then, older women may be said to have an advantage over older men. Older men may be more advantaged than older women in other ways, however, and it is necessary to consider a variety of common social characteristics in which they differ and which may affect the quality of their lives in significant ways.

Marital Status

Of the day-to-day determinants of life satisfaction and the long-term quality of life, marital status is one of the most important. As one of the fundamental social institutions in society, marriage has a major impact on spouses, children, relatives, and society in general. Men and women of all ages who are married have many advantages over those who never marry or whose marriages are dissolved through widowhood, divorce, or separation. Compared to single individuals of the same age, married persons generally enjoy a richer and more fulfilling social life, greater income, and better health. Although a high divorce rate in American society would suggest that marriage must have a downside for many people and, in any event, is a fragile institution, it is increasingly coming to be realized that a high rate of stable marriages is, perhaps, the major social flywheel in society. How do older men and women compare on this critical dimension of life?

As of 1993, nearly 75% of men 65 years of age and over were married and living with their spouses, in comparison with only 41% of elderly women (U.S. Bureau of the Census, 1995a). This reflects the commonplace observation among social gerontologists that the dominant marital status of older men is "married" whereas that of older women is "widowed." This is usually attributed to the shorter life expectancies of elderly men relative to elderly women and to the fact that women are generally younger than their husbands at age of first marriage.

Although it is debatable whether men or women benefit most from marriage, older men clearly have greater access to the institution than older women. Not only are a far higher percentage of older males than older females married, but it is easier for older men to maintain this status if they desire. For older men who outlive or divorce their wives, the greater number of older widows facilitates remarriage and, as of 1988, of all the remarriages that occurred in the United States, 5.2% were among males 65 years of age and over, whereas only 2.8% of remarriages were among older females. Presumably, remarriage extends the same benefits to older males and females as their original marriages may have done.

Living Arrangements

For both elderly men and women, marital status obviously affects living arrangements. Although in 1993 the vast majority of persons 65 years old and over were living in households, only 15.5% of elderly men were living alone, whereas 40.8% of elderly women lived by themselves. Not surprisingly, 73.7% of elderly men lived with their spouses, while only 40.1% of elderly women did so. It may be natural to assume that, for older women, living alone represents an unwanted situation brought on by the death of a spouse, divorce, or never having married. This may be true for some older women, but a brief aside may put this in a different perspective.

Several years ago, a group of advocates for older persons in Dade County (Miami), Florida brought a federal suit against the State Office on Aging alleging that the formula for the distribution of Older Americans Act (OAA) funds was flawed and discriminated against Planning and Service Areas (PSAs) with large poor and minority populations. Not only did the formula allegedly not sufficiently reflect economic need and minority status, it was also claimed that the use of the percentage of older persons living alone as a proxy measure of social isolation and loneliness was unwarranted. The plaintiffs, through their gerontological consultants, argued that rather than reflecting social isolation and loneliness, as assumed by the State Office on Aging, living alone mainly represented a desired lifestyle choice among those older persons, mainly women, who valued independence and had sufficient economic resources to maintain their own homes. Although there were counterarguments by the defendants, the federal court eventually ruled in favor of the plaintiffs and the OAA funding formula was modified. Several million dollars in OAA funds flowed out of such counties as Pinellas (the location of St. Petersburg) with either fewer poor or minority elderly and more living alone, toward Dade County, and others like it, with large minority populations and lower percentages of older persons (mainly older women) living alone. At the very least, this outcome called into question the traditional gerontological view of living alone as being socially undesirable for older persons.

Income

Although the financial sufficiency of older persons has been problematic throughout most of this century and a *cri de coeur* among gerontological advocates until quite recently, the economic situation of the elderly in the United States has gradually improved over the years. One indication of this is the percentage of families with members 65 years of age and over who are below the poverty level, in comparison with families of all ages. As of 1992, 7.8% of older families were below the poverty level, in comparison with 11.7% of all families. For older white families, the situation was even brighter, with only 5.9% of them below the poverty level. Older minority families, however, still experience a much higher rate of poverty than older whites, with older African-American families having a poverty rate of 24.9% and older Hispanic families having a rate of 16.3% in 1992.

For males 65 years of age and over in 1992, the median income was $14,548, while the comparable figure for older females was $10,791. Presumably, most of these individuals were retired and receiving incomes that were only a portion of their preretirement earnings. What of the situation of older workers who are still working on a year-round, full-time basis? In 1992, older males who were still working had average earnings of $38,719 while older female workers earned $19,932, on the average. In keeping with an earlier point about how demographic characteristics (such as education) affect one's life chances, these figures are enhanced considerably when income is viewed in relation to education. Older males with less than a ninth-grade education earned $21,258 in 1992 but those with a bachelor's degree or more earned $56,955, an amount second only to that of college-educated men 45 to 54 years of age—usually considered the peak earning years. By contrast, older females who were working on a year-round, full-time basis earned far less than comparable older males. Because of their small numbers in the population, figures were not available for older women with less than ninth-grade educations, but those with bachelors' degrees or more earned $26,508 in 1992, about 47% of the amount earned by older males. It should be borne in mind, however, that older males or females who are still working full-time are only a small minority of all older persons and, as workplace "survivors," may not be representative of older persons in general.

Education

Compared with younger persons, older Americans have long had an educational gap and, therefore, a social status gap in an education-oriented society such as the United States. This situation has improved in recent years, and the median number of years of school completed by older persons is approaching that of younger persons. Still, there are considerable variations between elderly men and women in the amount of formal education they have had. Generally, higher percentages of older women than men have completed high school, 37.4% vs. 29.7% as of 1993. Older males, however, are slightly more likely to have had 1 to 3 years of college than older women, 14.3% vs. 13.9%, and they are considerably more likely to have had 4 or more years of college than older women, 16.1% vs. 9.0%. These general patterns have held for a long time and are mainly a function of the social norms surrounding the labor force participation of males.

Men have traditionally been expected to be the sole or main family breadwinners in American society and higher education has, for them, long been viewed as a means to this end. Older women have typically been less involved and less socially expected to be involved in work outside the home during their adult lives than men, and higher education has been seen as more of a social adornment than an occupational instrumentality. Indeed, until recent times, many occupations requiring a college degree were essentially closed to women, and those women with college degrees often could expect to have jobs that did not usually require degrees (e.g., secretarial work). Currently, these patterns are changing and women are involved in higher education as much as or, in some fields, even more than men and, in the future, there may be no appreciable differences between men and women in amount of formal education.

Labor Force Participation

The labor force participation of older males has declined dramatically during this century. In 1900, nearly 70% of older males were in the labor force (Aiken, 1995), a fact that is sometimes interpreted to mean that the past was more hospitable than the present to older workers. In reality, however, paid employment in the past was a simple economic necessity for most men. Social Security, company pensions, and retirement as a normative social institution were not yet part of the "warp and woof" of American society. If a man and his family wanted to survive, and if there were no other sources of income, he had to work. Even older men had to work, unless they were willing to live with and be supported by relatives or, occasionally, live on a county poor farm. Times have been changing, however, and except for the period during World War II, the percentage of older male workers has been steadily declining since 1900. As of 1993, it stood at 15.9% of the older male population. For older females since 1900, the percentage in the labor force has been low and fairly stable; currently, 7.9% of them are employed. Older persons who are still working are usually in part-time and often low-paying jobs. As noted earlier, however, those older persons, especially college-educated older men, who are still working full-time, year-round, have substantial income from earnings.

THE LOCATION OF ELDERLY MEN
IN DEMOGRAPHIC SPACE

Twelve major demographic characteristics have been reviewed in the interests of locating elderly men in demographic space. Based on these characteristics, it can be said in a summary fashion that, on the negative side of the ledger, the demographic space of elderly men in the United States is one in which they are a numerical minority among older persons, a fact that is reflected in a low sex ratio. Their life expectancy is considerably less than that of women of the same age as a result of their mortality rates being higher. Their health is somewhat poorer than that of elderly women, and they are much more prone to commit suicide and considerably more prone to die from accidents and violence. On the positive side of the ledger, however, elderly men are more likelier than elderly women to be married and living with a spouse, to have higher post-retirement incomes than single older women, to have more formal education than older women, and to have greater involvement in the labor force.

This is an admittedly simplistic conceptualization of the demographic space of elderly men. All concepts are abstractions, but the concept of demographic space may be more abstract than most, creating difficulties in adequately characterizing it for older men. It also involves an inherent dynamism; demographic space varies both with the social environment being described and with time. For instance, the demographic space of elderly men in the United States in 1900 was very different from that of elderly men in the 1990s; men from the two time periods might be biologically equivalent, but they would be very different in a sociodemographic sense. This is simply part of the more general problem in gerontology of "getting a fix" on older persons, including elderly men; our descriptions of them, even when extensive and intensive, tend to be static, while their defining characteristics are constantly changing. As has been said of social scientists, we are always dealing with snapshots of social reality when we should be dealing with motion pictures.

ARE ELDERLY MEN DEMOGRAPHICALLY ADVANTAGED OR DISADVANTAGED IN RELATION TO ELDERLY WOMEN?

In this final section, an attempt will be made to determine whether elderly men are demographically advantaged or disadvantaged in relation to elderly women. Many feminists would probably argue that, even in the 1990s, this is hardly a question that needs to be asked; men are still the more privileged sex. This may be true in relation to such factors as income and social power in the workplace but, in some other ways, women seem to have a clear advantage. It is desirable, therefore, to consider all the reviewed demographic characteristics and to attempt to judge the degree to which each represents an advantage for elderly men in relation to elderly women. The results of this attempt are shown in Table 2.4.

The bottom line of Table 2.4 is that elderly men in the United States are currently more demographically "disadvantaged" than elderly women. This assertion, coming from a male author in a book on elderly men, may seem more than a little disingenuous, but the scores on which it is based resulted from an honest, if necessarily subjective and method-ologically crude, process whose outcome was unknown in advance and which was not deliberately contrived to win sympathy for older men nor to minimize the plight of many older women. The following discussion reviews the process which led to the total advantage score of 27 for elderly men and the higher score of 34 for elderly women.

In earlier thinking about how to determine whether or not a particular demographic characteristic could be construed as an advantage or a disadvantage for elderly men in relation to elderly women, a tentative decision was made to simply list the characteristics after discussing them and to make a quick "yes or no" judgment in this regard. It later became apparent, however, that "advantageousness" was not only relative, but also a matter of degree for elderly men and women rather than an absolute "yes or no" phenomenon. This led to the use of the 6-point scales for men and women shown in Table 2.4, and an attempt to use a sort of *Verstehen* approach to judging advantageousness. The term *verstehen* is a German word meaning "understanding." It was used by Max Weber and Wilhelm Dilthey to refer to a method of interpreting

TABLE 2.4   Selected Characteristics of Elderly Men and Women and Inferred Degree of Advantage of Each Characteristic

Characteristic	Degree of Advantage to Men						Degree of Advantage to Women					
	0	1	2	3	4	5	0	1	2	3	4	5
Number in U.S. population	X									X		
Sex ratio				X			X					
Life expectancy	X											X
Mortality	X											X
Health status		X								X		
Suicide	X											X
Deaths from accidents and violence	X									X		
Marital status					X					X		
Living arrangements					X					X		
Income					X					X		
Education			X									
Labor force participation			X					X				
	Total score = 27						Total score = 34					

social interaction that involves putting oneself in the place of another (Vogt, 1993).

The fact that there are considerably more older women than men in the U.S. population led to the supposition that, in a democracy, superior numbers usually produce an advantage in the form of social power. Since older men are in the numerical minority, their numbers, alone, confer no power and they have been scored "0" on this characteristic. Women, because of their numerical superiority, have greater potential power but, until they attain full equality with men, it cannot be realized. Thus, they were scored a "3" rather than a "5" on this characteristic. Next, men are believed to derive a high degree of advantage from a low sex ratio which, even though it is based on the number of males and females in a population, reflects a different dimension of social reality than sheer numbers alone. Older men are assumed to benefit from a "surplus" of older women, as possible marriage or remarriage partners or companions, whereas older women are presumably disadvantaged financially, socially, and even sexually by a deficit of male age peers.

Older women would appear to be the clear beneficiaries of greater life expectancy than older males, while they would appear to benefit slightly more than men from their somewhat better health.

The apparent advantage of greater life expectancy and better health for women may be more illusory than real, however. Katz et al. (1983) argued that elderly men of all ages have a higher percentage of total remaining years of life that are independent than do elderly women of comparable ages. While a more sophisticated approach here might produce unanticipated findings and interpretations for some of the characteristics, men would appear to be at a decisive disadvantage with respect to mortality rates, suicide rates, and death rates from accidents and violence. With respect to the remaining demographic characteristics, elderly men would seem to benefit relatively more than elderly women, on the grounds that it is generally more socially and financially satisfying to be married than not married; generally more satisfying to live with someone than alone; better to have more rather than less income; better to have more formal education; and relatively more satisfying, for a man, to be working.

Elderly men, in this analysis then, are not invariably masters of the universe vis-à-vis elderly women. They, too, are humans whose societally conferred strengths may be more than counterbalanced by their peculiar vulnerabilities.

REFERENCES

Aiken, L. R. (1995). *Aging: An introduction to gerontology.* Thousand Oaks, CA: Sage.

Brown, A. S. (1996). *The social processes of aging and old age.* Upper Saddle River, NJ: Prentice Hall.

Duensing, E. E. (Ed.). (1988). *America's elderly: A sourcebook.* New Brunswick, NJ: Center for Urban Policy Research, Rutgers, The State University of New Jersey.

George, L. K. (1996). Social factors and illness. In R. H. Binstock & L. K. George (Eds.), *Handbook of aging and the social sciences* (4th ed.) (pp. 229–252). San Diego: Academic Press.

Katz, S., Branch, L. G., Branson, M. H., Papsidero, J. A., Beck, J. C., & Greer, D. S. (1983). Active life expectancy. *New England Journal of Medicine, 309,* 1218–1224.

National Center for Health Statistics. (1992). *Current estimates from the National Health Interview Survey, 1991.* Washington, DC: U.S. Government Printing Office.

Treas, J. (1995). Older Americans in the 1990s and beyond. *Population Bulletin, 50,* 1–46.

U.S. Bureau of the Census (1995a). *Statistical abstract of the United States, 1994.* Washington, DC: U.S. Government Printing Office.

U.S. Bureau of the Census (1995b, November 22). *On-line PopClock projection of the U.S. population.* Available: World Wide Web: http://www.census.gov/cgi-bin/popclock.

Vogt, W. P. (1993). *Dictionary of statistics and methodology.* Newbury Park, CA: Sage.

B.   Special Settings

CHAPTER 3

Breaking New Ground: Older Men and the Workplace*

Donna L. Wagner, Ph.D.

INTRODUCTION

The workplace, long a bastion of men who, upon attaining the "venerable" age of 65, are rewarded with a pension, a watch, and leisure time, has changed considerably over the past two decades. Older men have been both the victims and beneficiaries of these changes as well as the architects of the change. Today's cohorts of older men are a pioneering group of individuals who are reshaping the role of the older person in literally every social system within our society, including the workplace. For the first time in history, there are good odds of living a relatively healthy life for 20 years or more after the age of 65. This change alone has many implications for the workplace and how society views and values older persons, as well as the future norms regarding retirement, leisure time, and family roles in late life. Changes in the workplace pose significant challenges to older men of today. The one-career, one-employer path is largely a thing of the past. Older men have been caught in the middle of these changes and are seeking ways to manage the effects of these changes in their own personal lives.

* A special thanks to the men who provided their views to the author.

This chapter will review some of the current myths about older men in the workplace, the meaning of work in the lives of older men, the status of men in the workplace, and current trends affecting older men and the workplace in the future.

MYTHS ABOUT OLDER MEN AND THE WORKPLACE

Myths have an influence over not only the way we think about the world, but individual behavior as well. The myths associated with older men and the workplace are barriers to change, and can influence the opportunities for older men both as a result of the employer's behavior and the behavior of older men themselves.

Myth 1: Older men who are out of the workplace *chose* to exit paid work in order to pursue other activities

Research has shown that the corporate downsizing of the 1980s had a disproportionate effect on older workers. This occurred for two reasons—the type of companies who were most active in the downsizing of their workforce were mature companies who employed higher levels of older workers; and the downsizing strategies employed were often centered around early retirement packages directed at mature workers.[1]

Myth 2: Older men are not interested in working

While the demographic trend during the past 20 years has been earlier retirement on the part of older men, this tells only part of a bigger story. Older men have left the workplace due to a complex, and not yet well understood, set of dynamics including underemployment, unemployment, personal situations, and attitudes, and financial incentives for retirement. A study of older persons for the Commonwealth Fund conducted by Louis Harris and Associates (1993) found that an estimated 5.4 million older nonworking adults are ready, willing, and able to work. As a result of limited training opportunities and the persistence of negative attitudes about older workers, work remains an elusive goal for many.

Myth 3: There are too many costs associated with hiring an older worker

In a meta-analysis of research related to the job performance of older workers, Sterns and McDaniel (1994) conclude that there is little evidence to support the idea that older workers are a burden on those who employ them. Older workers are less costly than young workers in terms of turnover, voluntary absences, and on-the-job accidents. Also, overall job performance appears to be positively related to age. The authors also point out that, according to recent research, human resource departments express high levels of satisfaction with older workers—despite the fact that a negative stereotype regarding older workers persists. Health insurance costs, a factor more related to the national health care system than to the individual worker, remains a valid concern.

Myth 4: Older men are more difficult to manage in the workplace and resent being supervised by younger persons

Romondet and Hansson (1991), in their study of personal control in the workplace, found that older workers reported few job control concerns, less job stress, and high levels of satisfaction and work involvement. In contrast, those workers between the age of 30 and 49 were likely to express job control concerns. The ability to accept supervision in a constructive fashion is likely to be directly related to the older worker's experience over time, and highlights just one very positive contribution to the workplace of older worker involvement.

THE MEANING OF WORK

The meaning of work is not only a very personal thing for older men, but an important factor in their continued participation in the work environment. In addition to the more obvious benefits of work for an individual's sense of self-esteem, productivity, and personal competence, work provides a social structure in which the older man derives a feeling of connection to others and an opportunity for teamwork and comradery. In short, the meaning of work extends far beyond those factors associated with the financial rewards of work.

Some suggest that the increasing numbers of older men choosing early retirement in the past 20 years is a function of financial options available to them through pensions and Social Security. However, there is ample evidence to suggest that these options are a relatively small part of the equation. For example, a study of the effect of Social Security on retirement decisions found that the Social Security system had contributed to the demographic trends of increasing numbers of workers retiring between age 62 and 65, but this influence was due more to altering the social norms than to financially-based decisionmaking (Leonesio, 1993).

Many factors influence the meaning of work, both while an older man is working and after his retirement. Structural changes affecting the economy and the workplace provide a lens through which the individual worker assesses the meaning of work. Changing work environments with new demands placed upon workers and inadequate opportunities for training of older workers can, for example, influence the extent to which the older worker feels comfortable in the workplace, and able and interested in continuing to work. Downsizing and restructuring, as well as the larger economic trends that directly affect the small businessman or entrepreneur, influence the extent to which older men can and will continue in the marketplace as well as the meaning they attach to the workplace.

Bill, a 73-year-old retired sales manager, speaks of his feelings about work:

> When the recession hit the construction industry hard I was 62 and self-employed after working with one company for more than 20 years. I felt relief at the prospect of taking an early retirement and looked forward to walking away from the difficulties of making a sale in a bad market. And, for the first couple of years, it was good. I got involved in the golf course and was very active with many friends at the club. But, now I miss work very much. Work gave me self-satisfaction and I was very proud of the fact that, even though I didn't have a lot of formal education, I was able to get things done and support my family. I loved the thrill of making a "big deal," the status of working for a good company, and the respect of others who worked with me. The worst

part though, is not feeling connected to the world. When the Census Bureau was hiring enumerators, I decided to apply and got a job. It was exciting and fulfilling to be back in the world and to feel like I was contributing to something bigger than myself. If the economy had been better, I would have continued to work and, I think, feel better about things.

CURRENT PARTICIPATION IN THE WORKFORCE

Aggregate data on workforce participation (Manheimer, 1994) show that the participation of older men in the workforce has been steadily declining. In 1972, 71% of the men between the ages of 60–64 were employed compared to 56% in 1992. Participation of those between the ages of 65–69 was 35% in 1972 and 27% in 1991, and for men over 70 years of age the participation rates were 16% in 1972 and only 11% in 1992.

These aggregated data, however, obscure the fact that there are many changes taking place among older men. In the past two decades, the American workplace has undergone a significant transformation. New technology has reshaped the way we work and the types of jobs available to workers. Economic changes have occurred which have resulted in growth in certain sectors, like the service sector, and decline in other sectors, such as the production and manufacturing sectors. As pointed out earlier, these structural changes affecting the workplace have also affected older workers in disproportionate ways. These trends include the following dynamics:

- The downsizing and reorganization of large corporations has resulted in a negation of the social contract between worker and employer in regards to lifetime employment.
- The rapid change in technology and limited opportunities for retraining of the older worker has posed barriers to continued employment for older workers.
- The shift from production-based employment to service and high-technology bases has left many older workers behind.
- An increasing reliance upon "contingent" workers has created a competitive workplace with diminished job security for the older worker.

These trends are a backdrop against which the aggregate data regarding increasing numbers of older men leaving the workforce must be interpreted. It is likely that these structural changes within the work environment have played a very large role in the lives of older men who are now being counted as "opting" for early retirement.

George, a 69-year-old soft drink distributor, describes his situation:

> I worked for a metal fabricating plant for 35 years and, at the end, was trained to use a new "state of the art" machine which was designed to do the work of what used to take 15 men. Then came the lay-offs. We were organized and the union took the strike vote on a Saturday night—I'll never forget it. We were all frightened about what might happen, but felt we were right in fighting the lay-offs, so I supported the strike. We were all on the picket lines every day for six weeks. It was tough for my family because the strike benefits didn't cover our bills and they were worried about what would happen to us if nothing worked out. Then we learned that the company decided to close the plant and move everything to another site in the South. I knew I'd never get another job doing what I knew how to do—there weren't any other companies left. I was unemployed for more than two years before I found this job. . . . it's not a great job, but it's money. I went through it all—feeling like a bum, getting mad about things and just knowing I was a failure because I couldn't support my family. But, they stuck with me and now things are better because we have the money coming in. I still miss the machines though and often think about all of the fellows at the plant. I may retire next year . . . my youngest will finish college then. I just hope it's better for him.

If George had been a few years older when his employer left the area, he might have chosen an early retirement option available under Social Security for those aged 62. Instead, he showed up in the Department of Labor Statistics as an unemployed worker. The statistics available from the Department of Labor suggest that older workers have a lower unemployment rate than other age groups. However, this may be an artifact of the "discouraged" worker phenomenon coupled with the option of aging into the early retirement provisions of Social Security. Even though older workers have lower unemployment rates, when older workers become unemployed, they remain unemployed longer than younger workers. And, while the passage of the Age Discrimination in Employment Act (ADEA) has made discrimination based upon age illegal, proving age discrimination is not an easy task. For the

50-plus unemployed worker, rising above attitudes and perceptions about older workers can be a significant challenge in the search for a new position.

In contrast to the data which indicate the continuing decline of older men in the workplace, Herz (1995) identifies a new trend which has important implications for our understanding of the labor force participation of older men—the re-employment of men after retirement. She analyzed data from men who were receiving a pension and participating in the workplace and discovered a large increase among men aged 55–61 years of age. For this group, participation rates were up from 37% in 1984 to 49% in 1993. Between the ages of 61–64, rates had increased from 19% in 1984 to 24% in 1993. Part-time work accounted for more than half of the workplace arrangements of these pensioners. Herz suggests that both negative and positive economic trends have influenced this return to work, including downsizing and early-out arrangements as well as more flexible work opportunities.

The percentage of persons over the age of 65 who are involved in part-time work has increased. In 1989, of employed men over the age of 65, 48% were employed part-time. Many public opinion polls have also indicated that older persons would prefer to work part-time. However, when this question is posed to unemployed older workers, the majority of respondents reply that they are looking for full-time—not part-time—employment. Self-employed older men have the most flexibility when it comes to part-time options. Fred, a 72-year-old plumber, describes his situation:

> I've been a plumber for more than 50 years and have had my own plumbing business for 40 of those years. My wife and I talked about selling the business a few years ago and moving to North Carolina to be closer to our children. I really like my work and like being able to solve problems for my customers—many of them are elderly and have been with me since I started the business. I didn't want to go someplace new and have nothing to do. I don't play golf or fish or any of the things you're supposed to do when you retire. So, we compromised. I agreed to take two weeks off of work every four months and we go down to visit the grandkids and take a little vacation. Also, I don't really take new customers anymore so I usually only work only five or six hours a day. When we go off on a vacation, I leave a message on my answering machine telling my customers who to call and everyone is happy—especially me.

While men have been retiring at younger ages, middle-aged women's participation in the labor force has been steadily increasing (Manheimer, 1994). In 1989, 70.5% of the women between the ages of 45–54 were in the labor force, double the participation of this age group in 1950. The workforce participation of women over the age of 60 has remained stable and is less than that of older men. For women over the age of 65, the participation rate in 1992 was 8.3% compared with 16% for men. However, given the dramatic increase in participation of women between 45 and 54 years of age, there is every expectation that the participation of women over the age of 60 will increase as these women grow older.

Older men are a heterogenous group and can be found in all sectors of the workforce. Older men are well represented in executive, managerial, and sales occupations and less represented in the service occupations. A different pattern of employment is present for women, who are heavily represented in the service occupations and less well represented in executive or managerial occupations. Similarly, older men are well represented in semi- and unskilled labor categories. Perhaps most interesting, rates of self-employment are highest for older men, exceeding those for younger men and older women.

Race and ethnicity play a role in the participation of older men (as is the case with all workers in this country). Correlates of race and ethnicity, such as education and training, are factors in explaining workforce opportunities. McIntosh (1994), for example, points out that African-American men have more work interruptions throughout their work life, due to the nature of their occupations as well as their health. These interruptions can play a role not only in their retirement income levels, but in the options they have for continued employment and the extent to which they *need* to continue working into late life. Older African-American men are less likely than white men to be working in late life and those who are working are more likely to be engaged in part-time work than are white men. Older African-American men are also more likely than white men to express a desire to work more than they are working now (McIntosh, 1994).

From an individual perspective, the skills of older men play an important role in the opportunities available to them in late life. Although surveys of older people indicate an interest in and willingness to participate in training programs to improve skills, the opportunities for these workers are limited. Hall and Mirvis (1994) undertook a survey of 400 employers to ascertain their investments in training of employees. They found that there was a decreasing investment in employees as they aged. The highest investment was made in those workers age 35 and younger.

Continuing education courses are an alternative for older men who are not receiving training from employers. In fact, there has been significant growth in both the offerings in continuing education directed at career changes and upgrading of skills, and in the numbers of midlife and older persons participating in the courses. But, as pointed out by Kanter (1994), we are still behaving as if the primary investment in human capital is needed during the younger years. She suggests that the late-life equivalent to "Junior Achievement" is lacking and we still assume that economic participation of older persons should revolve around the mentoring and counseling, on a volunteer basis, of younger persons.

Harold's story illustrates this point:

> I retired officially from an educational testing company when I was 69 years old. The company's attitude towards me and my place within the company had been changing for several years prior to my retirement. Management had stopped giving me the lead on new projects and had assigned others to develop proposals for funding in areas which had previously been my areas of expertise. It was as if they were already phasing me out and a not-too-subtle hint to me that there would be fewer interesting opportunities for me in the future. After retiring, I joined up with a civic group in town that was developing a mentoring program for ghetto youth and helped them plan and acquire funding for the program. During the planning phase I felt useful and productive and was happy to be making a volunteer commitment to such an important project. When the work started, paid staff managed the project and the only role open to me was to become a volunteer mentor. I took on one young man and continue with him to this day. It just wasn't enough for me, however. I wanted to be more proactive in the program and more creative in my contributions and had hoped that I could have been involved in the program management as a paid staff, even if on a part-time basis. Now I'm busy shopping my credentials around to consulting firms hoping to find a paying job in program development. I'd even take a volunteer job developing a new program, but don't know how to find such an assignment on a volunteer basis. So, I spend my time FAXing out my resume, spending time with my young friend, reading and waiting for something more interesting to come along.

FACTORS INFLUENCING WORKFORCE PARTICIPATION OF OLDER MEN

There are structural factors, workplace factors, and personal factors influencing the participation of older men in the workforce. Structural factors can be viewed as barriers to "productive aging" and include, in addition to the larger economic trends affecting the workplace, financial incentives for retirement, unemployment, the mix of available full- or part-time work, compensation patterns, and employer attitudes (Quinn & Burkhauser, 1993). Employer attitudes shape the workplace factors which influence the participation of older men. These attitudes directly affect the training and retraining opportunities of the older worker and the design of flexible work arrangements which can accommodate the needs of older workers, as well as policies and practices around retention and recruitment of older workers.

Less well-understood are the personal factors influencing participation of older men in the workplace. In addition to personal preferences and lifestyle choices, and the resources available to support these choices, family situations and health are factors in workforce participation.

In a pilot study, Bailey and Hannsson (1995) explored the psychological obstacles to career change in late life. They found that age-related norms in the workplace and the extent to which older men have internalized these norms, concerns about obsolete skills, and older men's perception of their own aging are obstacles to changing jobs or careers.

Family situations can play an important role in whether an older man decides to continue or seek new employment, and affect their preferences for full- or part-time work. A husband caring for a wife with a chronic, debilitating illness may prefer a part-time position in order to have some respite from caregiving and yet continue to provide the ongoing needed care. A grandfather raising his grandchildren alone may prefer to remain at home with the children but, in order to meet the financial obligations of the family, must seek or retain full-time employment. A growing number of grandfathers and fathers are raising children, many of them alone. Although many large employers have embraced a work-family agenda which fosters a more "family-friendly" work environment, for the most part this agenda has primarily targeted younger workers with small children. Only recently has the work-family agenda been expanded to include caregivers for the older person; yet, responses to this employee population have been limited.[2]

Although the health status of older persons has improved significantly over the past two decades, health still currently influences the decisions of many men. For some men, though, work decisions are based upon the availability of health insurance. Joe, a 57-year-old communications specialist, explains:

> It wasn't too long after taking my current job that I knew I would not be happy here. I started sending out my resume about a year after beginning the job but never was successful in getting a new position. My wife has her own small business in the communications area and I would much prefer working with her on a full-time basis. However, because I have a chronic illness which requires substantial medical care to manage, I don't have that option. It is impossible for me to get health insurance to cover this condition as an individual purchaser—I must be in a group to get the health care coverage I need. Only five more years and I'll be eligible for Medicare and able to work with my wife on a full-time basis. I've stopped looking for another job and am trying to hang on here until that time.

VOLUNTEERISM

Volunteering is another way in which older men participate in the workplace. Studies of volunteerism have demonstrated the significant contribution made to society by such activities. The Marriot Senior Living (1991) survey, for example, estimated that 40% of the elderly were involved in some volunteer work, contributing more than 3.6 billion hours of their time on an annual basis. Older men's participation as volunteers has been increasing over time and Chambre's (1987) study estimated that 24% of older men were involved in volunteer work, although most older volunteers are women (55%). Correlates of volunteering include higher education levels, higher income, and being married. Chambre's work suggests that there are different patterns of volunteerism between men and women. Men are more likely to link work with volunteerism; when retiring from work, they also retire from volunteering. Women, on the other hand, appear to view volunteer work as a substitute for paid employment.

Religion plays an important role in volunteering. Not only does the belief system associated with religious organizations support the ethic of service to the community, but religious organizations provide an avenue to volunteer opportunities for many older men. There are also volunteer patterns associated with different religious organizations. Jews are more likely than any faith to volunteer, Protestant faiths follow, and the lowest volunteer rates can be found among Catholics (Chambre, 1987). These differences may be attributable, however, to educational attainment levels between faith groups. Educational and socioeconomic factors may also play a role in the observed differences in volunteerism between whites, African-Americans, and Hispanics, with lower rates of volunteering observed in the latter two groups.

In contrast to the public investment in training programs to expand paid opportunities of older men, there has been significant public investment in programs which recruit, train, and involve older persons in volunteer activities. These programs include the Retired Senior Volunteer Program (RSVP), Foster Grandparent Program, Senior Companion Program, Volunteers in Service for America (VISTA), and the Service Corps of Retired Executives (SCORE), as well as other programs sponsored by the public and private sectors.

How an older man incorporates volunteer work into his life is influenced by the opportunities available to him, as well as his history in volunteer work and interest in continuing with this activity over time. For the older man who has never been a volunteer, there may be attitudinal barriers to the initiation. Bill, the 73-year-old retired sales manager referred to earlier in this chapter, explains:

> I never thought of volunteering, maybe I should have. But, I'm not sure what I have to offer in this area. Everything was changing so much in the workplace when I was working and I felt a little off-kilter about these changes then. I really can't use a computer and don't think there's much call for volunteer sales managers. I guess I just don't know what good I'd be now to some group that is looking for volunteers.

FUTURE TRENDS AFFECTING OLDER MEN IN THE WORKPLACE

At the beginning of this chapter, older men were referred to as the pioneers in the area of work. The courses charted by these pioneers will open up new opportunities for all older workers and, hopefully, dispel some of the persistent myths about gender, older workers, and the role of older men in the family. In this section, trends will be identified which affect older men in the workplace as a result of changing demographics, changing employer attitudes and opportunities, and changing family roles.

Demographic and Structural Changes

The workforce demographic changes significantly favor the older worker in the future. Although analysts began to forecast a labor shortage as a result of fewer young workers in the 1980s, the consequences of this shortage were obscured by economic downturns. The forecasted demand for older workers did not materialize as a result of these downturns. If the economy stabilizes and remains stable over time, we can expect to see significant increases in the demand for older workers due to the shortage of younger replacement workers. This demand will undoubtedly result in new and improved efforts in the area of training and retention of older workers in all sectors of society.

To this end, we have recently seen changes in the recruitment of older workers in certain industries—most notably the service sector. McDonald's has aggressively recruited older workers in certain areas of the country and has a national media campaign directed at older consumers (with an older worker message as well). Will, however, the demand for older workers provide opportunities that are meaningful and meet the needs of the older men who wish to continue in or return to the workforce?

The increasing use of contingency workers in the marketplace is a well-documented trend which is anticipated to accelerate over time. Kanter (1994) points out that not only were more than half of all new jobs created between 1980 and 1988 designed for contingent workers, but by the year 2000, 80% of all American jobs are expected to be within the service sector—a sector which relies heavily on contingency workers. The use of contingency workers is not limited to the service sector. Government, corporations, and nonprofit organizations use contingency workers—both on short-term and long-term assignments. By the very nature of the relationship between the employer and the contingent worker, there is little to suggest that employers will feel any responsibility to provide all but the most basic training to the worker. Rather, those workers selected will have the skills and qualifications needed by employers in an increasingly competitive marketplace. Staying competitive in this marketplace may be problematic for older men who do not have training opportunities or continuing service paths within the contingency worker market.

As a nation, we are facing a paradox when it comes to older workers. On the one hand, we are acknowledging the capacity of older workers and the need to include them in the workforce (when we debate increasing the retirement age from 65 to 70). On the other hand we have not, as a society, embraced a "productive aging" philosophy for older Americans.[3] The Senior Community Service Employment Program (SCSEP), which offers training to low-income older persons, is experiencing cutbacks in funding (as are other job training programs). This program served more than 100,000 older, low-income Americans in 1994, 40% of whom were men. Other publicly supported training programs are primarily targeted at young workers and offer little to the older man. With the exception of a portion of the Job Partners in Training Act programs (JPTA), the public training investment has largely overlooked the older worker. Remaining competitive in a contingent workforce, outside of the service sector, may be a function of the older man's ability to purchase the continuing education and training needed over time.

Employer Attitudes and Practices

Many employers have discovered that older workers can be of significant benefit to the workplace. Rife (1995) identifies several large corporations that have reshaped their policies and practices in order to attract and retain older workers. Some of the strategies these corporations have used include the development of a job bank of retirees, revisions in the pension system in order to permit part-time work, retraining of both older workers and retirees who wish to return to work, and flexible work schedules and locations.

In a study of private sector companies with more than 20 employees, Hirshorn and Hoyer (1994) found that nearly half (46%) of the surveyed firms hired retirees. Larger companies were more likely than small firms to hire retirees and more likely to have flexible options for the retirees. Most of the surveyed companies indicated that they did not have written policies in place regarding older workers, but had hired the retirees because they qualified for the job for which they had applied. The researchers also found that two factors were related to the willingness of the employers to hire retirees: reliability, and the fact that they had the skills needed for the job.

It is likely that, as demographic shifts occur, employers will seek out ways to attract older workers and modify policies which work against the older worker. It will be important to provide employers with accurate information about older workers to ensure that the policies and practices which emerge over time reflect both the preferences of older workers and the flexible options which allow these preferences to become a reality for the older worker.

Kanter (1994) suggests that a new social contract of "employability security" is needed between employers and employees. This contract should offer flexibility to make change when it is needed, not only to the employer but the employee as well. As Kanter (1994) states: "A society that encourages investment in human capital via continuing education, training, and support for new venture creation can help people feel secure even when they move across companies or invent their own jobs" (p. 28). And, we can add, this investment in human capital must span the lifespan in order to realize the promise of older workers and their contributions to America.

Older Men and Their Families

Several changes are taking place in the American family which have implications for older men and their participation in the workplace. The most dramatic change, observed during the past two decades, has been the increasing labor force participation of middle-aged women. Approximately 70% of the women between the ages of 45 and 54 are now actively participating in the workforce. The commitment of a spouse to continued labor force participation may become more of a factor in an older man's decision to either remain or re-enter the workforce after retirement. The issues associated with a retired husband and fully employed wife, who is not particularly interested in retirement, have just recently begun to be explored. It is also likely that this phenomenon accounts for at least part of the male retirees who are returning to work in increasing numbers.

The increasing numbers of grandparents who are raising grandchildren may also play a factor in the work decisions of older men, presently and in the future. There has been a 40% increase in grandparent-headed households during the past 10 years and, according to the U.S. Census, there were 3.4 million children being raised by grandparents in 1993. It is estimated that 40% of the grandparents raising grandchildren are men. The grandparent-headed households are found in all communities and within all ethnic and racial groups. An estimated 68% of the grandparents raising a grandchild are white and 57% of the households can be found in the southern part of our nation (U.S. Census, 1994). The specific effect of this new role for the older man depends on his situation. For some, this role will require returning to work in order to support the expanded household; for others it may provide the impetus to retire early in order to care for the new family members.

Alfred describes his difficult decision:

> My wife died 2 years ago. I had just retired at the age of 64 and had too much time on my hands. So I started helping out with the baseball teams in the park and driving some of my neighbors to do their shopping . . . you know, just to keep busy. Then my son got put in jail and his wife was on the drugs. I think my son was pretty much taking care of the grandkids and when I saw how they were living without him there, I knew I had to take them in. So now I have three little ones and don't have time to even sleep. I had to take a part-time driving job to get enough money to feed them. That's the thing—when I didn't really need to work, I didn't have anything much to do; when I had too much to do with the children, I had to go back to work to make ends meet.

Alfred is one of the grandfathers who has undertaken the sole responsibility for their grandchildren. Other grandfathers are participating in this venture with their wives. It is estimated that 76% of the grandparent-headed households include two adults. While single grandparents have the most difficult task ahead of them, work-related decisions may be a part of the adjustment to child-rearing responsibilities in the two-adult households as well.

Many family roles are important to older men and older women. An older man may be a caregiver for a disabled spouse or a disabled adult child. The caregiving role, no matter what it entails, will play some factor in the preferences of older men regarding the workplace. The preferences of a spouse or partner will also come into play when an older man is deciding whether to work full-time, part-time, or retire.

A final emerging trend among men also has implications for the future. There are increasing numbers of men who are not in the workforce and are not looking for work—an estimated 4.6 million men between the ages of 25–54 in 1994. While many of these men could be classified as "discouraged" workers, there is a growing group of men who are out of the workforce because they are too busy doing something else. Increasingly, the "something else" is keeping house and raising children. There was a 26% increase in men in this category between 1990 and 1994. These men may have started out as discouraged workers, segued into students, then moved into what we might term the "disinterested worker."

Peter, aged 39, tells his story:

> When I got married to my wife, she had a very high earning capacity— much higher than I had ever imagined would be in my own future. We decided that this might be a good time for me to return to school, finish a degree and do some graduate study. While I was finishing school we had three children. After I graduated I began to look for work as I had always planned to do. This search for work continued for about 8 months and then one day I just woke up and said: "I don't really want a job." Maybe I was rationalizing my way through job defeat, I don't know. Anyway, I'm done looking and very happy with my life at the moment. I love being "Mr. Mom" when the kids come home from daycare and there are plenty of things to do around the house and in the community. Actually, after I worked through the stigma thing and got over the embarrassment associated with telling people I wasn't working and wasn't looking, I can honestly say that this is just about the best time I've had since I became an adult. Maybe I'll start a business or work someplace someday. But, for now, this is where I want to be.

We can only speculate on the future involvement in the workplace of these "disinterested" workers and the growth in their numbers. Certainly, however, their work lives will be different than those of current cohorts of older men. For many, the contingency workforce may afford appropriate options and, for others, a change in their family status (such as a divorce) may predict diminished financial futures during their work years as well as in their retirement years.

CONCLUSION

The status of older men in the workplace has been, and will continue to be, affected by changes in society, the workplace, and the family. As a nation, remaining globally competitive will, in part, be based upon how well we can manage the aging of America. Hall and Mirvis (1994) point out: "A combination of future labor and skill shortages, if coupled with advantages gained from being wiser about older worker issues, will make innovation in the management of older workers a factor in achieving competitive advantage" (p. 90).

In order to make the transitions which will not only ensure a competitive economy but also maximize the personal choice and preferences of older men, there are areas which need to be improved. These include training and a lifelong education philosophy which embraces the productivity of older persons, a flexible workplace which accommodates individual situations and preferences, and a revision in the way we view the appropriate role of older persons.

ENDNOTES

[1] For a discussion of this and other trends affecting older workers, see Auerbach, J., & Welsh, J., *Aging and Competition: Rebuilding the U.S. Workforce* (Washington, DC: National Planning Assoc., 1994).

[2] For a review of corporate programs for employed caregivers to the elderly, see Wagner, D., & Neal, M. (1994). "Caregiving and Work: Consequences, Correlates, and Workplace Responses." *Educational Gerontology, 20*(7), 645–663.

[3] For a comprehensive review of the issues around productive aging, see *Achieving A Productive Aging Society*, S. Bass, F. Caro, & Y. Chen (Eds.), Westport, CT: Auburn House, 1993.

REFERENCES

Bailey, L. L., & Hansson, R. O. (1995). Psychological obstacles to job or career change in late life. *Journal of Gerontology: Psychological Sciences, 50B*, 280–288.

Chambre, S. M. (1987). *Good deeds in old age: Volunteering by the new leisure class.* Lexington, MA: Lexington Books.

Hall, D. T., & Mirvis, P. H. (1994). The new workplace and older workers. In J. A. Auerbach & J. C. Welsh (Eds.), *Aging and competition: Rebuilding the US workforce* (pp. 58–92). Washington, DC: National Planning Association.

Herz, D. E. (1995). Work after early retirement: An increasing trend among men. *Monthly Labor Review, 118*(4), 13–20.

Hirshsorn, B., & Hoyer, D. (1994). Private sector hiring and use of retirees: The firm's perspective. *The Gerontologist, 34,* 50–58.

Kanter, R. M. (1994). U.S. competitiveness and the aging workforce: Toward organizational and institutional change. In J. A. Auerbach & J. C. Welsh (Eds.), *Aging and competition: Rebuilding the US workforce* (pp. 7–30). Washington, DC: National Planning Association.

Leonesio, M. V. (1993). Social Security and older workers. *Social Security Bulletin, 56,* 2, 47–57.

Manheimer, R. J. (1994). *Older Americans Almanac.* Detroit, MI: Gale Research.

McIntosh, B. R. (1994). Understanding labor markets and productive activity through race and gender. In J. A. Auerbach & J. C. Welsh (Eds.), *Aging and competition: Rebuilding the US workforce* (pp. 166–183). Washington, DC: National Planning Association.

Quinn, J. F., & Burkhauser, R. V. (1993). Labor market obstacles to aging productively. In S. A. Bass, F. G. Caro, & Y. Chen (Eds.), *Achieving a productive aging society* (pp. 43–60). Westport, CT: Auburn House.

Rife, J. C. (1995). *Employment of the elderly: An annotated bibliography.* Westport, CT: Greenwood.

Romondet, J. H., & Hannsson, R. O. (1991). Job-related threats to control among older employees. *Journal of Social Issues, 47,* 4, 129–141.

Russell, C. (1995). Find the missing men. *American Demographics, 17*(5), 8.

Sterns, H. L., & McDaniel, M. A. (1994). Job performance and the older worker. In S. E. Rix (Ed.), *Older workers: How do they measure up?* Washington, DC: AARP.

U.S. Department of Commerce, Bureau of the Census (1993). Statistical abstract of the United States, 1992. Washington, DC: Author.

U.S. Department of Commerce, Bureau of the Census (1994). The diverse living arrangements of children. Washington, DC: Author.

CHAPTER 4

Elderly Men of the Inner City

J. Kevin Eckert, Ph.D. & Lucy Geissler Repaci, M.A.

INTRODUCTION

In contrast to the general population, more ethnic and elderly populations are likely to live within cities (National Research Council, 1994). What Clark (1971) noted 25 years ago remains true today: The aged cannot join the flight of some younger affluents to suburbia to avoid the noise, smog, dirt, and other social tensions associated with city life. Both minority and aged groups are locked into the urban environment by a complexity of factors, including inexpensive housing provided by tenements, cheap hotels, and furnished rooms (Eckert, 1980). Brice (1970) suggests that the urban aged, too poor to join the rush to the suburbs, remain trapped in inner-city neighborhoods where they are exploited by landlords, robbed by thugs, and ignored. Despite hardships and hazards, some center cities still provide compensations not readily available to the aged poor in other locations. For example, cities often provide elements that make life easier and more pleasurable for the elderly, such as public transportation and an infrastructure of necessary services (Golant, 1992).

This chapter will focus on the life circumstances of elderly men residing in urban areas alternatively defined as "inner-city," "urban," and "center-city." After discussing general trends affecting urban elderly males and the problems and benefits associated with urban life, the chapter will conclude by reviewing research on specific "inner-city" settings housing older men and identifying knowledge gaps in the literature.

TRENDS AFFECTING INNER-CITY, ELDERLY MEN

Trends associated with urban America—such as poverty, public safety, changing urban neighborhoods, and publicly funded city services—affect the lives of urban men.

Poverty

Historically, the elderly experienced higher rates of poverty than other age groups; however, this trend changed with the introduction of programs such as Medicare and the Older Americans Act. Between 1959 and 1990 there was a two-thirds reduction in elderly poverty, which exceeded the one-third reduction in the general population poverty level. However, certain elderly groups, such as women (15.4%) and African-Americans (33.8%), experienced more poverty than men (7.6%) and whites (10.1%), with elderly African-American women having the highest incidence of impoverishment (38%) (Devine & Wright, 1993).

Unlike younger persons or more affluent elderly, poor elderly are unable to move to suburban areas (DeLeaire, 1994). For elderly men living in metropolitan areas and inner-cities, poverty continues to be a major problem, especially in African-American neighborhoods. Forty-two percent of America's poor reside in inner cities and greater than half of the urban poor (52%) reside in census-defined poverty areas, where the poverty rate is almost three times higher than the national poverty rate. Consistent with general elderly poverty, African-Americans and Hispanics experience more poverty and are concentrated in these inner-city areas. It is important to note that ghettoization of poverty is not only a problem that affects the often-studied large Northern cities, but affects American cities of any size (Devine & Wright, 1993).

Public Safety: Crime/Victimization/Violence

The elderly experience less of all types of crime than all other age groups, with certain groups of elderly experiencing more crime than others. For example, elderly African-Americans generally have increased rates of victimization compared to elderly whites. Elderly who reside in inner cities experience the highest victimization from all types of crime when compared to elderly residing in suburban or rural areas. Furthermore, different groups experience different types of crime. Lower-income elderly have higher rates of violent crime victimization than more affluent elderly. Renters are more likely to be victims of personal theft and violence, and owners are more likely to be victims of household crime (United States Department of Justice, 1994).

Like the public misperception of the number of elderly crime victims, the elderly's fear of crime is also often overstated; however, factors such as type of community (age-heterogeneous v. age-homogeneous), geographic location, health status, and sociodemographic variables mediate fear of victimization. For example, some elderly (women, low-income, never-married, living alone, having poor health) fear crime more than their corresponding counterparts (Akers, Sellers, & Cochran, 1987). Moreover, the urban elderly fear victimization more than rural elderly, and this fear increases as size of community increases. Lastly, elderly who reside in age-homogeneous communities fear crime less than those in age-heterogeneous communities; however, elderly who move to age-homogeneous communities may transfer their fear of crime from their community of origin with them (Akers et al., 1987).

Neighborhoods

The environment, and more specifically the neighborhood, is "a place that possesses a structure interrelating physical, social, and cultural properties to encourage certain behavior patterns" (Biegel & Farkas, 1990, p. 116). As the elderly age and become more mentally and physically vulnerable, they are more reliant on cultural, social, and physical facets of their environments. Beyond being the locus of social ties and informal support networks, the neighborhood is also the context for providing formal supports, such as human service agencies, schools, churches, and governmental agencies (Biegel & Farkas, 1990). When their environment includes safe neighborhoods, affordable and convenient transportation, and reasonable health care facilities, elderly persons are more likely to have higher life satisfaction than those who do not. Without the above features, elderly lose satisfaction and a sense of well-being (DeLeaire, 1994).

The decline of many urban neighborhoods is a concern among elderly, inner-city men. Golant (1992) discusses factors that older people, themselves, link to the desirability of their neighborhoods. The lack of convenient transportation, leisure, and recreational opportunities, coupled with high crime levels and poorly maintained housing and undependable public services, decrease the desirability of neighborhoods. Some of these problems are the result of declining neighborhoods that have lost their social and economic desirability.

A different set of problems may affect older men whose neighborhoods have become revitalized and gentrified. Older persons residing in such neighborhoods may experience increases in apartment rents, property taxes, and the cost of everyday goods and services. Some studies show that many older people (estimates reach as high as 30%) are displaced from their longstanding dwellings because of events linked to revitalization. Proponents of revitalization maintain that without rejuvenation, the neighborhoods would decline to a point at which most elderly residents would have to move away because of building decay, disinvestment, abandonment, and an exceptionally hostile living environment (Golant, 1992).

Whether through deterioration, abandonment, revitalization, or gentrification, the availability of low-rent housing for low-income elderly men is a problem. Although older men have benefitted from federally subsidized housing programs, there is substantial evidence of an inadequate housing supply of low-rent housing, creating a situation that will worsen with the disproportionate growth of low-income older renters. For example, since the 1970s, the federal government has shifted from a project-based approach to rental subsidization. As a result, the federal assistance for the construction or substantial rehabilitation of low-rent apartment units dropped sharply, since programs emphasized rent subsidies which were tied to existing housing stock in need of very little or no rehabilitation (Golant, 1992). Redfoot and Gaberlavage (1991) have argued that the older renter market is increasingly likely to be restricted to the oldest and poorest—those most likely to experience multiple income, health, and social service needs. Most experts agree that the current supply of affordable rental opportunities is inadequate and unlikely to keep pace with the disproportionate growth of low-income older renters (Golant, 1992).

The 1990 National Affordable Housing Act funded Section 202 programs for the elderly and nonelderly disabled (Section 811). Section 202 housing provides an important housing alternative for poor inner-city elderly men. By the end of the 1980s, the Section 202 program had elderly living in some 218,000 units and nonelderly physically and mentally disabled were living in 12,000 units (Golant, 1992). Experts consider Section 202 to be one of the more successful federal housing programs catering to the low-income elderly (United States House of Representatives, 1989).

Section 8 rental programs is another federal effort directed at all age groups, including the elderly. Under this program, older persons who are paying excessive rent in their present apartment are eligible for this rental assistance. Eligibility extends to those in shared housing accommodations, single-room-occupancy hotels, and rented manufactured housing. Section 8 rental programs are particularly important to inner-city, elderly men in single-room-occupancy hotels. Although rent subsidy programs help some elderly, older African-American persons may have their housing options limited to certain neighborhoods and, consequently, be forced to select from poorer quality rental units because of housing discrimination (Golant, 1992).

Residents of low-rent housing who have aged in place present management with new dilemmas. These initially healthy and independent tenants have grown older and become frail. Many hide their increasing frailty to avoid eviction. Especially vulnerable are those who live alone, depend on Social Security and Supplemental Security Income (SSI), and are members of racial minority groups (Golant, 1992). The owners and managers of these federally subsidized low-rent housing projects show a range of responses to their frail elderly populations. Since no uniformly acceptable service models exist, sponsors are free to interpret service needs however they choose (U.S. Senate, 1990). Moreover, it is not known whether service models consider the differential needs of older men in these settings.

Transportation

Inner-city elderly includes many people who are "transit-dependent" and accustomed to the high density of activities and neighborhood services that characterized urban neighborhoods of the early decades of this century. Many of the current cohort of elderly grew older in communities and never experienced the "automobile-centrism" of later generations who were more accustomed to suburban low-density living. Many urban, mobility-dependent elderly must rely on taxis, public transportation systems, and relatives or friends who drive (thereby reducing their freedom of choice and spontaneity) (Wachs, 1988).

Public transportation, in particular, has several problems. First, persons using public transportation are limited to choosing fixed destinations and to traveling at hours of the day when services are conveniently available. Wachs and Kumagai (1973) found transit-dependent elderly were particularly limited in the number of available hospitals and clinics (or parks, theaters, and educational facilities) reachable within acceptable access times. A second problem with public transportation is that it involves substantial physical barriers associated with the urban landscape and fixed routes. For example, many elderly must walk long distances and expose themselves to environmental elements (such as excessive temperatures, rain, hills, and busy streets). These problems become particularly acute for the elderly with functional deficits. A third problem involves victimization of people using public transit systems. "Many elderly people report that they are fearful of using public transit, especially after dark, and their fears appear to be well founded" (Wachs, 1988, p. 178). A study by Levine and Wachs (1985) found that the elderly were far more likely than members of other age groups to be victims of crime while traveling on public transportation.

ELDERLY MEN IN THE URBAN ENVIRONMENT

Housing options that allow poor, inner-city elderly men to live in community settings include inexpensive hotels, apartments, rooming houses, and—for those needing assistance—small board-and-care homes and foster homes. These housing alternatives have a great deal in common.

Although they respond flexibly to the atypical lifestyles of many inner-city elderly men, such housing is frequently perceived as incompatible with planning efforts to "revitalize" neighborhoods (with gentrification as the result) (Ehrlich, 1986).

While the plight of the urban aged has been expounded by many scholars, these high-density urban areas often provide the only places in which the aged and the poor can secure the goods and services necessary to continue independent living (Clark, 1971). Studies conducted over the past several decades provide a glimpse of life among aged residents of the inner city. For example, Lawton and Kleban (1971) and Clark (1971), in a two-part series for *The Gerontologist*, gave a useful overview of aged residents of the inner city and their patterns of aging. Lawton and Kleban (1971) concentrated on the lifestyles of poor Jewish tenants residing in a section of Philadelphia known as "Strawberry Mansion." The once prestigious area had become a low-income, high-crime area. They discovered that by almost all indices of well-being, the older residents were markedly deprived compared to members of their age cohorts in other areas of the city. The residents of Strawberry Mansion were more likely to be single or widowed, with grossly low incomes. Additionally, compared to other samples of older persons, they were deprived in health, neighborhood motility, leisure-time activity, peer interaction, morale, and housing satisfaction. These elderly persons were coping with their situation, but ordinary coping behavior required energy expenditures that reached near-upper threshold levels. Their life-chances were severely limited and they were locked into their environments due to low incomes and comparatively low rents. They also had few contacts with neighbors and relatives. The results of this study showed that environmental factors had a substantial and unique association with neighborhood motility and interviewers' ratings of vigor, interaction, and responsiveness.

Clark's 1971 article, "Patterns of Aging Among the Elderly Poor of the Inner City," gives rich insight about urban environments and their potential for promoting both human misery and human survival. She emphasized the important role that formal and informal structures play in the survival strategies of the inner-city elderly. This examination of informal structures and social support systems among inner-city elderly men was conducted among occupants of Single Room Occupancy hotels and the homeless.

Single Room Occupancy Hotels (SROs) and Rooming Houses

SROs consist of low-priced, furnished one-room rental units in transient hotels, residential hotels, and rooming houses located in inner-city, skid row, or commercial areas.

During the 1970s ethnographic studies in diverse metropolitan areas—San Diego (Eckert, 1980); St. Louis (Ehrlich & Ehrlich, 1982); Syracuse, New York, and Charlestown, West Virginia (Rubenstein, Schuster, & Desiervo, 1976); Detroit (Stephens, 1975); and New York (Siegel, 1977)—had shed light on this housing type and established it as an essential alternative to the survival of the inner-city elderly poor (Ehrlich, 1986). In reporting on research conducted in Chicago, Keigher (1991) suggests that SRO hotels are one of the most affordable and flexible types of housing for the inner-city poor, although the stock of SRO housing in Chicago, as in other places, is limited and rapidly shrinking. In spite of a 12% decrease in SRO housing stock during the 1970s, 397,000 elderly people were identified as residing in SRO accommodations (Haley, Pearson, & Hull, 1981). In the early 1980s, census-based research showed that more than 80,000 hotel units were occupied by people 65 years of age and older (Goode, Lawton, & Hover, 1980). It is suspected that the number of SRO units has continued to decline since the 1980s.

The elderly poor represent the largest single group of SRO residents. Haley et al. (1981) suggest a profile of the SRO elder as a white male with 8.7 years of schooling and a total personal income of $4,419 in 1980. The majority of elderly SRO residents lived in their rooms for 5 or more years, and over half never married. Ethnographic studies conducted in the mid-1970s (e.g., Stephens, 1975) identified the elderly population living in SRO housing as primarily male, single, mobile, nontraditional, and exhibiting independent and self-reliant lifestyles.

In recent years, there has been an increase in ethnic minorities seeking SRO housing. Keigher (1991) notes that in Los Angeles, the SRO population (historically middle-aged or older single, white men) has been supplanted by homeless families, and young, single men of color. Ex-mental patients, including those discharged from psychiatric institutions between 1965 and 1975, comprise the other large subgroup relying on SRO housing. In Chicago, Keigher's research shows that the number of persons over 65 in SROs is increasing, and that the residents remain largely men (Keigher, 1991).

SRO facilities share common characteristics, including furnished rooms with or without bathrooms, generally no kitchens, management services (24-hour desk clerks, housekeeping, linens, laundry), permanent residents, and older facilities in need of repair (Golant, 1992). The urban commercial area supplies older residents with important supports and services to meet their needs (Eckert, 1980). Such services as inexpensive restaurants, secondhand clothing stores, discount drug stores, soup kitchens, beauty and barber shops, laundromats, entertainment, and transportation are all combined with hotels to provide an infrastructure of supportive services required for continued independent living. However, many inner-city neighborhoods containing SRO hotels have witnessed declines in social, health, and nutritional services, which diminish the attractiveness of the SRO option (Golant, 1992).

In contrast to the earlier impressions that SRO residents lived thoroughly isolated lives, ethnographic studies have documented the presence of social relationships and supports essential for survival (Eckert, 1980, 1982). In a study of 27 SRO hotels in Chicago, Keigher, Berman, and Greenblatt (1991) reaffirm the importance of informal supports provided by hotel personnel and "special friends."

> Staff in the building—the owner, manager or desk clerk, but also the maid, bell man, superintendent, custodian, or security guard—provide what assistance there is, helping out with everything from incidentals to personal care. . . . The elder is also secure who has a "special" friend, usually a roommate, who will help out with personal care. Men tend to receive more help this way, as lots of girlfriends help out even if they only visit intermittently (Keigher, 1991, p. 171).

The census-based study conducted by Haley et al. (1981) included five urban community case studies in Massachusetts, New York, and Oregon. Their findings supported those of the ethnographic studies referenced above and attest to the value of the SRO housing type for low-income, single city residents. Golant (1992) noted that several communities (e.g., New York City, San Francisco, and Portland) have taken legal action to stem the loss of SRO units by establishing programs designed to preserve and rehabilitate current SRO units. Advocates argue that the cost of rehabilitating and subsidizing SRO hotels is less than the cost of providing new low-rent conventional apartments for single people (Franck, 1989). These efforts have been supported through federal rent subsidy and renovation programs. Despite the widespread recognition of the benefits of this private form of housing, the future of SRO housing is bleak. Urban redevelopment and gentrification, commercial encroachment and speculation, condominium and apartment conversions, and lack of substantial private or federal funds for renovations threaten this housing stock. Since the 1970s, more than one million SRO rooms in the United States were lost because of these actions (Golant, 1992).

Homelessness

Homelessness has been on the rise since the early 1980s (Snow & Anderson, 1993). As a group, the homeless lack permanent homes and find accommodations at night in public or private emergency shelters or places not intended to be shelters (such as train and bus stations or the street). Nationwide, persons over the age of 60 comprise at least 2.5 to 9.0% of the homeless (Institute of Medicine, 1988), with some estimates as high as 19% (Keigher, Berman, & Greenblatt, 1991). Homelessness grew dramatically in the 1980s and is expected to continue to grow in the future, as the nation's infrastructure of basic housing resources erodes and federal, state, and local budget crises undermine the social services safety net (Congressional Budget Office, 1988). Keigher and Pratt (1991) note that homelessness is increasing at least as fast among the elderly as among younger groups, but the elderly appear to have unique social and health vulnerabilities. The "new homelessness" is closely related to the general housing problems faced by the urban aged; namely, a growing shortage of low-income housing, federal program cutbacks, changing tax benefits, and prepayment and buyouts of federal mortgages on rent-subsidized building (Keigher & Pratt, 1991). Golant (1992) notes that studies of elderly homeless have produced conflicting findings about whether this group is dominated by men or women or by younger as opposed to older elderly persons. However, most studies find that elderly African-Americans are overrepresented (Golant, 1992).

The roots of homelessness, and its awareness as a mounting national problem, lie in several related societal dynamics: (1) a decline in the availability of low-cost housing, (2) a decrease in actual income or its purchasing power, and (3) a dramatic increase in U.S. unemployment since the early 1980s resulting from deindustrialization, job and income polarization, and governmental cutbacks (Snow & Anderson, 1993). Other factors include extreme poverty; impaired functional status (mental illness, alcoholism, drug abuse, depression, dementia); poor physical health; paucity of social resources (relatives and friends); history of eviction and relocations; and the demise of SROs, and decline in the availability of inexpensive, skid-row neighborhood services (e.g., "slop joints," used clothing stores) (Golant, 1992).

It appears that patterns of homelessness are different for urban African-American and white elderly persons. In one study completed in Detroit (Douglass & Hodgkins, 1991), homeless white elderly were more likely to be never married and experience homelessness for many years. Elderly African-American homeless tended to be widowed and homeless for 3 or fewer years. In addition, white homeless were more likely than African-American homeless to be former patients of state mental hospitals, and African-American homeless were more likely than white counterparts to have been incarcerated at some point in their lives. Thus, unlike African-Americans, white homeless elderly most reflect the traditional findings of homeless elderly, with many isolated or living in skid row. These differences have important implications for those funding and serving the homeless (Douglass & Hodgkins, 1991).

The Stewart B. McKinney Act, signed into law in 1987, is the federal government's major provision to help local governments and agencies in providing services for the homeless (U.S. Senate, 1990; Golant, 1992). Even with programs such as the McKinney Act and other programs that benefit the elderly, such as Medicare and Social Security, many elderly continue to be at risk of homelessness. Many programs are symbolic at best. For example, shelters only provide temporary housing without addressing permanent housing needs, and food pantries and soup kitchens offer only several meals a week and do not provide for basic nutritional needs. Only well-coordinated, permanent services can help prevent homelessness of the elderly (Martin, 1990).

Keigher (1991) summarizes the efforts of past governmental administrations:

> In short, the Administration's efforts of the last decade have been of symbolic importance at best, and at worst an effective comprehensive strategy to abandon any federal role in public provision of housing altogether. The prospects for federal maintenance of support for low income housing for elders, much less for the creation of new housing

resources to meet needs of rapidly aging populations, are bleak at best (p. 10).

Although the present Democratic administration is trying innovative approaches to the problem of scarce low-income housing, activitists maintain that the real bottom line is money. In fact, there is less money available for housing programs than in earlier administrations. To add to this problem, state and local agencies, which supported housing programs during earlier years, no longer have funds to make up the void. Stephen Banks, an attorney for the Homeless Family Rights Project, states: "For 12 years, the federal government was absent from the table, and now, although the federal government is at the table rhetorically, there aren't new dollars being put on the table" (Stanfield, 1993, p. 3001).

Residential Care

The need for supportive residential settings and services will be especially acute for older persons with limited financial and social resources, since society cannot rely on a profit-motivated marketplace to provide low cost alternatives (McCoy & Conley, 1990). Residential care facilities, commonly called board-and-care homes, are one community-based option being identified as a critical, yet largely untapped, resource for long-term care in the United States (Dobkin, 1989). The generic term "board-and-care" is used to describe a range of noninstitutional residential care arrangements, such as domiciliary care, adult foster care, assisted living, and small congregate housing (Conley, 1989). Most board-and-care providers are still small-scale operators, functioning primarily in facilities housing six or fewer clients (Baggett, 1989).

In general, board-and-care homes house vulnerable populations who often lack key resources. These populations are poor, have few or no kin and other social supports, and suffer from long-term disabilities, mental illness, mental retardation, and chronic physical conditions (Eckert & Lyon, 1991). Board-and-care homes typically provide shelter (room), meals (board), 24-hour supervision, housekeeping, laundry, personal care, recreation, and other services to residents (Morgan, Eckert, & Lyon, 1995). Furthermore, they serve as a bridge between independent living and nursing care (Chelseth & Serva, 1990).

Nationally, estimates of the number of board-and-care homes depend on how they are defined. A 1987 national industry survey identified about 563,000 board-and-care beds in 41,000 licensed homes in the U.S. (General Accounting Office, 1989). A more recent study found some 75,000 licensed and unlicensed homes serving a million people, including a half million disabled elders (GAO, 1992). McCoy and Conley (1990) estimate that there are nearly 70,000 licensed and unlicensed board-and-care homes housing nearly a million elders and others, and that an additional 3.2 million are estimated to be at immediate risk of board-and-care placement.

Older persons are estimated to compose 40 to 60% of the board-and-care population, with the largest category of residents being older, functionally impaired women (Dobkin, 1989). For example, in a survey of 670 residents in six states, Mor, Sherwood, and Gutkin (1986) found that 66% of the respondents were female and 40% were over age 75. More recently, in a study of 560 board-and-care residents in Cleveland, Ohio, and Baltimore, Maryland, Morgan, Eckert, and Lyon (1995) found that 32% of those age 65 and over were male. Low-income elderly men, although in the minority, represented many board-and-care home residents. Although frail older women who are widowed, never married, separated, or divorced are over-represented among older board-and-care home residents, a second major group is composed of predominantly male, deinstitutionalized mental hospital patients (Morgan et al., 1995). This later group is aging in place, suggesting an increase in the proportion of males residing in such facilities in the future.

Small board-and-care homes are most likely to be located in commercial or lower-income neighborhoods next to inner-city areas. They provide one of the few residential care settings for vulnerable elderly males unable to live independently in apartments, SRO hotels, rooming houses, or "on the streets." Golant (1992) noted that compared to the elderly population generally or in congregate housing and assisted living facilities, board-and-care facilities contain a disproportionate share of the poor who cannot afford the cost of full-time in-home assistance. Public opposition to this type of housing for dependent adults suffers from the NIMBY (Not In My Back Yard) syndrome, thereby forcing it into commercial districts and declining multifamily residential areas.

Unlike larger institutions that care for dependent adults, family-based "Mom and Pop" board-and-care homes are smaller (Hawes, Wildfire, Lux, & Clemmer, 1993), more personalized, less regulated, less regimented (Rubinstein, 1995), and less costly (Morgan et al., 1995). McCoy and Conley (1990) add that the primary purpose of board-and-care homes is to provide nonmedical personal care to physically and mentally disabled persons.

Studies of small board-and-care homes (e.g., Morgan et al., 1995) have found them to be much like typical informal settings in single-family homes. Most operators are self-selected, middle-aged women motivated to provide care for humanitarian reasons, including strong religious convictions, and a wish to keep elderly residents out of nursing homes (Sherman & Newman, 1988). Operators characterize their homes as family-like environments in which they share activities and affection with residents and give one-on-one care (Morgan et al., 1995). Similarly, residents identify the board-and-care atmosphere as homelike and emphasize its importance as a place of residence (Namazi, Eckert, Rosner, & Lyon, 1991). From their viewpoint, caring is enmeshed in the domestic domain of family and friends, rather than formal relationships and arrangements typical of organizations, such as nursing homes (Morgan et al., 1995). Finally, operators of small board-and-care homes play a pivotal role in the daily operations of their homes and in the lives of their residents (Morgan et al., 1995; Newman, 1989).

The public's perception of board-and-care homes is mixed. Sweeping conclusions based on media coverage of abuses and neglect, and congressional reports, characterize all such home operators as unscrupulous, uncaring, or worse (United States House of Representatives, 1989; United States Senate, 1989). Golant (1992) lists the problems associated with some board-and-care homes: inadequate fire protection, poor levels of cleanliness and nutrition, misuse and poor oversight of medication, neglect of residents' basic personal care needs, inability of operators to provide all the care residents need, and financial exploitation of residents. By contrast, there is ample evidence of responsibly operated and effective homes (Morgan et al., 1995). Dobkin (1989), in a critical look at board-and-care oversight and environments, was forced to note that residents reported high levels of satisfaction, despite some objective environmental problems discovered by researchers.

Although board-and-care homes provide essential services to vulnerable adult men (and women), their viability in the future is questionable. The need to assure optimal outcomes for residents of board-and-care homes drives national and local efforts for greater oversight and regulation of facilities. However, the difficulty in defining quality forces policymakers to fall back on aspects of the physical structure (e.g., staffing, building safety) and process features (e.g., residents' activities, autonomy) of the home as the basis for assessment (Segal & Hwang, 1994). Unfortunately, this approach overlooks the very dimensions of care and interpersonal relationships that are most important to the quality of life of the residents (Morgan et al., 1995). The failure to measure and understand what is central to quality care in board-and-care homes leaves it open to inappropriate regulatory models, such as that for nursing homes (Baggett & Adler, 1990). Regulations that are too bureaucratic and stringent will undoubtedly drive many small board-and-care operators out of business or underground (Applebaum & Ritchie, 1992).

SUMMARY AND CONCLUSION

Research and information focusing exclusively on inner-city elderly men is spotty at best. From a demographic perspective, it is known that inner-city elderly men are not a homogeneous group; however, the implications and meanings of these differences are not yet known. What does it mean for the individual and society, for example, that elderly African-American men are more likely to live alone than are white or Hispanic men?

Much of what is known—beyond basic demographic profiles of the elderly—is from case studies done in the 1970s and 1980s. Although beneficial, they do not help the understanding of the changing urban landscape, or the political and social realities facing inner-city elderly men in the 1990s. For example, it cannot be assumed that the experiences of vulnerable elderly, inner-city men will be the same in large Northeastern cities as smaller cities of the South and Southwest. To what extent are successive cohorts of inner-city, elderly men coping with crime, decreasing housing options, rising rents, and threats to the social services/health care safety net? To what extent are "charitable" and voluntary programs filling the gaps left by decreasing publicly funded programs? Are programs labeled "charity" accepted and used by elderly men in need, and at what personal cost? Acknowledging the extensive urban redevelopment and renewal efforts of the past several decades, to what extent do inner-city environments still provide an infrastructure of necessary services for those who remain?

Elderly, poor, inner-city men fit into the underclass of American society. The term "underclass" emerged in the 1960s to describe highly marginalized urban populations of low income and low social status, suffering from physical, social, and psychological isolation (Baca Zinn, 1989). The current debate on welfare reform, education, and health care shows that society has not come to terms with either the reasons that such populations exist, or what society should do about them (Morgan et al., 1995). The harsh reality is that many in America choose to continue to blame the victim and have become frustrated with federal and state programs to help those less fortunate. There is strong reluctance among taxpayers to support social programs for dependent adults, especially the most marginalized groups, such as the mentally ill. Similarly, funding for research on better understanding and serving inner-city elderly men has disappeared. Urban poverty, crime, declining neighborhoods, and diminishing low-rent housing stock, combined with unsympathetic public attitudes toward the underclass in America, suggest a worsening future for the poor, inner-city elderly.

REFERENCES

Akers, R. L., Sellers, C., & Cochran, J. (1987). Fear of crime and victimization among the elderly in different types of communities. *Criminology, 25*, 487–505.

Applebaum, R., & Ritchie, L. (1992). *Adult care homes in Ohio*. Oxford, OH: Miami University.

Baca Zinn, M. (1989). Family, race, and poverty in the eighties. *Signs: Journal of Women in Culture and Society, 14*, 856–874.

Baggett, S. A. (1989). *Residential care for the elderly: Critical issues in public policy*. New York: Greenwood Press.

Baggett, S. A., & Adler, S. (1990). Regulating the residential care industry: Historical precedents and current dilemmas. *Journal of Aging and Social Policy, 2*, 15–32.

Biegel, D. E., & Farkas, K. J. (1990). The impact of neighborhoods and ethnicity on black and white vulnerable elderly. In Z. Harel, P. Ehrlich, & R. Hubbard (Eds.), *The vulnerable aged: People, services, and policies* (pp. 116–136). New York: Springer Publishing Company.

Brice, D. (1970). The geriatric ghetto. *San Francisco, 12*, 70–72, 82.

Chelseth, R., & Serva, J. (1990). Assisted living: Matching health needs with care and living options. *Retirement Housing Industry, 1989*. Philadelphia: Laventhol & Horwath.

Clark, M. (1971). Pattern of aging among the elderly poor of the inner city. *The Gerontologist*, 7(1), 58–66.

Congressional Budget Office. (1988). *Current housing problems and possible federal responses*. Washington, DC: Congress of the United States.

Conley, R. W. (1989). Federal policies in board and care. In M. Moon, G. Gaberlavage, & S. J. Newman (Eds.), *Preserving independence, supporting needs: The role of board and care homes* (pp. 41–59). Washington, DC: AARP Public Policy Institute.

DeLeaire, R. N. (1994). *The inner-city elderly: How effective are their support structures*. New York: Garland.

Devine, J. A. & Wright, J. D. (1993). *The greatest of evils: Urban poverty and the American underclass*. New York: Aldine de Gruyter.

Dobkin, L. (1989). *The board and care system: A regulatory jungle*. Washington, DC: American Association of Retired Persons.

Douglass, R. L., & Hodgkins, B. J. (1991). Racial differences regarding shelter and housing in a sample of urban elderly homeless. In S. M. Keigher (Ed.), *Housing risks and homelessness among the urban elderly* (pp. 43–57). New York: The Haworth Press.

Eckert, J. K. (1980). *The unseen elderly: A study of marginally subsistent hotel dwellers*. San Diego, CA: San Diego State University Press.

Eckert, J. K., & Lyon, S. (1991). Regulation of board and care homes: Research to guide policy. *Journal of Aging and Social Policy*, 3, 147–162.

Ehrlich, P. (1986). Hotels, rooming houses, shared housing, and other housing options for the marginal elderly. In R. J. Newcomer, M. P. Lawton, & T. O. Byerts (Eds.), *Housing and aging society: Issues, alternatives, and policy* (pp. 189–199). New York: Van Nostrand Reinhold.

Ehrlich, P., & Ehrlich, I. (1982). SRO elderly: A distinct population in a viable housing alternative. In G. Lesnorr-Caravaglis (Ed.), *Aging and the human condition* (pp. 28–37). New York: Human Sciences.

Franck, K. A. (1989). Single room occupancy housing. In K. A. Franck & S. Ahrentzen (Eds.), *New households, new housing* (pp. 245–262). New York: Van Nostrand.

Golant, S. M. (1992). *Housing America's elderly: Many possibilities/few choices*. Newbury Park, CA: Sage Publications.

Government Accounting Office. (1989). *Board and care: Insufficient assurances that residents' needs are identified and met*. Washington, DC: United States Government Printing Office.

Government Accounting Office. House Committee on Aging (1992). *Board and care homes: Elderly at risk from mishandled medications* (HRD 92–45). Washington, DC: United States Government Printing Office.

Goode, C., Lawton, M. P., & Hover, S. I. (1980). *Elderly hotel and rooming house dwellers.* Philadelphia: Philadelphia Geriatric Center.

Haley, B., Pearson, M., & Hull, D. (1981, November). Urban elderly residents of single-room occupancy housing (SROs), 1976–1980. Paper presented at the 34th Annual Meeting of the Gerontological Society of America, Toronto, Canada.

Hawes, C., Wildfire, J. B., Lux, J. L., & Clemmer, E. (1993). *The regulation of board and care homes: Results of a survey in the 50 states and the District of Columbia.* Washington, DC: AARP Public Policy Institute.

Institute Of Medicine. (1988). *Homelessness, health, and human needs.* Washington, DC: National Academy Press.

Keigher, S. M. (1991). The effects of a shrinking housing resource on older communities in Chicago. In S. M. Keigher (Ed.), *Housing risks and homelessness among the urban elderly* (pp. 93–101). New York: The Haworth Press.

Keigher, S. M., Berman, R. H., & Greenblatt, S. T. (1991). Overview of the Chicago study of elderly persons at housing risk. In S. M. Keigher (Ed.), *Housing risks and homelessness among the urban elderly* (pp. 19–25). New York: The Haworth Press.

Keigher, S. M., & Pratt, F. (1991). Growing housing hardship among the elderly. In S. M. Keigher (Ed.), *Housing risks and homelessness among the urban elderly* (pp. 1–18). New York: The Haworth Press.

Lawton, M. P., & Kleban, M. H. (1971). The aged resident of the inner city. *The Gerontologist, 11,* 277–283.

Levine, N., & Wachs, M. (1985). *Factors affecting the incidence of bus crime in Los Angeles* (Report No. Ca–06–0195). Washington, DC: United States Department of Transportation.

Martin, M. A. (1990). The homeless elderly: No room at the end. In Z. Harel, P. Ehrlich, & R. Hubbard (Eds.), *The vulnerable aged: People, services, and policies* (pp. 149–166). New York: Springer Publishing Company.

McCoy, J., & Conley, R. (1990). Surveying board and care homes: Issues and data collection problems. *Gerontologist, 30,* 147–153.

Mor, V., Sherwood, S., & Gutkin, C. (1986). A national study of residential care for the aged. *Gerontologist, 26,* 405–417.

Morgan, L. A., Eckert, J. K., & Lyon, S. M. (1995). *Small board-and-care homes: Residential care in transition.* Baltimore, MD: The Johns Hopkins University Press.

Namazi, K. H., Eckert, J. K., Rosner, T. T., & Lyon, S. M. (1991). Psychological well-being of elderly board and care home residents. *Adult Residential Care Journal, 5,* 81–96.

National Research Council. (1994). *Demography of aging.* Washington, DC: National Academy Press.

Newman, S. (1989). The bounds of success: What is quality in board and care homes? In M. Moon, G. Gaberlavage, & S. J. Newman (Eds.), *Preserving independence, supporting needs: The role of board and care homes* (pp. 109–123). Washington, DC: AARP Public Policy Institute.

Redfoot, D. L., & Gaberlavage, G. (1991). Housing of older Americans: Sustaining the dream. *Generations, 15,* 35–38.

Rubenstein, D., Schuster, K., & Desiervo, F. (1976). *A study of older persons living in inner city SRO hotels and boarding houses: Final Report.* Syracuse, NY: School of Social Work, Syracuse University.

Segal, S. P., & Hwang, S. D. (1994). Licensure of sheltered-care facilities: Does it assure quality? *Social Work, 39,* 124–131.

Sherman, S. R., & Newman, E. S. (1988). *Foster families for adults: A community alternative in long-term care.* New York: Columbia University Press.

Siegel, H. (1977). *Outposts of the forgotten: N.Y. City's welfare hotels and single room occupancy tenants.* New Brunswick, NJ: Transaction.

Snow, D. A., & Anderson, L. (1993). *Down on their luck: A study of homeless street people.* Los Angeles: University of California Press.

Stanfield, R. L. (1993). Home economics. *National Journal, 25,* 2999–3002.

Stephens, J. (1975). Society of the alone: Freedom, privacy, and utilitarianism as dominant norms in the SRO. *Journal of Gerontology, 30,* 230–235.

Thompson, E. H., Jr. (1994). Older men as invisible men in contemporary society. In E. H. Thompson, Jr. (Ed.), *Older men's lives* (pp. 1–21). Thousand Oaks, CA: Sage Publications.

United States Conference of Mayors. (1986). *Adaptive reuse for elderly housing.* Washington, DC: United States Conference of Mayors.

United States Department of Justice. (1994). *Elderly crime victims.* March, NCJ-147186.

United States House of Representatives. Select Committee on Aging. Subcommittee on Health and Long-Term Care. (1989). *Board and care homes in America: A national tragedy* (No. 101–711). Washington, DC: Government Printing Office.

United States Senate. Special Committee on Aging. (1988). *Aging America: Trends and projections.* Washington, DC: Government Printing Office.

United States Senate. Special Committee on Aging. (1989). *Board and care: A failure in public policy* (Serial No. 101–1). Washington, DC: Government Printing Office.

United States Senate. Special Committee on Aging. (1990). *Developments in aging, 1989* (Vols. 1 and 2). Washington, DC: Government Printing Office.

Wachs, M. (1988). The role of transportation in the social integration of the aged. In *The Social and Built Environment in an Older Society* (pp. 437–456). Committee on an Aging Society and Institute of Medicine and National Research Council. Washington, DC: National Academy Press.

Wachs, M., & Kumagai, T. G. (1973). Physical accessibility as a social indicator. *Socio-Economic Planning Sciences, 7,* 437–456.

CHAPTER 5

Elderly Men in Retirement Communities

Burton D. Dunlop, Ph.D.,
Max B. Rothman, J.D.,
& Chandra Rambali, M.H.S.A.

INTRODUCTION

A retirement community (RC) is a relatively recent addition to housing choices in the United States. Special housing for elders, from which retirement communities have evolved, dates back only to the 1920s (Bowers, 1989). Unfortunately, but not surprisingly, research on RCs has been limited and rarely rigorous. The existing literature raises far more questions than it answers. No reliable source of information exists on the size of the total RC resident population in the United States, but there probably are several million individuals residing in these settings that, although widely disparate in organization, philosophy, and ambiance, categorize themselves as RCs. The most is known about Continuing Care Retirement Communities (CCRCs), a type of RC with a broad array of services and that, in reality, constitutes a form of health insurance. In this chapter, RCs will be defined and described prior to a discussion of the roles, behavior, and attitudes of men who reside within these settings.

RETIREMENT COMMUNITIES

RCs can be defined as planned neighborhoods of age-segregated individuals or married couples, usually retired, 60 years of age or over, and typically—though not always—middle-class. These entities are commonly referred to as retirement housing, retirement villages, life-care communities, and CCRCs. The literature varies widely in its definition of these entities and tends to use these designations interchangeably.

Although naturally occurring retirement communities emerge where concentrations of middle-age neighbors "age-in-place," the vast majority of RCs are planned, developed, maintained, and operated for retirees by either nonprofit or, increasingly, for-profit sponsors. In the past, most RCs were operated on a nonprofit basis and often by religious organizations. Today, a considerable number of RCs are operated for profit, and it appears that proprietary sponsorship will continue to grow as a proportion of RC settings.[1] As of 1995, for example, the Marriott Corporation had built approximately 14 RCs and had plans to open between 10 and 12 similar facilities each year for the next 7 years (Scruggs, 1995).

The characteristics of an RC may change over time (Hunt, Feldt, Marans, Pastalan, & Vakalo, 1983). As its resident population ages, an RC which began as a residential community may add services to address the increasing needs of residents—in effect, becoming an RC of a far different type than when it began.

In contrast to past cohorts, who often sought retirement housing in their own locales, contemporary retirees are somewhat more likely to venture beyond their familiar environs (Bowers, 1989). It has been found that California, Florida, Illinois, and Ohio account for more than one-third of all CCRCs in the country (Scruggs, 1995).

The 1996 edition of the directory of RCs, which includes CCRCs, Adult Congregate Living Facilities (ACLFs) and Independent Living Facilities (IFS) in the United States, lists approximately 22,000 entrants (HCIA, 1996). The American Association of Homes and Services for the Aging (AAHSA, 1995) reports that, as of 1994, approximately 350,000 older adults were living in 1,174 CCRCs in 42 states and the District of Columbia. In addition, there are an estimated 200 to 250 for-

---

[1] Although their numbers could not be determined, apparently there are at least a few government-sponsored facilities for elders that categorize themselves as RCs, as well.

profit CCRCs (Scruggs, 1995). The number of residents in these latter facilities could not be determined.

Perhaps the most important distinction among RCs lies in whether or not ongoing personal assistance or health services are provided or available on-site, in addition to housing alone or with other limited services (such as maid services or congregate meals). RCs that provide health-related services, such as assistance with personal care or a skilled nursing unit, not only offer greater potential for the residents to age-in-place, but also fall under considerably more state regulatory authority. Most of those with skilled nursing units would be CCRCs or, as they are sometimes referred to, life-care communities. Some RCs that are not life-care communities provide assistance to meet the needs of frail residents up to the level of skilled nursing care (i.e., personal care, homemaker, and even home health aide services). Clearly, leisure-oriented RCs (i.e., those facilities without extensive supportive services) are vastly more numerous. Even in Florida, which has a large number of CCRCs compared to most other states, 83% of households living in retirement communities reside in RCs that offer no supportive services (Berry & Henretta, 1996).

CCRCs

As indicated, the health care component of CCRCs, in part, distinguishes them from other forms of RCs. These settings offer, in addition to a variety of social and recreational activities (Cohen, Tell, Batten, & Larson, 1988), housing options on-site that range from fully independent apartment dwellings to a skilled nursing home residence (Sherman, 1990). Independent living units are usually governed by the same regulations as other housing; however, units that provide such services as assistive and nursing care are governed by more stringent state and federal regulations. The only accrediting body for CCRCs (as total entities) is the Continuing Care Accreditation Commission (CCAC), which is sponsored by the AAHSA. The CCAC accredits only nonprofit CCRCs and accreditation is voluntary for CCRCs.

The particular health insurance arrangements vary somewhat across CCRCs. The residents may contract for health-related services that cover a specified period or for life (AAHSA, 1995). Residents receive whatever services they need (e.g., personal care or nursing home) and would not pay any additional costs (Cohen et al., 1988). That is, the CCRC guarantees continued residence and services other than on-site hospital care, and regardless of the level of need that develops. In other CCRCs, residents pay a set monthly "rent" for basic services, or perhaps for basic services plus assisted living, and then—during whatever period they need the next level of care (e.g., assisted living or nursing home)—they pay an additional monthly amount.

All CCRC entrants pay a monthly "rent," or maintenance fee, based on the size of the living unit. Also, in most cases, when they join a CCRC, residents pay a separate admission fee, a "founder's fee" or "insurance endowment" which varies widely, depending on the type of facility and amenities offered (but it is at least several thousand dollars). Virtually all CCRCs, as well, require that admittees possess Medicare eligibility or comprehensive medical insurance to cover the costs of hospital, physician, and ancillary medical services.

The health care component of the arrangement between residents and management may be likened to commercial health insurance where there is pooled risk. Consequently, management of these communities, like their counterparts in the insurance industry, employ selection criteria for accepting enrollees. Residents, for example, must be fully independent at the point of admission and able to manage by themselves in an apartment unit.

Other RCs

Information obtained by the authors directly from three RCs which provide independent living arrangements, and two that provide both independent and assisted living arrangements, reveal that the communities of the first type are significantly larger in size. Rossmoor in New Jersey, Century Village in Pembroke Pines, Florida, and Sun City West in Arizona have 2,300, 6,200, and approximately 14,500 housing units, respectively. On the other hand, Carlyle on the Bay and Epworth Village, two South Florida communities that provide both independent and assisted living arrangements, have only 286 and 300 housing units, respectively. As could be expected, the age of residents upon entry is different for these two types of RCs. Independent living facilities (such as Rossmoor) tend to attract a younger population and some (Century Village, for example) accept a lower age limit of 18 years old, while facilities that offer both independent and assisted living tend to attract individuals about 75 years and older. Unsurprisingly, as well, the proportion of married couples is higher in the former than in the latter.

Residents at Century Village, Rossmoor, and Sun City West own their units, while those at Carlyle on the Bay and Epworth Village rent on a month-to-month basis. The price range for purchased units is between $60,000 and $300,000, while that for monthly rental in independent/assisted living facilities is between $598 and $2,900. These prices are reflective of factors such as size of unit, location of community, and offered services and amenities. Also, the two RCs offering assisted living have units for rent only. Managers of RCs that offer ownerships typically do not maintain information on residents such as age, gender, and marital status. For example, Century Village was able to provide only the age of residents recorded at the time of sale. RCs that offer assistive and health care services had this information readily available.

Maintenance fees cover such services as water, sewer, and trash collection, outside maintenance of building and landscaping, basic cable TV, and 24-hour security and medical emergency service. The organization of security services may vary. For example, Rossmoor and Century Village have paid security personnel to patrol their facilities, while Sun City West has the Volunteer Sheriff's Posse, which boasts a team of 200 members. Medical services are provided on an emergency basis and are usually minimal. The 24-hour services of the two registered nurses at Century Village are included in the maintenance fee. Century Village allows Humana Health Plans and some emergency medical groups to operate at their facility. Likewise, a medical clinic at Rossmoor operates on a pay-as-you-go basis.

While there are several different activities on the calendars of RCs, some of which have minimal costs, many can be considered quite expensive. Bus trips to various attractions range from $3.00 (to a restaurant) up to $692.00 (to Las Vegas with air fare included) from Rossmoor. Recreation facility membership fees at Sun City West are $126.50 per person annually. Annual golf and cart permits are available at a cost of $890 annually, while bowling costs $1.35 and $1.75 per game for residents and guests, respectively.

DEMOGRAPHICS

The age of residents in RCs varies widely, but is considerably older, on average, in CCRCs. In the 10 RCs examined by Hunt and colleagues (1984), age ranged from 61 to 85; while an AAHSA profile of the CCRC population, exclusively, shows the mean age to be 75 years (Scruggs, 1995).

The average age of residents in these facilities is increasing. Seguin noted as early as 1973 that the median age of residents in her study had risen from 73.5 years to 80 years within a 10-year period. Bowers (1989) also found that the entry age of residents of the 19 CCRCs in her study had increased from 75 years to 79 years, on average, from the time the facilities first opened. Bowers attributes this increase to the fact that residents of RCs are staying longer; that is, living longer. Longevity for elders, in general, continues to increase, so that the median age in RCs can be expected to continue rising, at least slightly, in the foreseeable future.

Initially, more married couples than single individuals join RCs, and these couples are usually made up of men who are older than their wives. Thus, in a newly-opened RC, the male population will usually be older than the female population. However, given the significantly higher mortality rate of men, RCs—over time—come to house a greater proportion of single females who tend to be older than the incoming male population (David, 1990; Sheehan & Karasick, 1995; Stacey-Konnert & Pynoos, 1992). A typical male/female ratio in RCs is 1:3 (AAHSA, 1995), compared to 5:7 for whites 60 years and older in the general population (United States Census Bureau, 1990).

The large proportion of men in RCs who are married reflects, first of all, the dominance of married couples among RC admittees. In addition, however, as is true for married men in general, the recently-widowed older male has to deal not only with a tremendous emotional loss, but also with unfamiliar roles such as taking responsibility for household chores. This combination contributes to widowed men choosing to re-marry rather quickly (Van Den Hoonaard, 1994). An added factor in RCs that undoubtedly contributes to the high number of married men is the large number of single women in close proximity from which widow-ers can select another spouse. A better understanding of the marital dynamics of the population in RCs could be gained from data on the frequency of marriages and remarriages. This information, unfortunately, is not available in the literature.

HEALTH

There is overwhelming evidence that residents in RCs are generally healthy, a finding that may be explained in large measure by the selective nature of this population. The choice to live in an RC that provides health services, although entrees are considerably older, on average, does not necessarily mean that residents use these services immediately after enrollment. Rather, enrollment in a facility that offers such supportive services may well reflect anticipated future needs. As long as 2 decades ago, Seguin (1973) found that 66% of elders were in good functional health. Seventy percent of RC elders in another more recent study (Stacey-Konnert & Pynoos, 1992) rated their health as either excellent or good. In a report on a study of residents in a Florida RC, Van Den Hoonaard (1994) captures the general mindset of residents in RCs: "Their days are filled with leisure activities that fulfill their image of what successful retirement is like" (p. 123).

One study (Longino & Lipman, 1981) of residents in two Midwestern RCs found only a 2% difference between married men and married women who considered themselves in good health (66.9% and 65.1%, respectively). However, among those who were unmarried, more women than men considered themselves to be in good health (65.9% and 58.9%, respectively). In a recent study of an exclusive RC, Free (1995) found that older men reported somewhat better health than their female counterparts, but suggests that this difference may be apparent rather than real, and could reflect the stoical socialization of that generation of males which leads them to downplay health problems.

EDUCATION AND INCOME

RCs are the homes of a significant number of highly educated professional men who were trained as lawyers, physicians, engineers, accountants, and the like. This segment of the population is the focus of much of the literature. However, the vast majority of residents in RCs have received somewhat less formal education, and were engaged in such occupations as teaching and medium-sized business ownership and management (Seguin, 1973). Men in RCs studied by Longino and Lipman (1981), approximately 15 years ago, had less education than female residents, although their income level was higher.

Income levels in RCs vary considerably, although they tend to be significantly higher than among elders in the general population. The mean income in one RC (Stacey-Konnert & Pynoos, 1992) was $35,000. Eighty-four percent of 100 couples in eight RCs scattered across the U.S. (Lauer, Lauer, & Kerr, 1990) reported annual incomes of over $20,000. Married men in the RCs, studied by Longino and Lipman in 1981, claimed the highest earnings ($12,548), while the lowest earnings ($8,486) were reported by unmarried women. Income has been found second only to health as a factor that determines satisfaction with retirement in general (Seccombe & Lee, 1986).

THE DECISION TO MOVE

For both men and women, the decision to move from their own homes to an RC seems to reflect a great deal of deliberation made over a considerable period of time. The decision calculus probably is quite complex in most instances. Two defining events in the life cycle that appear to precipitate, or at least often precede, movement to an RC are retirement and the death of a spouse. Tripple, McFadden, and Makela (1992) suggest that men tend to change their living arrangements upon retirement, while women tend to do so upon becoming widowed. Thus, the timing of the move of a large proportion of married couples probably coincides with the husband's retirement; the entry of single women may well occur soon after widowhood commences.

The explanation for the timing of the admission of single men into RCs, however, is less easy to surmise but may be as equally tied to widowhood as it is for women. Widowers have been found to be three times more likely than widows to leave the home they shared with their spouses (O'Bryant, 1995). Moreover, Loomis, Sorce, and Tyler (1989) found that men were twice as likely as women to identify widowhood as the reason for relocation. Other research, cited earlier, has shown that widowed men move to RCs primarily to get help with unfamiliar tasks, such as housekeeping.

It is important to note that, as mentioned earlier, the age of admission to CCRCs is much older than that for other RC settings. Therefore, the decision process involved in joining a CCRC undoubtedly is quite different from that involved in joining most RCs, which appeal primarily to younger retirees and typically offer fewer supportive services. That appeal seems to be the availability of multiple leisure activities and the proximity of other individuals in the same stage of life with whom these activities and interests can be shared conveniently. In at least three studies, availability of medical or health care and support services at the facility were cited most often by both men and women as important factors in their decision to join the RC (Cohen et al., 1988; Sheehan & Karasik, 1995; Tripple et al., 1992). Married persons reported that the most important reason to join was the availability of health care for a spouse, should the need arise. An accompanying consideration in the move to settings with health and supportive services seems to be the strong desire to avoid becoming a burden on one's children when dependency arrives. VanderHart (1995) suggests that demographic considerations override financial ones in the decision to move to an RC.

Several researchers (Johnson-Carroll, Brandt, & McFadden, 1995; Lucco, 1987; Sheehan & Karasik, 1995) suggest that elders who decide to move generally still prefer to relocate to RCs in their current geographic areas; indeed, the longer the tenure in a locale, the stronger seems to be the determination to remain there. However, this preference clearly is outweighed by other factors among movers to Sunbelt states, particularly for those who have vacationed over the years in these states.

Research findings which describe the reasoning of elderly men in their decisions to relocate to RCs are virtually nonexistent. This state of affairs reflects not only the relative recency of the RC phenomenon, but also (as alluded to earlier) the highly complex nature of this decision process, making measurement extremely challenging. One consideration which cannot be ignored is the willingness to reside in an age-segregated setting. Probably relatively few older men would prefer it, and a significant proportion, perhaps, would not give such an environment any serious consideration. Thus, men who reside in RCs represent a highly self-selected population and those factors, as well as the relative weights of those factors, that play out in such decisions almost surely differ greatly depending on the type of RC under consideration.

ADAPTATION TO THE RETIREMENT COMMUNITY LIFESTYLE

Given that relocation to an RC often appears to correspond to the timing of men's retirement and, therefore, appears to reflect heavily on their preferences, it is not surprising that men adapt better in a retirement setting than their female counterparts. To older men, the RC seems to function as an extension of their places of rest, very much like their former homes. In contrast, women experience more difficulty adjusting because, in this new home environment, they neither have the volume of work nor the amount of space which they were accustomed to in their former homes (Free, 1995). Elders entering RCs carry over the roles they held prior to joining (Free, 1995; Stacey-Konnert & Pynoos, 1992). Men's roles in this new environment reflect to a high degree their previous occupations. Their self-image is based largely on the level of prominence and respect commanded in their working years. It is not unusual, then, to find that men hold most of the leadership positions in RCs, while women assume auxiliary roles such as organizing bake sales and craft fairs (Stacey-Konnert & Pynoos, 1992). For example, male residents may become involved in various stages of facility construction, such as fundraising and contract negotiations for a new wing (Seguin, 1973). Wan and Odell (1983) have observed that the loss of the work role exerts a stronger effect on older men than even the loss of a spouse. In response to this finding, they recommend pre-retirement education for men that stresses their need to develop formal and informal support networks.

Although carrying over pre-retirement roles probably brings considerable satisfaction to most men residing in RC settings, possessing a professional background can become a curse of sorts. Those retired from professions such as law, medicine, and accounting, in fact, may feel themselves virtually forced into social isolation in order to avoid the frequent requests for professional advice that come from other residents (Crandall, 1991). Seccombe and Lee (1986) argue that, in general, it is really not the type of occupation held prior to retirement that contributes to satisfaction in the retirement years, but rather the level of income and wealth associated with an occupation that is key.

Overall participation in activities in the RC appears to contribute positively to residents' physical and social well-being. Typically, multiple social clubs and activities are available. Some RCs, for example, boast some 200 clubs and organizations for their members. Interestingly, clubs in RCs tend to be very gender-specific (Stacey-Konnert & Pynoos, 1992), with the arts, sewing, and ceramics classes comprised almost entirely of women, and the wood shop and lapidary clubs composed almost exclusively of men.

Representatives from all five of the RCs contacted said their facilities offer about an equal number of activities for men and for women. The gender-specificity of activities, as noted in the research literature, was not that apparent in the sales packets received from the three leisure-oriented RCs described earlier. Only three activities could be found that were clearly gender-exclusive, namely: "Golf-Men" and "Golf-Women," "Men's Social Club" and "Women's Social Club," and "Forever Fat Free Classes (men only)." It appears that most of the gender-specificity of formal activities results from resident preference rather than the design of RC management.

Apart from the gender-specificity of clubs, activity patterns also differ by marital status. While activities in one RC, for example, were open to all, and although singles constituted the larger population in the total community, activities were predominantly couple-oriented. This caused singles to feel excluded. The isolation of single men, as well as of single women, often was further intensified by their waiting to be invited by their married friends to social affairs instead of their initiating an invitation (Van Den Hoonaard, 1994).

While the tasks with which men occupy themselves and the availability of female companionship in RCs may serve to reduce their loneliness (Stacey-Konnert & Pynoos, 1992), men in RCs—like those in the larger community—still take longer to recover than their female counterparts from the loss of a spouse. Therefore, it would appear that the factors which seem to reduce loneliness do not necessarily serve to shorten the grieving process for men in RCs. Men's "passivity" may be a factor in the process (Free, 1995). That is, because men often conceal their emotions, they take longer to recover. Research needs to address whether involvement in activities actually diminishes or just masks emotions, and what can be done in the context of the RC to alleviate the longer grieving period of widowers.

A day in the life of an RC resident depends on several factors. Physical ability might be a major constraint in taking part in activities. Other factors include financial affordability and climate. Physical incapabilities may result in residents becoming shut-ins where they do little or no outdoor activities. Their typical day may be restricted to activities that they are able to perform within their apartments. Depending on the degree of their physical restrictions, this group might have friends or paid help perform daily activities for them. Shut-ins also include the less sociable who choose to live in seclusion or those who, as mentioned earlier, feel that others prey upon their professional expertise (Crandall, 1991). While most RC residents are relatively well-off, they may still be concerned about their financial security. This sometimes results in their avoiding activities that incur costs.

It is well to remember that the shut-in male resident's day is quite different from that of active residents and might include going outdoors only occasionally to obtain groceries or to visit the barber. A typical day for active male residents might start at about 8:00 a.m. with a review of investment opportunities in the newspapers over breakfast, then a round of golf or jogging. Most RCs provide a jogging trail on campus. In the midmorning hours, residents might choose to attend classes in current events, world affairs, or philosophy. A game of pool or bridge might precede lunch and the midday news, followed by a game of tennis or croquet or the pursuit of a hobby such as woodwork, stamp collecting, or photography. After dinner and the evening news, there might then be a commitment to a regular meeting of the RC's finance, planning, or building committee followed by a social engagement, such as a dance or movie. The evening news, a TV documentary or reading might close out the day at about 11:00 p.m.

ALCOHOL CONSUMPTION

Alcohol consumption appears to play a prominent role in the lives of many men in RCs. One survey (Alexander & Duff, 1992) of 932 residents in Florida RCs revealed that RC residents drink "considerably more" than their counterparts in the general population. Observable levels of consumption, according to Alexander and Duff, seem to correlate positively with degrees of sociability, but negatively with the religiosity of residents. However, it could be hypothesized that consumption is highest among single men in RCs, and especially the recently widowed—a possibility that Alexander and Duff do not address.

RELIGION

Initially, many RCs were organized by religious denominations to care for their elders. For example, Epworth Village in South Florida was founded by a member of the United Methodist Church who donated her home to house 12 elderly women. Epworth still retains its Methodist affiliation, but has evolved into a much larger operation, providing both independent and assisted living arrangements, with the Suzanna Wesley Nursing Home annexed to it. Daily devotional services are convened in the chapel. Epworth postures itself as nondenominational and invites ministers from other Christian denominations to deliver sermons in its chapel. Some RCs might be distinguished along religious lines, although not formally so. For instance, the Hermitage, an exclusive RC for the very wealthy, is basically Christian in orientation, while another nearby RC is predominantly Jewish (Free, 1995).

The literature is sparse on information about the extent of religious involvement of elders. Crandall (1991) attributes this to several factors, one of which is the difficulty in measuring religiosity. While at one time religiosity was measured by church attendance, now factors such as praying in the privacy of one's home, listening to religious programs on the radio, or watching religious programs on television are considered additional indicators. The frailty factor must also be considered when examining the religious involvement of this population. It is assumed that RCs sponsored by religious organizations provide formal opportunities for spiritual growth and development of residents.

Retirement community residents could also be active contributors to the RC by offering companionship to fellow church/synagogue members, comfort to those in distress, and even assistance with religious services. These religiously based groups also may function as proxy support systems for those lacking family or other informal support networks. This might be true especially for men in RCs, given their typical restricted informal networks. To what extent men in RCs are drawn to religious affiliation as a means of informal support, or upon the loss of a spouse, could not be determined from the literature and remain empirical questions.

TRANSPORTATION

Access to transportation would appear to have highly significant implications for patterns of activity and, indeed, for the overall quality of life of most RC residents. Prospective RC residents appear to recognize this importance. In studying a sample of persons interested in (and financially eligible for) RC living, Parr, Green, and Behncke (1989) found that 88% regarded transportation as an important service. The present cohort of RC residents is made up of men who started driving in their teens and 20s and women who started in their 30s (Persson, 1993). Therefore, the inability to drive might have a greater effect on men in RCs than their female counterparts. Additionally, married men in this group undoubtedly still feel the need to "provide" for their spouses, and the availability of transportation is an important means to such an accomplishment.

Most RCs studied in this report provide transportation (including buses or vans) within their communities to doctor's offices, grocery stores, shopping centers, and places of entertainment. For some residents, essential transportation may be provided by other residents who still drive, by churches, or by relatives living nearby. These informal sources, however, may tend to counter feelings of independence, so that these individuals may seek, or strongly prefer, formal means of transportation that they can access independently. Older residents, such as those in assisted living facilities, may be very dependent on transportation services offered by the facility.

Even in RCs that provide only independent living, there is emphasis on reducing the need for residents to travel great distances. For example, Century Village in Florida allows an HMO-sponsored doctor's office on-site, thus reducing the need for residents to go elsewhere for medical services. The office is staffed by a primary care physician and is equipped with examination rooms and laboratory facilities for the exclusive use of residents of Century Village. Likewise, a local bank provides services on the premises on certain days of the week. Most RCs also have gift shops where residents can purchase such items as greeting cards, candies, and even food items such as milk, juice, and snacks. Male residents interviewed at Epworth Village expressed pleasure in being able to walk to a small shopping mall to obtain food items and toiletries, to dine out, or just to pass the time.

A large number of both male and female residents join RCs for security reasons. Therefore, public transportation services might not be considered an acceptable option. Government-run special transportation systems for the elderly and disabled can provide an alternative for residents, but the cost and inconvenience attached to this service could limit use.

INFORMAL SUPPORT SYSTEM

The various losses that older men experience in the process of aging appear to exert an adverse effect on their health status. For example, O'Bryant (1995) reported research showing that one in five widowers died soon after the death of a wife, a rate 10 times that of recently bereaved widows. Support systems may serve to cushion such effects (Query & James, 1989). Support provided by family and friends usually is defined as primary or informal support, while that provided by such groups as housekeepers, nurses, and other professionals and paraprofessionals is defined as secondary or formal support (Longino & Lipman, 1981). In their study of elderly married men and women in household settings, Antonucci and Akiyama (1987) found for both that the quality of support given them was more important to their well-being than the quantity. However, the quantity of primary support was found to be more important to the well-being of women than men.

The average number of persons that RC members turn to for primary support is 10 (Longino & Lipman, 1981). However, single men have the smallest support systems. In addressing this issue, at least two different studies found that elderly men in the general community were happy with (and, therefore, not interested in extending) the size of their primary networks (Antonucci & Akiyama, 1987; Levitt et al., 1985). This may well be the general case in RCs, as well, although it still would be helpful to know whether the RC setting itself functions to enlarge the primary networks of elderly men, at least a little. Attempts to answer this question, of course, would have to control closely for the influence of self-selection in the RC population in order to explain any difference in the size or nature of the informal support network of RC residents versus older men in the general population.

MEN IN RETIREMENT COMMUNITIES OF THE FUTURE

It is unclear whether RC residences will continue to grow relative to the size of the aging population in the United States, although continued expansion seems likely in Sunbelt states like Arizona, Florida, and North Carolina. With the overall rising wealth of the elderly in the United States, more should be able to afford RC living. On the other hand, more may be able to purchase services that allow them to remain in their homes. Inability to perform homemaker and maintenance services are among the reasons that elderly persons move to RCs.

RCs of the future are likely to be more varied in both socio-demographic composition and culture. To date, RCs have been occupied almost exclusively by whites, reflecting not only their greater wealth but, perhaps, also a stronger cultural norm supporting independent residence of the generations. In the future, minorities will comprise a significantly larger proportion of the total retired population. Asians represent the fastest-growing minority group among the population 65 and over in the United States. This trend is sustained through 2050 (the period reviewed for these statistics) with the highest increase of 96% occurring between the period 1990 to 2000. Second to Asians is the Hispanic population (all races) which would experience the greatest increase during the same period. While the percentages for both whites and African-Americans peak during the period 2010 to 2020 at 33 and 41%, respectively, these increases are much smaller than those for Asians and Hispanics. The overall elderly population is increasing at a decreasing rate, with the greatest decreases occurring over the period 2030 through 2050 (Day, 1993).

Future cohorts of minority elders also are likely to experience increased wealth, allowing them more discretion in their living arrangements. This, together with a loosening of the norm of common multigenerational residence that, heretofore, has accompanied improved economic status of elders in the United States, suggests that the future will find increasing numbers of African-Americans, Asians, and especially Hispanics in RCs—perhaps in segregated RCs.

Specialized RCs organized by or for male or female homosexuals also are conceivable. When asked, "Would you consider moving into a CCRC for older homosexuals?" 88 and 95% of homosexual men and women, respectively, polled in a non-random volunteer sample in 1987 responded in the affirmative (Lucco, 1987).

Finally, with the increasing educational, occupational, and income levels of females in U.S. society, future male RC residents may find themselves sharing more of the leadership roles with female residents than is currently the case. Would such a loss of unique roles and any accompanying diminution of prestige make men significantly less satisfied with RC living?

Although the vast majority of RCs operate within the private sector and have seldom come under the purview of public policy decisions, perhaps policy makers should look more closely at this arrangement to see if there is any good reason for encouraging their expansion, or for shaping them differently in the future. If, for example, research determines that RCs foster the development of informal support systems among residents that, at least to some degree, take the place of extended family members and allow residents who become impaired to remain outside of a nursing home longer, policy makers may want to encourage RC living by offering tax incentives to residents or to RC sponsors. If CCRCs are found to be particularly effective in reducing nursing home days because they offer immediate arrangements, should public policy encourage this type of RC arrangement (perhaps with fewer amenities) to the elderly of lesser means? Should the public sector seek to effect improved access to RCs for older men of minority status? Is there any benefit to be gained from specifically encouraging minority-sponsored and operated RCs (or CCRCs, in particular) that would attract older cohorts of elderly from minority groups?

The trend toward nonreligiously sponsored organizations has the potential of decreasing religious involvement within RCs. Ready access to a place of worship within a facility can be a significant incentive to participate. The necessity of going outside of the facility to do so might entail hardships such as negotiating transportation arrangements.

Strategies for future RCs with regard to transportation should consider either locating them in close proximity to shopping malls, doctors offices, theaters, etc., or having such amenities on the premises. Urban rather than rural settings seem to be better suited for RCs because they put residents in close proximity to services that they might be able to access independently. The extent to which RCs use elder advocacy groups to assist with the transportation problems of their residents needs to be explored.

While aging-in-place might seem the best proposition for elderly persons, RCs might not have adequate resources to facilitate the process. Bowers (1989) talks about the "reluctantly accommodating model," where management effects changes on a reactive/crisis basis as individual needs arise instead of on a proactive basis to address the changing needs of the entire community. Of course, this decision might be a financial one rather than a case of ill-management. It is estimated that facilities need to be renovated approximately every 10 years in order to keep up with technological advances. The AAHSA recommends that older communities that have been able to build up equity over the years consider loan refinancing for renovation purposes in order to keep pace with the industry and to facilitate the aging-in-place process of their clients (Scruggs, 1995).

As is apparent from what has been just discussed, consideration of virtually all of these policy issues hinges on getting answers to some relatively fundamental empirical questions. Remaining research questions will be articulated in the following section.

SUMMARY AND ISSUES FOR FUTURE RESEARCH

The findings reported in this chapter are based largely on a review of the research literature and are restricted by the various definitions of facilities and age groups of elders examined by these sources. Most of the research fails to make distinctions in types of RCs that are needed in order to better understand older men in these environments. With seemingly interchangeable references to entities as diverse as Sun City and CCRCs, the picture that emerges is very unclear and likely reflects "a wash" of reality. The lack of specification in studies to date contributes to an array of apparent contradictions. These studies, however, do allow some tentative conclusions and serve to raise several important questions for future research.

RCs are a relatively new phenomenon in the U.S. and take on widely varying forms. Probably the most important distinction among these privately sponsored environments is whether or not they offer health care as well as housing. There appear to be approximately 22,000 facilities that qualify as RCs, with an unknown number of residents. About 1,200 of these are CCRCs with an estimated 350,000 residents. Except for RCs in Sunbelt states, residents tend to relocate from surrounding areas. Residents of CCRCs are considerably older than those of RCs generally and the average age upon admission in all RCs has been increasing. Men are usually married and older than women upon entry. Over time, however, as the men die earlier than the female residents, older women come to dominate the ranks of residents. Some facilities expand their service options to allow their residents to "age-in-place." Overall, men in RCs report better health than both women residents and men in the general population. Average income varies greatly across RCs.

The decision to join an RC is undoubtedly complex and may well vary enormously depending on the type of RC being considered. The two most common factors in a move to an RC are retirement and the death of one's spouse. Men appear to adapt better than women to the RC environment, although (like men in the general population) they grieve longer than women when their spouses die. Men appear to adjust more readily than women because they tend to carry over their pre-retirement reputation and leadership roles. Single men, however, tend to be somewhat socially isolated, owing to the dominance of married couples in social activities.

Finally, men—even in RCs—appear to have far smaller primary support systems than their female counterparts. Finances, as well as proximity to relatives, are factors that determine choice of RCs. Facilities that are located in areas where elders age-in-place might experience a lesser need to provide for services, such as transportation and social support. These services might be undertaken by relatives and friends. On the contrary, facilities that are located away from residents' former homes (e.g., in Florida or Arizona) might find that their residents are much more dependent on them for transportation and for informal, as well as formal, support.

While there are a few preliminary answers, a number of questions beg further study or deliberation. These include very basic issues:

1. How many of each type of RC are there in the U.S.?
2. Should the conventional definition be expanded to include public-sponsored housing for elders or single room occupancy hotels

(SROs), in which the majority of units are occupied by older persons, usually men (Rollinson, 1991)?

3. How many men of what ages live in RCs? By type of RC?

A number of questions surrounding the decision to relocate to an RC remain unanswered:

1. What self-selection factors determine which men relocate to RCs and which do not?
2. What are the principal factors that men consider in the decision to relocate to an RC? How does this differ for single versus married men?
3. How do those considerations vary by type of RC, especially according to whether or not the RC offers health services?

What are the effects of living in an RC on critical areas of men's lives (Dunlop, 1980)?

1. How does the health status of men in RCs compare with that of women residents? With men in the general community after self-selection is accounted for?
2. To what extent do men who become widowers after moving to an RC leave the setting, remain and remarry, or remain and stay single?
3. What effect does RC residence have on the grieving process for men who lose their spouses just prior to relocation? For those who lose their spouses after becoming an RC resident? Which particular aspects or activities exert an effect?
4. What influence does residence in an RC have on the primary support systems of older men who are married? On those who are single?
5. How involved are male residents with religion, and to what extent does religious involvement help male residents deal with loss?
6. How does having a church or synagogue on the premises affect the fulfillment of male residents' need for worship and fellowship?
7. Are informal support groups more readily formed in RCs that are sponsored by religious denominations?
8. Does the quality of informal support provided by religiously sponsored RCs differ from that provided by other types of sponsorship?

9. Do men lose unique leadership roles and prestige to increasingly well-educated and professionally experienced female RC residents?
10. How does this loss affect men's satisfaction with RC living, and even the likelihood of their joining an RC?

Finally, there are a series of outstanding issues with respect to the dynamic aspects of RCs, particularly related to their adaptation to the changing needs of their residents:

1. To what extent does, or should, management target services to men, especially widowed or single men, because of their more limited social support networks?
2. To what extent do RCs encourage the development of informal supports? To what degree is it the responsibility of RC management to do so?
3. Does living in a facility that is located within close proximity to relatives increase/decrease caregiving and quality time? Is living near family members more a source of security and peace of mind than a means of daily assistance?
5. How does the social milieu of RCs change as the residents become older and predominantly female?
6. How many RCs add services to cope with the changing needs of aging male residents?
7. What is the responsibility to address the needs of male residents according to the particular sponsorship, management, or contractual arrangements of an RC?
8. Do men fare better under some arrangements than others?
9. To what extent should government encourage the building of RCs within close proximity to services, such as shopping centers, theaters, and banks?
10. How would the trend toward home health care affect the RC industry? Would more elders elect to receive care in their own homes? Could services be delivered at less cost for both the government and residents in a community setting?
11. How many RC residents are forced to relocate because they come to need services not provided by the RC?

CONCLUSION

Answers to the above questions, undoubtedly, will surface a series of more specific inquiries that will need to be undertaken. This iterative process is the normal pattern by which all empirical knowledge becomes more highly specified or detailed. However, careful research to address several of these more basic questions will go a long way toward understanding the lives of older men in these particular settings. It will also aid substantially in understanding what stance policy makers should take toward these thoroughly modern institutions that have emerged as yet another byproduct of post-industrial society.

REFERENCES

Alexander, F., & Duff, R. W. (1992). Religion and drinking in the retirement community. *Journal of Religious Gerontology, 8*, 27–44.

American Association of Homes and Services for the Aging. (1995). Continuing Care Retirement Communities. Washington, DC: Author.

Antonucci, T. C., & Akiyama, H. (1987). An examination of sex differences in social support among older men and women. *Sex Roles, 17*, 737–749.

Berry, B. M., & Henretta, J. C. (1996). Comparing the older population: Florida and the U.S. *Aging Research and Policy Report, 3*, 23–28.

Bowers, B. J. (1989) Continuing care retirement communities' response to residents aging-in-place: The reluctantly accommodating model. *Journal of Housing for the Elderly, 5*, 65–81.

Cohen, M. A., Tell, E. J., Batten, H. L., & Larson, M. J. (1988). Attitudes toward joining continuing care retirement communities. *The Gerontologist, 28*, 637–43.

Crandall, R. C. (1991). *Gerontology: A behavioral science approach* (2nd ed.). New York: McGraw-Hill.

David, D. (1990). Reminiscence, adaptation, and social context in old age. *International Journal on Aging and Human Development, 30*, 175–189.

Day, J. C. (1993). Population projection of the United States by age, sex, race, and Hispanic origin. (Current Population Reports no. P 25-1104). Washington, DC: *Bureau of the Census.*

Dunlop, B. D. (1980, February). *Retirement communities: Existing knowledge and needed research.* Paper presented at the Annual Meeting of the Southern Gerontological Society, Atlanta, GA.

Free, M. M. (1995). *The private world of the Hermitage: Lifestyles of the rich and old in an elite retirement home.* Westport, CT: Bergin & Garvey.

HCIA. (1996). *Directory of Retirement Facilities.* Baltimore, MD: Author.

Hunt, M. E., Feldt, A. G., Marans, R. W., Pastalan, L. A., & Vakalo, K. L. (1984). *Retirement communities: An American original.* New York: The Haworth Press.

Johnson-Carroll, K. J. A., Brandt, J. A., & McFadden, J. R. (1995). Factors that influence pre-retirees' propensity to move at retirement. *Journal of Housing for the Elderly, 11,* 85–105.

Lauer, R. H., Lauer, J. C., & Kerr, S. T. (1990). The long-term marriage: Perceptions of stability and satisfaction. *Aging and Human Development, 31,* 189–195.

Levitt, M. J., Antonucci, T. C., Clark, M. C., Rotton, J., & Finley, G. E. (1985). Social support and well-being: Preliminary indicators based on two samples of the elderly. *Aging and Human Development, 21,* 61–77.

Longino, C. F., Jr., & Lipman, A. (1981). Married and spouseless men and women in planned retirement communities: Support network differentials. *Journal of Marriage and the Family, 43*(1), 169–177.

Loomis, L. M., Sorce, P., & Tyler, P. R. (1989). A lifestyle analysis of healthy retirees and their interest in moving to a retirement community. *Journal of Housing for the Elderly, 5,* 19–35.

Lucco, A. J. (1987). Planned retirement housing preferences of older homosexuals. *Journal of Homosexuality, 14,* 35–57.

O'Bryant, S. L. (1995). *An investigation of widowhood and remarriage of older men: Do gender roles explain behavior and well-being?* (*Final Progress Report prepared for AARP Andrus Foundation.*) Columbus: The Ohio State University, Department of Family Relations and Human Development, Ohio State University.

Parr, J., Green, S., & Behncke, C. (1989). What people want, why they move, and what happens after they move: A summary of research in retirement housing. *Journal of Housing for the Elderly, 5,* 7–33.

Persson, D. (1993). Elderly driver: Deciding when to stop. *The Gerontologist, 33,* 88–91.

Query, J. L., & James, A. C. (1989). The relationship between interpersonal communication competence and social support among elderly support groups in retirement communities. *Health Communication, 1,* 165–184.

Rollinson, P. A. (1991). Elderly Single Room Occupancy (SRO) hotel tenants: Still alone. *Social Work, 36,* 303–308.

Scruggs, D. W. (1995). *Dare to discover: The future of continuing care retirement communities.* Washington, D.C.: American Association of Homes and Services for the Aging.

Seccombe, K., & Lee, G. R. (1986). Gender differences in retirement satisfaction and its antecedents. *Research on Aging, 8,* 427–440.

Seguin, M. M. (1973). Opportunity for peer socialization in a retirement community. *The Gerontologist, 13*, 208–214.

Sheehan, N. W., & Karasik, R. J. (1995). The decision to move to a continuing care retirement community. *Journal of Housing for the Elderly, 11*, 107–123.

Sherman, S. R. (1990). Housing. In A. Monk (Ed.), *Handbook of gerontological services* (2nd ed.) (pp. 477–507). New York: Columbia University Press.

Stacey-Konnert, C., & Pynoos, J. (1992). Friendship and social networks in a continuing care retirement community. *The Journal of Applied Gerontology, 11*, 298–313.

Tripple, P. A., McFadden, J. R., & Makela, C. J. (1992). Housing environment important for retirement. *Journal of Housing for the Elderly, 10*, 93–115.

U.S. Department of Commerce, Bureau of the Census. (1994). *1990 Census of Population and Housing: Special tabulation on aging.* (Report No. CD90-AOA-US) [CD-ROM]. Washington, DC: Author.

Van Den Hoonaard, D. K. (1994). Paradise lost: Widowhood in a Florida retirement community. *Journal of Aging Studies, 8*, 121–132.

VanderHart, P. G. (1995). The socioeconomic determinants of the housing decisions of the elderly homeowners. *Journal of Housing for the Elderly, 11*, 5–35.

Wan, T. T. H., & Odell, B. G. (1983). Major role losses and social participation of older males. *Research on Aging, 5*, 173–196.

CHAPTER 6

Elderly Men in Prison

William A. Formby, Ph.D.
& Christopher F. Abel, M.A.

INTRODUCTION

When the problem of crime in America is considered, the perception of most people involves an image of a young, male offender. Similarly, when one refers to inmates in our prisons, the image again is often that of young males. The reason for these stereotypes is the fact that most crime is committed by young men, and they represent the largest portion of the inmate population. While offenses against the elderly seem commonplace, we are simply unaccustomed to thinking of the elderly as offenders. The perception overlooks the fact that the elderly can and do commit crimes, and they do represent a portion of America's prison population. In 1990, an estimated 19,160 persons aged 55 or older were incarcerated in state and federal correctional institutions in the United States. In 1992, the figure had risen to 23,025, and as of June 30, 1993, this figure stood at an estimated total of 25,004 (U.S. Department of Justice, 1993). America is, by all accounts, clearly aging. People are staying healthy longer, and living longer. As the population continues to move toward an older society, the number of older offenders increases. This, coupled with the prevalence of determinant sentences—mandatory minimum periods of imprisonment and extended prison terms without benefit of parole—produces a growing group of elderly male inmates. These individuals will spend a significant portion of their adult lives in a correctional institution, and some are likely to live out the remainder of their lives in a correctional setting (Sabath & Cowles, 1988). The fact that elderly inmates represent such a small percentage of the prison population, coupled with their double minority status as elderly and criminal, renders them low-priority status in society and within the prison structure.

Though they represent a minority in the prison system, other factors—not the least of which is the rising cost of health care—are attracting the attention of prison officials. A study of elderly inmates in Maryland, for example, showed that they each suffered an average of three chronic illnesses during their incarceration. The cost of their individual prison care averaged $69,000 annually, three times the expense of a younger inmate ("The Aging Prison Population." 1990). This chapter will review the status and problems of elderly offenders in prison and programs for them.

PRISON HOUSING AND ENVIRONMENT

Prison systems in the United States consist of a variety of types of institutions. Each is designed to fulfill a specific purpose based upon the characteristics and risks posed by its population. Most states and the federal jurisdiction traditionally classify their institutions as maximum-, medium-, and minimum-security institutions. Within these security classifications, the correctional system may operate specific programs based on the needs of the inmates.

Maximum-security institutions are, as the name implies, the most secure of the prison systems. Frequently they are massive buildings, with high masonry walls or electrified fences, and a primary emphasis on security. Prisoners are under constant surveillance, and their movements are severely restricted. In many cases, some of the inmates are required to remain in their cells most of the day. Outdoor recreation is minimal and visits, when allowed, are often conducted by telephone with a glass partition between the prisoner and the visitor. The inmates in these facilities usually have been convicted of the most serious offenses, such as murder, rape, and robbery, or are considered to be high escape risks.

Medium-security institutions are usually less ominous than the maximum-security facilities. They tend to focus more on rehabilitation programs and counseling. Inmates in these facilities have either been reclassified from maximum-security institutions, or were convicted of less serious offenses, and are considered less of a threat to escape. Many of the medical and drug rehabilitation facilities are operated as medium-security institutions.

Minimum-security prisons, on the other hand, are often built on a campus-like arrangement, allowing prisoners a higher degree of autonomy and options within the bounds of the institution. Security is a low priority, and visitation is allowed to a greater extent. There is more emphasis on programs which prepare inmates for release back into society.

Whether housed in a maximum-, medium-, or minimum-security facility, the elderly inmate faces numerous obstacles in the prison environment. From the physical structure to the social setting, the elderly are often disadvantaged. The physical layouts of most facilities were primarily designed for control of the inmates and administrative convenience of the prison staff. In fact, much of the discussion about prisons emphasizes that they are for punishment and should not be comfortable. Most of the facilities within the prison are secured in a fixed position. This becomes a problem for the elderly inmate who, because of reduced physical flexibility, may have difficulties with the standard seating, raised sleeping arrangements, abundance of stairs, a lack of ramps, and the distance between the elderly inmate's cell and prison and program functions. The young offender is usually able to adapt to these physical barriers. Also, the lack of privacy may be frustrating to the elderly, particularly if they enter prison at an advanced age. These conditions, along with the fear of victimization from the younger and more aggressive inmates, reduces the elderly inmate's physical movement and increases his isolation. The result may be that medical or mental help is necessary (Vito & Wilson, 1985).

THE PROFILE OF THE ELDERLY OFFENDER IN PRISON

Elderly inmates are those persons who have committed criminal offenses, have been found guilty of those offenses, have been officially sentenced, and are serving time in a penal institution. However, a discussion of the elderly male in prison requires several distinctions to be made. The population of penal institutions generally tend to be young; thus, inmates may be considered "old" at the age of 25 to 30 years of age. Yet, even though these individuals may be old by inmate standards, they would not be considered elderly—at least not in the outside world.

Defining an elderly inmate by social standards may also present some difficulties. Because of the previous lifestyles of many of these inmates (drugs, alcohol, poor eating habits, living on the streets, and stress from the lifestyle), they have aged at a much faster rate than the normal or "free" population. There may be as much as a 10-year difference between the overall health of elderly inmates and that of age peers in the general population. Therefore, a 55-year-old inmate will often have the health problems of a 65-year-old person on the outside. There may be two exceptions. First, inmates who enter criminal lifestyles, or commit their first crimes, at an advanced age may have "normal" health and aging problems. Secondly, inmates who enter prison at an early age on a long-term sentence may be even healthier than the norm on the outside, due to a life of regular exercise, diet, and readily available medical care. However, since these two categories represent a small proportion of the total elderly male prison population, this discussion will utilize age 55 as being elderly.

Based on various research efforts, it is difficult to develop a generalized profile of the elderly male in prison. The findings in the area of the elderly inmate tend not to be consistent in certain areas. On the one hand, Weigand and Burger (1979) claim that the elderly inmate is competent, responsive, quick, and shrewd. These qualities are necessary, since the elderly inmate must survive in a prison setting with younger, more competitive, and physically stronger inmates. On the other hand, Panton (1977) finds that the aged inmate functions at a lower intelligence level than the other inmates and has a significantly lower educational achievement level. Furthermore, he states, the number of mentally defective older inmates is twice that of their younger counterparts.

The elderly prisoners are more likely to have histories of poor health, more likely to be widowed or divorced and unemployed, and have a high incidence of involvement with alcohol. The aged have also served a greater percentage of two or more prior sentences. This is, in part, due to their age and the time span available for the opportunity to partake in criminal activity. Further, the physical and mental conditions of elderly inmates have been found to deteriorate rapidly during incarceration (Bergman & Amir, 1973). The elderly inmate is at the mercy of the younger, more aggressive, prisoners who frighten and even harm them. As a result, the elderly become depressed, anxious, and consequently dependent on the prison staff for protection.

As is true of most research, one must consider the characteristics of the samples studied. For example, inmates who remain in integrated custody tend to be much like their younger counterparts in terms of intellect. Their health is usually dependent upon their past health history. Many of them have adapted to the prison lifestyle, though they may be more prone to depression and isolation than younger inmates. Other elderly inmates may be housed in special units within the institution, or in special institutions. Such inmates have been classified as not being able to survive in the general population of prisons. Inmates, such as those in the Aged and Infirmed Unit of the Alabama Department of Corrections, are physically and/or mentally unable to cope with normal prison life. There is strong evidence that as prison sentences tend to get longer, special units will become more commonplace for aged inmates.

TYPES OF ELDERLY INMATES

Traditionally, there have been two types of elderly inmates, based on their incarceration history. There are those who are first-time inmates, and those with multiple incarcerations. The multiply-incarcerated or chronic offender may spend many years in and out of prison, and resembles the younger inmates in terms of crime classification. The first-time incarcerated, on the other hand, seem to be older persons who commit a first offense after a lifetime of being law-abiding citizens. They are more likely to be sentenced for crimes against the person. In recent years, however, with the emphasis on longer sentences and life without parole sentences, a third type has emerged. These long-term prisoners grow old in prison.

Goetting (1983) further divided the typology into four classifications. The first type consisted of those inmates who lived normal lives for the majority of their life, but were incarcerated for the first time after the age of 55. These inmates were labeled as "Old Offenders." The second type were listed as "Old Timers," which consisted of those inmates who had been incarcerated at an early age and have grown old in prison. The third type consisted of recidivists who had a long history of offenses and incarceration, and whose first incarceration came before the age of 55. They were labeled as "Career Criminals." Lastly, there were those short-term first offenders who were incarcerated before the age of 55 and had turned 55 while in prison (excluding the "Old-timers").

Contrary to expectations, Baum and Berman (1984) reported that most elderly inmates were not in prison for crimes committed when young, but had received their sentences after the age of 50. In 1980, over two-thirds of the prisoners sentenced after the age of 50 were first-time offenders. The Baum and Berman (1980) study further reported that the crimes committed by these individuals tended to be more severe than those committed by the general population.

Alston (1986) estimated that up to half of the elderly inmates were serving time for first-time offenses, and added that most of the first-time offenders were more likely to have been sentenced for violent, interpersonal offenses, while older multiply-incarcerated offenders were more likely to have been sentenced for property offenses. Due to the differences among the incarcerated elders, it is necessary to divide them into typologies like those stated above. Prior incarceration experience and length of incarceration are important variables available to classify the elderly inmate. Older first offenders are more likely to suffer from the shock of imprisonment and withdrawal from their usual lifestyle. On the other hand, the multiply-incarcerated, and those who grew old in prison, are more likely to exhibit symptoms of prisonization and to be assimilated into the prison culture.

Seip (1990) stated that elderly inmates may be sorted into one of three categories. First, those who have the mental and physical capabilities to live within the general population. They may have health ailments, but they are still able to function "independently" without any special accommodations. These inmates are usually mainstreamed. A second group consists of those elderly inmates who are not totally dependent, but have limitations in their ability to function independent of support from the prison. Their needs range from assistance with one or more basic activities to environmental support, such as elevators or ramps to help navigate the prison. Seip refers to the third group as the "dependent inmates." These inmates have chronic health problems that require the assistance of the prison staff for virtually all of their daily needs. In these instances, the prison staff take on the long-term care with nursing and therapeutic programs similar to the ones available on the outside.

THE EFFECTS OF IMPRISONMENT
ON THE ELDERLY

Incarceration can have serious negative effects on the elderly male, particularly the first-time offender, who suddenly finds himself removed from his family and friends and placed in the strictly regulated and confined environment of the prison. This move to a prison setting is a radical environmental change bound to have profound effects on the individual. Research shows a rapid deterioration in the physical and mental condition of elderly inmates. Often they were found to be at the mercy of the younger inmates and ridiculed and threatened. As a result, elderly persons become depressed, anxious, and consequently rely upon the warden and prison staff for protection. There is also a higher degree of insecurity, more expressed fear of pain, a constant fear of illness, more fear of correctional officers (and of authority in general), and a heightened fear of young African-American inmates (Fattah & Sacco, 1989).

Additionally, many of the elderly inmates have a fear of the future. This evolves from the uncertainty of their lives on the inside, and their fear of having no place to live on the outside when they are released. The reliance of the elderly inmate on the prison staff, and the desire to stay within the system, demonstrates his tendency to become dependent on the institution. Institutional dependency is influenced by the severing of ties to the outside community. The elderly inmate loses contact with family and friends due to deaths, being placed in an institution a great distance from family, and being abandoned by family who are ashamed of him. He must then look within the prison structure for emotional support from other inmates and the warden and prison staff.

Although the effects of imprisonment on both young and elderly inmates are overwhelmingly negative, the prison may have some positive effects on a few of the older men. The prison environment provides new contacts for those who were lonely on the outside. For those who were living in unhealthy, substandard conditions, or who were leading self-destructive lives (such as through drug addiction and chronic alcoholism), the prison generally offers a healthier, regulated, and less-destructive environment. Being in prison removes these individuals from the enticement of life on the street which often involves alcohol, drugs, prostitution, and other illegal activities. The prison environment provides them with regular meals, medical care, regular sleep patterns, and the opportunity to keep fit. Another positive effect of imprisonment, particularly for the first-time offender, is the fact he no longer has the worry and responsibility of day-to-day living and surviving on the outside.

CARING FOR THE ELDERLY

Prison is one type of domiciliary institution where the residents live together 24 hours a day, 7 days a week, within a circumscribed space under a scheduled routine administered by a staff. Furthermore, the prison environment may share some of the qualities characteristic of military bases, mental hospitals, certain kinds of schools, and—one might add—nursing homes. Regardless of the purpose of incarceration, the institution is responsible for the care of the inmates. When society removes people from its midst, it assumes the responsibility for their care and well-being. This responsibility for the older prisoner depends on society's degree of caring.

Of all the domiciliary institutions, the prison is unique in that its functions revolve around the control of inmates who have been convicted and sentenced as criminals. The first priority is to protect society, and then to worry about the needs and care of the inmate. This, coupled with the small number of elderly inmates in each institution, makes it difficult to accommodate the needs of the elderly inmate. However, as previously discussed, the number of elderly males in prison is likely to expand significantly in the years to come. This will continue to bring the needs and care of elderly inmates to the forefront of prison administration.

The care of older prisoners may take several forms, depending upon where the inmate is incarcerated. Each state and the federal system operates within its own guidelines and policies, and the interpretation of "caring" for inmates is, therefore, subject to differing views. McCarthy and Langworthy (1988) note three types of care for the elderly prisoner:

(1) humanitarian care, (2) therapeutic care, and (3) custodial care. *Humanitarian* care primarily focuses on the concern of society, the state, and the prison that elderly inmates adjust and adapt to the prison environment. Elderly persons are among the primary interests of humanitarian care because of their vulnerability and because they are perceived as less of a security risk. The differential effects of penal incarceration on elderly inmates involves the distinction between those who have aged in prison and those who have received their first incarceration at an older age. The major aim of humanitarian care would be to focus on the shock of abrupt confinement for the older first offender. Although incarceration has an impact on the long-term prisoner as well, humanitarian care may overlook those who have aged in the prison or have been in and out throughout their lives. These individuals seem to have gradually adjusted or adapted to the inmate subculture and are not perceived as needing as much attention as the first-time offender.

Therapeutic care revolves around effecting change in the elderly inmate. Priority is given to the change of those attitudes, aptitudes, and capacities of the inmate which are believed to be part of the explanation for the committed offenses. Under this interpretation of care, the feelings of the inmate are pertinent, and rapport between the inmate and the therapeutic environment is essential. The rapport serves as a means of correcting or effecting change in the person. The institution provides counseling, medical care, and other forms of therapeutic intervention to assist in adjusting the inmate to confinement and preparation for possible post-release conditions. The type of therapeutic care provided depends largely on the inmate's situation. If the inmate is to be released at a specified time, the focus is on preparation for reentering society and how best to get by on the outside. If the aged inmate has an unspecified or indeterminate sentence, or one such as life without parole, the focus would be on assisting him with coping with prison life.

The concept of *custodial* care, perhaps, best describes the current situation of elderly inmates. These men have been defined legally as not being desirable residents of society. Thus, the primary focus of institutions holding these inmates is to insure that they do not escape or harm anyone while in prison. This view centers around the management of the institution in order to meet the basic needs of their residents as physical organisms and human beings. The institutions are obligated, by law, to provide for their basic human needs such as food, shelter, clothing, and medical attention. This is, perhaps, the ultimate form of "warehousing" offenders. The state, however, is obligated to provide care for the health of the inmate. To what degree will the state provide medical care to keep the inmate alive and at what cost—should the inmate suffer the onset of a chronic, life-threatening illness? How will constrained prison budgets be expanded to provide a long-term care system (parallel to state and private nursing homes) for dependent prisoners in need of chronic nursing care? In some cases, the state has maintained the care of the individual up to, but not including, extraordinary care that maintains life support for the inmate. In other cases, the state has opted to release those individuals not serving sentences of death or life without parole. This, of course, simply shifts the burden of care back to the family (if the inmate still has family willing to assume responsibility for his care). If family care is not available, the released inmate simply becomes another indigent elderly man for whom society assumes responsibility.

AGE INTEGRATION VERSUS AGE SEGREGATION

The issue of age-integrated (mainstreaming) versus age-segregated environments is as prominent in the field of corrections as it is in the field of gerontology. Those who argue for age segregation believe that it is necessary to protect elderly inmates from victimization, exploitation, and harassment by younger, more aggressive inmates. Elderly inmates are viewed as vulnerable, and the institution should focus on their safety and well-being. This could best be accomplished by separating the elderly inmates from the other inmates. By housing them in separate units or facilities, they can benefit from care and services congruent with their needs. Additionally, these units can be constructed to accommodate individuals with reduced mobility. Besides these needs being met, age-specific groups in institutions can contribute to the mental health of elderly inmates. Participants in age-specific groups experience increased self-respect, diminished feelings of loneliness and depression, reactivated desire for social exchange, reawakened intellectual interest, a sense of identification between members and shared historical legacy, and increased capability to resume community life.

However, age segregation may have a detrimental effect on the inmate resulting from isolation from the general population. Although age segregation is often justified and in the best interest of the elderly inmate, it could easily be turned into age discrimination. Elderly inmates, because of their smaller numbers, might easily be deprived of some of the services and opportunities that are available to the general prison population. They might also suffer from undue paternalism and the stigma of being old, weak, helpless, and in need of special care. Communication with the prison environment will be reduced, their lives will become idle, and institutional dependency will likely be enhanced. By removing elderly inmates from the general population, their sense of inadequacy is only heightened.

In addition to challenging the need for segregating elderly inmates, proponents of age integration stress the benefits of such a policy to both the institution and the elderly inmate, and they suggest that dispersing elderly inmates throughout the prison can have a stabilizing effect on the general prison population (Fattah & Sacco, 1989). Proponents also suggest that older inmates have a calming effect, and note the general lack of problems from the elderly inmates. To counter this argument, one might point out that "old-timers" can also have a negative effect on younger, inexperienced criminals by teaching them the "tricks of the trade." In either case, it would seem appropriate that the interests of the elderly inmate should prevail over administrative considerations.

POLICY AND PROGRAMS FOR THE ELDERLY

As noted previously, the small number of elderly inmates does not accord them high priority for consideration of special programs to meet their needs. As often occurs in the outside world, most facilities and activities focus on the bulk of the population who are younger and more able. A major difference between prison and the outside world is that there are no advocacy groups lobbying for changes for incarcerated elderly. In prisons, inmates have little freedom or a voice in their situation. As a first step in program development, institutions must recognize the elderly as a special needs group. They must also be aware that the facilities and programs inside the walls are designed for the younger offender. They must realize that older men are placed at a serious disadvantage and, in some cases, without attention to their needs.

Specific suggestions for housing include placing elderly inmates in a separate wing or unit away from the younger inmates. This is not to suggest total isolation or segregation, but to permit for physical structural designs that would be more conducive to the elderly. Certainly, if an elderly inmate chooses to be placed in the general population, and has no mental, physical, or social limitations, he should be allowed to do so. Separate housing should have minimal drafts and dampness which can aggravate the physical conditions of many elderly inmates. Also, the facility should have restrooms and bathing facilities which are designed to safely accommodate the less physically able. Stairs should be kept to a minimum, distances from various facilities in the institution should be minimized, and facilities should be made more accessible to those with problems in ambulation with the use of ramps.

Similarly, educational, vocational, recreational, and rehabilitation programs should be expanded to meet the needs of the elderly. Older inmates should be encouraged to participate in these programs. Separate basic education classes for the elderly, for example, would allow the tempo of the class to be paced to elderly learners. Having books and other material printed in large print should be provided for those with vision problems. Providing separate classes for the elderly would reduce the embarrassment and frustration they might feel because of an inability to keep up with younger inmates.

Vocational programs for the elderly should be pragmatic and have utility in the outside world. Recreational programs should include activities that take into consideration the limited physical ability of the elderly. For example, activities that are popular among elderly inmates are cards, board games, checkers, movies, and music. Additionally, walks, shuffleboard, and horseshoes are popular activities that provide limited physical activity to overcome a sedentary prison life.

As for rehabilitative programs, the staff should receive training in the special needs of older persons so that they will be more attuned to the special needs and problems of elderly inmates. Services which should be provided in a geriatric unit include special diets and nutrition monitoring, special exercise, personal hygiene, attention to declining sight, hearing, and memory, and monitoring health conditions.

THE POSSIBILITY OF PAROLE AND THE ELDERLY OFFENDER

Parole is a major issue for habitual and chronic offenders who have spent a majority of their adult lives in a correctional setting. Generally, parole is used for inmates who have reformed and are not considered a risk to society. Many elderly offenders are not considered to be a risk to the public. Yet, there may be a commendable motivation of prison officials and parole boards not to release some of these offenders who have developed an institutional dependency and who may reject the possibility of parole when offered. These older prisoners have decided that life within the institution is "good" and that the prison is their home and the only safe and secure place they know.

For example, consider a case observed by one of the authors of a man imprisoned in North Carolina for murder at age 19 and released 45 years later. His ability to become responsible for his own life in an environment representing 45 years of technological change should have been severely questioned. Frequently, this situation results in one of two results: 1) the parolee commits another offense to return to his secure life; or 2) he commits suicide. In such situations, the inmate usually has no support from family or friends on the outside, as he has probably long since lost contact with them. Additionally, men sentenced to prison at a young age have not had time to develop even a Social Security base of financial support. They usually have no marketable skills, or they are unable to work as a result of health problems. Thus, they are forced to accept menial jobs for minimum wages, or they end up on public assistance.

Although first-time elderly offenders are very different from habitual or chronic offenders, their chances of parole are not very good. As noted earlier, they are often incarcerated for serious or violent crimes. As they still have a life on the outside, the change of environment, the deprivation of liberty, the pains of imprisonment, and the problems of adjusting to life inside the walls all mean that the first-time offender is counting the days until the parole hearing. As opposed to the chronic offender, the first-time inmate is likely to be unfamiliar with the parole process and may, therefore, be unprepared when the time comes for appearance before the board. Because of the seriousness of their offenses, these inmates are often rejected on their first and subsequent parole attempts.

They become depressed and disillusioned at the process, and eventually fall into an institutional mode of adaptation.

CONCLUSION

While elderly inmates constitute only a small, select population within prisons, they still present unique, important, and unexplored challenges. As the elderly inmate population continues to grow, prisons in the United States will be faced with a problem as well as an opportunity. To become a problem, prisons simply have to continue to ignore the present situation of increasing numbers of aging inmates. Prisons have begun to pay attention to the needs of the elderly. Continued concern should lead to better treatment. However, the growing number of elderly inmates presents correctional institutions with an opportunity. As the population grows, it will become not only increasingly necessary, but increasingly justifiable, to implement specialized programs and facilities to accommodate elderly prisoners. It will become most difficult to ignore this elderly constituency in corrections who, like the rest of society, will reflect the "graying of America."

REFERENCES

The aging prison population: Inmates in grey. (1990, August). *Corrections Today*, 136–141.

Alston, L. T. (1986). *Crime and older Americans.* Springfield, IL: Charles C Thomas.

Baum, S., & Berman, H. (1984). Older prisoners: Who are they? *The Gerontologist, 24,* 160.

Bergman, S., & Amir, M. (1973). Crime and delinquency among aged in Israel, an experience model. *The Israel Annals of Psychiatry and Related Disciplines, 11,* 33–48.

Fattah, E. A., & Sacco, V. F. (1989). *Crime and victimization of the elderly.* New York: Springer-Verlag.

Goetting, A. (1983). The elderly in prison: Issues and perspectives. *Journal of Research in Crime and Delinquency, 20*(2), 406–416.

McCarthy, B. R., & Langworthy, R. (1988). *Older offenders: Perspectives in criminology and criminal justice.* New York: Praeger.

Panton, J. H. (1977). Personality characteristics of aged inmates within a state prison population. *Offender Rehabilitation, 1,* 203–208.

Sabath, M., & Cowles, E. (1988). Factors affecting the adjustment of elderly inmates to prison. In B. McCarthy & R. Langworthy (Eds.), *Older offenders: Perspectives in criminology and criminal justice* (pp. 178–195). New York: Praeger.

Seip, D. E. (1990). The forgotten elderly: Inside America's prisons. *Contemporary Long-Term Care, 13,* 30–32.

U.S. Department of Justice (1993). *Sourcebook of Criminal Justice Statistics, 1993.* (DOJ Publication No. NCJ–148211). Washington, DC: U.S. Government Printing Office.

Vito, G. F., & Wilson, D. G. (1985). Forgotten people: Elderly inmates. *Federal Probation, 49,* 18–24.

Weigand, N., & Burger, J. C. (1979). The elderly offender and parole. *The Prison Journal, 59,* 48–57.

C. Special Populations

CHAPTER 7

Rural Older Men: A Neglected Elderly Population

John A. Krout, Ph.D.,
B. Jan McCulloch, Ph.D.,
& Vira R. Kivett, Ph.D.

INTRODUCTION

Over the years, a growing body of research has examined residential differences in the status and needs of older adults. Overall, studies have reported a substantial rural disadvantage in areas such as health, income, housing, and service availability (Krout, 1986, 1994). Researchers also have acknowledged considerable within-group variation among rural elders when these and other issues have been examined. Relatively little attention has been focused on examination of these acknowledged differences within rural older populations, however. In recent years, some researchers have directed attention to the characteristics and life status of older rural women (Kivett, 1990). However, little is known about the lives of older rural men. This paucity of information about rural elderly men contributes to the current lack of understanding about the role gender plays in the lives of persons aging in rural environments. It remains unclear whether gender differences in health, economic security, and social and informal support interactions reported for the older population in general characterize the rural older population.

Our knowledge of the relationship of gender to the life status of persons aging in rural areas, therefore, remains incomplete. This chapter provides a springboard for expanding an understanding of the role of gender in the life circumstances of rural elders by focusing attention on the status, experiences, and service needs of men. The interest is not only in rural gender differences among elders, but also in rural/urban differences between older men. A number of topics traditionally examined by gerontologists are examined here: health, economic status, poverty, marital status and living arrangements, family relationships, informal network interactions, work and employment, retirement satisfaction, community involvement, and service needs. Attention also is given to the diversity among older men within nonmetropolitan areas, especially nonfarm-versus-farm differences. The intent of the chapter is to synthesize the existing research on older rural men and to highlight existing gaps in the understanding of this neglected population subgroup. In this vein, research gaps in the knowledge of older rural males are identified, as well as gaps in public policy and in the delivery of services to this group.

DEFINITION OF "RURAL"

Although the term "rural" evokes many images and would seem to be fairly well understood, an acceptable and agreed-upon definition of the term has escaped academicians and policy makers for years (Krout, 1986; U.S. Senate Special Committee on Aging, 1992). Two issues emerge when examining the operationalization of "rural." First, the operationalization of residence as rural/urban sets up a false dichotomy, one that implicitly assumes homogeneity among elders living in either rural or urban areas (Krout, 1986; Rowles, 1991). As defined by the U.S. Bureau of the Census (1992), "rural" refers to any community that is not urban. Rural communities are designated as those with 2,500 or fewer residents—a definition appropriate for persons who live in small areas and areas of low population density (U.S. Senate Special Committee on Aging, 1992; Van Nostrand, 1993). The extensive urbanization of America and the growth of huge cities surrounded by sprawling suburbs, however, has reduced the utility of simply categorizing areas as rural or urban. Additionally, Rowles (1991) emphasizes the importance of controlling for rural diversity when he states that each rural community "provides a distinctive physical, demographic, economic, social and cultural context, and each one has a unique and ongoing history that has conditioned the lifestyles, values and expectations of its elderly residents" (p. 386).

Second, the terms "rural" and "urban" frequently have been used synonymously with the terms "nonmetropolitan" and "metropolitan." Although there is considerable overlap between counties that are defined as rural and nonmetropolitan, all counties cannot be categorized as falling into both designations. For example, approximately one-third of elders categorized as living in nonmetropolitan areas live in communities that do not conform to rural classification—a community of 2,500 or fewer residents (U.S. Senate Special Committee on Aging, 1992). In addition, researchers differentiating between rural farm and nonfarm populations have found significant differences, although such a distinction confounds residence and occupation (Coward, Bull, Kukulka, & Galliher, 1994).

Defining the term "rural" in so many different ways has, predictably, created problems in the comparison of results across studies. In this chapter, the term "rural" will be used generically, but efforts will be made to be clear as to the nature of the community and sample when reporting research findings.

DEMOGRAPHICS OF RURAL OLDER ADULTS

Data from the 1990 Census reveal that 8.2 million elders live in nonmetropolitan areas, a number that represents 26% of the total older population. Comparatively, 23 million older persons live in metropolitan areas (U.S. Senate Special Committee on Aging, 1992). Approximately 90% of rural elders live in rural small towns and villages or in nonfarm open country, underscoring the fact that the term "rural" no longer indicates farm residence. As of 1988, about 700,000 persons, or 2.5% of the total older population, lived on farms.

Generally speaking, the percent of the population 65 years of age and older increases as the population of a location decreases. In 1990, approximately 15% of the population in nonmetropolitan areas was over the age of 65, as compared to 12% of the metropolitan population (U.S. Senate Special Committee on Aging, 1992). The higher proportion of elders found in small towns has been attributed to several factors, such as the outmigration of young adults, the "aging-in-place" of middle-aged cohorts, and the movement of retired farmers and especially the widows of farmers to somewhat larger communities (Krout, 1986).

Gender Composition

It is well-known that there are more older females than males. Generally, this is illustrated by the use of the "sex ratio"—the number of male elders per 100 female elders. Data from the 1991 census reveal higher sex ratios for rural elders—69.6 for metropolitan versus 76.9 for nonmetropolitan areas, with metropolitan central cities reporting the lowest ratio, 64.1 (Coward et al., 1994). These residential sex ratio differences may partially be attributed to the sex-specific migration patterns of widowed rural elderly females who move to larger communities when their health status and/or ability to live independently declines, especially in sparsely populated areas. McLaughlin and Jensen (forthcoming) analyze 1990 Census Public Use Microdata Sample (PUMS) data and find that these sex ratios decrease with age, but are still higher for rural farm and nonfarm dwellers than for urban elders. For those persons 85 years of age and older, the sex ratios are .69, .53, and .35 respectively for rural farm, nonfarm, and urban categories. Thus, although rural areas exhibit a gender composition similar to the rest of the nation, there are proportionately more older males as compared with the proportions found in urban areas.

Marital Status and Living Arrangements

It could be expected that the rural/urban differences in sex ratios for older adults are mirrored by residential differences in marital status and living arrangements. Such patterns are displayed when 1991 census data are used. Coward et al. (1994), for example, report that nonmetropolitan older persons in every age category are more likely to be married (and less likely to be widowed, divorced, or separated) than central city elders. Living arrangements, likewise, show corresponding residential differences. Nonmetropolitan elders in every age category also are more likely to be living in husband-wife households than those living in central cities and, concurrently, are less likely to live in female-headed households (Coward et al., 1994). Data from the 1991 PUMS reveal that approximately 60% of rural nonfarm elders are married and live with a spouse, versus 72% of farm elders and 49% of urban elders. Additionally, data from the 1980s show that about one-third of rural elders are widowed, with rates that are higher for women and increase with age. After the age of 84, 40% of rural men versus 82% of rural women are widowed (Coward et al., 1994). Both older men and women, however, might be further disadvantaged by widowhood as more traditional gender roles, financial problems, more limited social support services, and fewer social contacts due to geographic distance make coping with the loss of a spouse more challenging in rural areas.

These data suggest that older rural males, especially those living on farms, have an advantage when compared to older urban men when it comes to the availability of one of the first lines of support—a surviving spouse. Rural males also are advantaged when compared with rural women. For example, 1990 census data show that 6.7% of non-metropolitan elders are men living alone while 24.6% are women living alone. This "front line" support is a major factor in avoiding or delaying the institutionalization of frail elders as well as providing higher levels of overall quality of life among older persons (Coward et al., 1994).

PHYSICAL AND MENTAL HEALTH

Physical Health

In rural/urban comparisons, many studies indicate an individual health status disadvantage for older rural adults, as well as community-level disadvantages, regarding the availability and accessibility of health care professionals and services (Coward et al., 1994; Krout, 1986, 1994). For example, rural elders report poorer objective and subjective health, including greater incidences of chronic illnesses, even though rural and urban older adults are reported to have similar physical health problems (Coward et al., 1994; Krout, 1986, 1994). In addition, rural elders have greater incidences of specific diseases, such as visual and hearing difficulties, heart disease, hypertension, arthritis, emphysema, ulcers, and kidney and thyroid problems (Coward et al., 1994). Few studies provide direct and comprehensive gender comparisons of rural elders' physical health status. The scholarly examination of the influence of gender relations on men's health and illness, especially in the case of rural men, is in its infancy. The health issues of older rural men typically are presented as referents for focal discussions of older rural women's health status and/or illness.

National as well as international data examining gender differences in older adult health show that men and women have different patterns of health. Available data also provide support for the argument that older rural men have a different health status than older rural women. For example, striking gender differences among farm elders were noted in Stallone's (1990) examination of Kentucky farm injury rates. For males, the average annual injury rate was 110.1 per 100,000, compared with 3.1 for females. A publication of the U.S. Department of Health and Human Services (Van Nostrand, 1993) reports that 44% of non-metropolitan women as compared with 33% of nonmetropolitan men had high blood pressure, 22% of nonmetropolitan women versus 10% of men were overweight, and nonmetropolitan men were four times more likely to report being heavy smokers (25 or more cigarettes a day, 27% versus 7%). In addition, nonmetropolitan males are much more likely to report being heavy drinkers (at least five drinks per day at least five times in the last year, 20% versus 1%).

It is reasonable to assume that these gender differences in the health of older rural adults are related to a combination of biological differences, gender-specific lifestyles, and occupational histories that present greater health risks to men than women *in certain areas.* For example, the agricultural occupations of rural men, and some rural women, are known to be particularly dangerous and involve long exposures to the elements, long hours of physically demanding labor, machinery operation, and exposure to manmade toxins. However, few studies have examined gender differences in the impact of these occupational risk factors or those more prevalent among rural residents who are not directly affected by farming.

As a specific rural occupational group, farm elders are more likely to report acute health conditions as compared to persons living in other residential settings and also are more likely to view their health as poor compared with urban elders. Conversely, farm elders, who are more likely to be male, consistently report fewer activity limitations and medical conditions when compared with nonfarm rural dwellers. Two possible reasons have been posited for these seemingly contradictory findings. First, farm elders may be in poorer health but they also are more likely to continue daily activities, especially strenuous farm labor during peak production times such as planting or harvest, even when they recognize that they should seek medical attention (Coward et al., 1994). Second, it has been hypothesized that severely injured or disabled farm elders may relocate and are subsequently classified as nonfarm, small town or village, or urban residents, reducing the proportion of rural elders reporting limitations and/or medical conditions. When specific health risks are examined, farming consistently is reported as stressful and has been classified as one of the most hazardous occupations, even though farmers and their families work in an environment that largely continues to be exempt from state or federal labor regulations (Purschwitz & Field, 1990). However, little is known about gender differences among farmers for these specific risks.

Mental Health

As with physical health, mental health differences within rural areas have been identified. Recent hardships in some rural areas—especially in areas relying heavily on mining, forestry, and farming—have been directly linked to increases in the incidence of mental health problems (Buckwalter, Smith, & Caston, 1994). Buckwalter et al. note that, although greater effort should be concentrated in this area, the mental health needs of rural elders are diverse, complex, and multidimensional. Some suggest that increasing economic difficulties and lack of appropriate services result in higher rates of mental illness among rural as compared to urban residents. For example, structural as well as cultural barriers affect not only the availability of services and qualified professionals, but also the willingness of rural residents to partake of services (McCulloch & Lynch, 1993).

The stress associated with economic hardships in rural areas is linked to increases in depression, anxiety, withdrawal, suicide, spouse and child abuse, and substance abuse (Beeson & Johnson, 1987). Beeson and Johnson underscore the economic and familial stress which rural farmers have experienced when they note that today's farmer, compared with 30 years ago, must generate eight times the gross income to realize the same net income. Even though farmers express satisfaction with their lifestyles and communities, their rates of mental distress are significantly higher when compared with urban and nonfarm rural residents.

INCOME AND ECONOMIC SECURITY

Numerous studies have shown that rural elders have lower incomes than their urban counterparts (Krout, 1986; Rural Sociological Society Task Force on Persistent Rural Poverty, 1993), with recent studies indicating that poverty is increasing for elders in rural areas. Indeed, older rural adults are reported to have incomes that are approximately 20% lower than those of metropolitan elders, an economic disadvantage that reflects lower Social Security payments, smaller savings, less widespread coverage by private pensions, few opportunities for part-time work, and infrequent enrollment in SSI (Supplemental Security Income) (Krout, 1986). For example, rural elders are reported to have monthly Social Security Benefits that average $60 less than those for urban elders (U.S. Senate Special Committee on Aging, 1992). Approximately one-half of elders in rural areas live in families that are classified as poor, near poor, or low-income (U.S. Senate Special Committee on Aging, 1992).

For individuals 65 years of age and older, the median 1992 income from all sources for nonmetropolitan elders was $9,229 as compared with $10,351 for their metropolitan counterparts (U.S. Bureau of the Census, 1993). As one would expect, there are gender differences within these groups. Differences in wages, work histories, and employment opportunities result in older men having considerably higher incomes ($9,148) than older women ($7,148) in rural areas (comparisons for nonfamily households). In addition, rural nonfarm incomes for both men and women are considerably lower than those for farm dwellers (U.S. Senate Special Committee on Aging, 1992).

Poverty rates for older adults follow the same residence pattern as that found for income. In 1992, 14.8% of nonmetropolitan elders were poor versus 12.2% of metropolitan elders (U.S. Bureau of the Census, 1993). Data from 1990 reveal that older rural males are much less likely to be poor than females, with poverty rates of 11.2% and 18.3%, respectively. Males make up to 30.5% of the older rural poor, while females make up 69.5% (McLaughlin & Jensen, 1993). It should be noted, however, that compared with metropolitan older males, rural men make up a slightly higher percentage of the elderly poor, possibly because of the generally lower economic status of rural men and the higher marriage rates of nonmetropolitan women (McLaughlin & Jensen, 1993).

WORK AND RETIREMENT

Recent examinations of the labor force experiences of nonmetropolitan residents indicate that male/female differences occur *within* and *across* different forms of work. Data from the 1990 census show that for those 65–69 years of age, 23% of rural nonfarm males versus 14% of females are in the labor force. For farm dwellers, these proportions are 54% for males and 18% for females. Among elders 70 years of age and older, the proportion of rural nonfarm dwellers in the labor force includes 10% of the male and 4% of the female populations; among farm dwellers, 32% of the male population are in the labor force, as compared with 7% of females (Dorfman, forthcoming). The rates for rural nonfarm residents are lower than urban rates for males and females in both age categories. Thus, among farm dwellers, formal involvement in the labor force continues to be an important aspect of daily life for a relatively large proportion of the male population. This, of course, reflects the nature of farming, where older adults, both men and women, often continue to own land and participate in farm work and management as adult sons and/or daughters increase their roles in these areas over time.

Harris (1950) describes this pattern as an "agricultural ladder," whereby manual labor on the farm is increasingly replaced by management functions, making age and retirement less abrupt events compared with the retirement patterns in other occupations. For example, Dorfman and Rubenstein (1994) report that one-half of a sample of rural Iowa men and almost one-third of the women retired gradually. Some rural elders continue to work even in "retirement." Few data, however, are available on this topic—a knowledge gap that makes generalizations difficult. Dorfman and Rubenstein (1994) note that 22% of a sample of retired rural Iowa men and 15% of women said they were working, with 53% of females and 43% of males reporting that they participated in unpaid volunteer work now that they were retired. Older rural men, especially those living on farms, have available to them social roles that provide social status and avenues for continued community involvement.

The gerontological literature indicates that most older adults anticipate retirement will be a positive experience and most are satisfied with this life-cycle stage. Rural elders appear to be no exception (Krout, 1986). For example, 81% of the 252 males and 80% of the 199 females from a retirement subsample of the "Iowa 65+ Rural Health Study" responded that retirement was generally good for people (Dorfman & Rubenstein, 1994). This study also found that rural elders were, on average, satisfied with retirement. Similar rural/urban scores were found on a scale that assessed satisfaction in retirement with activities, health, finances, and interpersonal associations. A minority of respondents reported losses, mostly to do with missing work, colleagues, and the satisfaction derived from working. Thus, existing data indicate that most rural elderly males anticipate and experience retirement with positive feelings and that male farmers appear to retire more gradually than those in other occupations.

Functional health and perceived health were found to be significant predictors of retirement satisfaction in the Iowa 65+ study, but this also holds for urban elders (Dorfman, forthcoming). Dorfman also writes that pulmonary disease and heart attack are the strongest predictors of dissatisfaction with retirement for males, while arthritis is the strongest for females. In addition, the quality—not the quantity—of relationships, frequency of aid from confidants and relatives, involvement with organizations, good health, and adequate income are the most important factors in the prediction of retirement satisfaction.

Studies conducted during the 1960s and 1970s suggest that formal social participation (i.e., clubs, churches, etc.) may make a stronger contribution to the well-being of rural as opposed to urban elders (Krout, 1986). The community structure of small communities may make such participation easier, as might expectations that elders stay involved in their communities. For example, among older rural Iowans, increases in volunteer organization use after retirement contributed to satisfaction for rural retired men, even more than women (Dorfman, forthcoming). Thus, rural residence may provide older males with some advantages, including a more gradual transition from work to retirement and more opportunities for social integration.

FAMILY AND KINSHIP

Kin networks are primary sources of assistance in later life, especially in rural underserved areas. Although most older men in all categories of residence and old age categories share the gender advantage of having a spouse, they share a disadvantage in the extent to which they are embedded in kin relationships and exchanges. This latter observation is generally attributed to the differential socialization of the sexes. Women are more likely than men to be kin keepers or caregivers and to be socially dependent. Despite limitations of gender and outmigration, older rural retired men have been found to be well integrated into kin networks (Dorfman & Mertens, 1990).

Data are equivocal regarding the rural/urban related advantages of kin availability and dynamics of older men. Older farm men are more likely than other older rural and urban adults to have a child living nearby (within one mile) and to visit a child at least once a week. Dorfman and Mertens (1990), in their study of retired men from small rural towns and farms, found that this rural advantage, however, did not translate into more assistance from children. Overall, they found few differences between farm and nonfarm men in kin relations. Strong gender differences were found in several aspects of kinship relations, however. Rural retired women had significantly more contact with siblings than men, and they also received more telephone calls from children and help from kin. Unmarried males were particularly vulnerable to insufficient interaction with kin during retirement.

Saliency and Satisfaction of Kin Relationships

Little is known of the saliency of older rural men's family roles or the predictors of their association with kin. Limited evidence has shown that rural men report a similar number of males and females as kin of most contact. Kivett (1988), in an analysis of 127 men 65 years or older living in a rural-transitional county, found that male kin, whether they be blood kin or related by marriage, played only minimal roles in the lives of older men as seen through association and assistance. The results of this research showed the elusive nature of rural men's kin relationships with selected primary kin. For example, the usual correlates of kin relations (such as proximity, race, health, income, kin affection, consensus, and normative expectations) did not predict older father-son association, support received from sons, or help given to sons.

Sociohistorical factors may impact older rural men's relationships with family members. Elder, Rudkin, and Conger (1994) studied the older father-son relationship with regard to the farm crisis (financial crises and farm loss) in rural Iowa, and found no evidence of negative effects upon the relationship between older fathers and sons who were displaced farmers (from the perspective of the sons). A childhood history of father-son conflict was associated with older father-son conflict in the case of the son's loss of the farm. Elder et al. (1994) observed little continuity in the relationships between older rural fathers (both farm and nonfarm) and sons across the life span. These researchers suggested this finding may be related to the lack of general lifespan stability in male family roles.

The saliencies of older rural men's family roles vary according to ethnicity. Although some roles (such as that of grandfather) have been found to be ranked similarly in importance by white and African-American older rural men, cultural differences are observed in the role (Kivett, 1991). Older rural African-American grandfathers have been found to have a higher household density, more grandchildren and great-grandchildren, higher association with grandchildren, higher grand-filial expectations, greater expressed affection for grandchildren, and provide more assistance to grandchildren than white rural grandfathers. Other research has shown ethnic differences in the centrality of older males' roles in the family. Strong sex-role distinctions are reported for Mexican-American families, with women's roles growing stronger with age than those of men (Kivett, 1993). Similarly, the family roles of older Native American men, most of whom live in rural areas, are less salient than those of older Native American women.

Older rural males have been found to have high satisfaction with family life (Dorfman & Mertens, 1990). Gender differences are found in kin affect. Although older rural men report high levels of affective closeness and value consensus with family members, levels are lower than those of older rural women.

Family Support

Contrary to popular stereotypes of rural life, there is little evidence that older rural adults have more extensive kin networks to provide support than urban adults (Krout, 1986; McCulloch, 1995). Rural elders have more children, but they have a smaller number of geographically proximate kin, due to rural outmigration. Regardless of the availability of formal services, older rural men, due to their strong values of self-reliance and individualism, usually turn to family members, not services, in times of need (Dorfman & Mertens, 1990). Despite the observation that older rural men's interaction and exchanges with a variety of kin are minimal, these men hold relatively high expectations of kin support in time of need, especially in illness.

Limited research shows that older rural men's relationships with family are more affectional than functional (Kivett, 1988). As a result, they are more disadvantaged in family support than older women. Dorfman and Mertens (1990) found, despite the observation that older rural adults appeared to be well-integrated into kinship networks, that older men were more disadvantaged than women in proximity to kin, frequency of contact, and receipt of aid. Other research has shown limited support to older men from primary relatives. Kivett (1988) found adult sons were only marginally incorporated into the support network of older rural men as viewed through frequency of association and helping. Some research has shown that older married rural men receive less assistance from children than urban men, even given the closer proximity to a child (Scott & Roberto, 1987).

In summary, limited research suggests that older rural men are well integrated into the family, as viewed through their marital status, satisfaction with family life, and proximity to a child. The extent of their integration varies according to ethnicity and gender. Gender differences in family integration and relationships are more pronounced than urban/rural differences. Older rural women are more advantaged than men because of greater kin involvement and support and greater continuity of family roles over the life span. The literature suggests the elusive nature of older rural men's family relationships, as seen through the equivocacy of research findings and the difficulty in predicting their family outcomes.

RECOMMENDATIONS FOR FUTURE RESEARCH

It is clear that large gaps exist in the knowledge of the characteristics and circumstances of older rural men. What little is known is based on a small number of case studies conducted largely in the Midwest and South, or has been extracted from large national data sets that include sex in analyses of a wide range of variables. Such data sets are useful for secondary analyses that reveal national level findings, but they do not provide the depth necessary to adequately identify and explain the meaning of any gender or residence differences that are revealed. The existing research is also largely atheoretical, so little in the way of conceptual guidance is available to frame research problems and interpret the available data.

This situation suggests several recommendations for future research activities on older rural males. The first is to work toward a research agenda that is better anchored in gerontological theory. A life-cycle approach might be particularly appropriate and productive. Without more attention to conceptual issues, research on older rural males will remain descriptive and not move beyond the rather limited state in which it now exists. The second is to conduct more research on population subgroup differences based on type of community, occupation, marital status, and race for all the topics reviewed in this chapter. For example, few older rural males come from a farm background, but much of the existing research has focused on farm communities, and almost no literature is available on nonwhite older rural males. Also, there is a need to focus attention on how other factors such as age, income, race, and occupation affect the impact of gender on the circumstances and needs of rural elders.

Another area in need of considerably more investigation is that of the need and demand for existing health and social services among older rural males, especially acute and long-term care. Information on supportive services, in areas such as transportation, housing, and income maintenance, is also sorely lacking. Such research should also focus on uncovering service modalities that are most appropriate for, and acceptable to, older rural males. In addition, virtually no attention has been given to identifying and examining the individual and community factors that differentiate rural older men who seek services from those that do not, or the factors that differentiate older rural men and women in this regard. Existing data are not sufficient to support informed policy and practice decisions aimed at meeting the needs of this population. More information is needed about the direct and indirect effects of community factors, such as population density, economic resources, and formal services (homebased services, etc.), on quality of life of the elderly and their ability to live independently within their communities.

Finally, there clearly is a need for a vigorous research effort to document the dimensions of aging as experienced by older rural males. This includes such issues as physical and mental health, interaction with family and friends, economic security, and housing. It is also extremely important to gain a better understanding of the social roles available to older rural males in the larger community and in kin networks. Volunteer and caregiving roles and opportunities for productive aging need to be identified and studied. Increasing the knowledge in all of these areas will require different methodological approaches including qualitative work at the individual and community level, primary survey research, and the examination of data available in large secondary data sets or from agency records.

CONCLUSIONS

It is concluded that there is a paucity of information on the characteristics, experiences, and needs of older rural males. Very few researchers have focused on either comparing older rural males with their female counterparts or with older urban males. There have been some studies of this population; however, they have generally been restricted to small, geographically limited samples, focused on rural elders who have been involved in farming as a primary occupation, or they have consisted of rather superficial examinations of national census data. Clearly, there is much need for a systematic research program on this population. The research that does exist indicates some significant gender differences among older rural adults in areas of income, health, and family and kinship, as well as important residential differences among older males, especially based on former occupation and ethnicity. For example, rural areas have higher sex ratios among older adults than those found in urban areas, and rural older males are more likely to be living in husband-wife households as compared to both their urban counterparts and to older rural females. However, research indicates that many of the gender differences in family relationships found for older adults hold in rural areas and findings on rural-urban differences in kinship relationships are equivocal.

Significant gender differences with implications for program planning, provision, and policy are suggested by existing research in areas of health, income, and retirement; but almost no attention has been paid to how policymakers and practitioners should respond to these differences programmatically. Gender differences in specific health problems of older rural adults have been found, as have differences for older rural adults based on occupation and ethnicity. Thus, the health service needs of subgroups of rural elders can be significantly different and require both acute and chronic care service modalities that are appropriately targeted and funded. The dictum that "one size does *not* fit all," when it comes to simply taking models of health service delivery designed for urban elders and using them in rural areas, is also true for older rural adults who differ in gender as well as other characteristics that interact with gender, such as ethnicity or income. Finally, it *is* clear that older rural males are better off financially than their female counterparts, but worse off than older urban males. Thus, poverty is more of a problem for older rural males than would generally be suspected, and requires particular attention by policymakers. These, and the many other issues concerning the status of older rural males, require and deserve considerably more attention by gerontological researchers.

REFERENCES

Beeson, P. G., & Johnson, D. R. (1987). *A panel study of change (1981–1986) in rural mental health status: Effects of the rural crisis.* Paper presented at the National Institute of Mental Health National Conference on Mental Health Statistics (May), Denver, CO.

Buckwalter, K. C., Smith, M., & Caston, C. (1994). Mental and social health of the rural elderly. In R. T. Coward, C. N. Bull, G. Kukulka, & J. M. Galliher (Eds.), *Health services for rural elders* (pp. 203–232). New York: Springer.

Coward, R. T., Bull, C. N., Kukulka, G., & Galliher, J. M. (1994). *Health services for rural elders.* New York: Springer.

Dorfman, L. T. (Forthcoming). Economic status, work, and retirement among the rural elderly. In R. T. Coward and J. A. Krout (Eds.), *Rural elders.* New York: Springer Publishing Company, Inc.

Dorfman, L. T., & Mertens, C. E. (1990). Kinship relations in retired rural men and women. *Family Relations, 39,* 166–173.

Dorfman, L. T., & Rubenstein, L. M. (1994). Paid and unpaid activities and retirement satisfaction among rural seniors. *Physical and Occupational Therapy in Geriatrics, 12,* 45–63.

Elder, G. H., Jr., Rudkin, L., & Conger, R. D. (1994). Intergenerational continuity and change in rural America. In V. L. Bengtson, W. Schaie, & L. Burton (Eds.), *Adult intergenerational relations: Effects of societal change* (pp. 30–78). New York: Springer.

Harris, M. (1950). A new agricultural ladder. *Land Economics, 26,* 258–267.

Kivett, V. R. (1988). Older rural fathers and sons: Patterns of association and helping. *Family Relations, 37,* 62–67.

Kivett, V. R. (1990). Older rural women: Mythical, forebearing, and unsung. *Journal of Rural Community Psychology, 11,* 83–101.

Kivett, V. R. (1991). Centrality of the grandfather role among older rural black and white men. *Journal of Gerontology: Social Sciences, 46,* S250–258.

Kivett, V. R. (1993). Informal supports among older rural minorities. In C. N. Neil (Ed.), *Aging in rural America* (pp. 204–215). Newbury, CA: Sage.

Krout, J. A. (1986). *The aged in rural America.* Westport, CT: Greenwood Press.

Krout, J. A. (1994). *Providing community-based services to the rural elderly.* Thousand Oaks: Sage Publications.

McCulloch, B. J. (1995). Aging and kinship in rural context. In R. Blieszner & V. H. Bedford (Eds.), *Handbook of aging and the family* (pp. 332–354). Westport, CT: Greenwood Press.

McCulloch, B. J., & Lynch, M. S. (1993). Barriers to solutions: Service delivery and public policy in rural areas. *Journal of Applied Gerontology, 12,* 388–403.

McLaughlin, D. K., & Jensen, L. (Forthcoming). The rural elderly: A demographic portrait. In R. Coward & J. Krout (Eds.), *Rural Elders.* New York: Springer Publishing.

Purschwitz, M. A., & Field, W. E. (1990). Scope and magnitude of injuries in the agricultural workplace. *American Journal of Industrial Medicine, 18,* 179–192.

Rowles, G. D. (1988). What's rural about rural aging? An Appalachian perspective. *Journal of Rural Studies, 4,* 115–124.

Rowles, G. D. (1991). Changing health culture in rural Appalachia: Implications for serving the elderly. *Journal of Aging Studies, 5,* 375–389.

Rural Sociological Society Task Force on Persistent Rural Poverty. (1993). *Persistent poverty in rural America.* Boulder, CO: Westview Press.

Scott, J. P., & Roberto, K. A. (1987). Informal supports of older adults: A rural-urban comparison. *Family Relations, 36,* 444–449.

Stallone, L. (1990). Surveillance of fatal and non-fatal farm injuries in Kentucky. *American Journal of Industrial Medicine, 18,* 223–234.

U.S. Senate Special Committee on Aging. (1992). *Common beliefs about the rural elderly: Myth or fact?* (Serial No. 102–N). Washington, DC: U.S. Government Printing Office.

U.S. Bureau of the Census. (1992). Census of the population and housing, 1990: Public use microdata sample of U.S. technical documentation. Washington, DC: Author.

U.S. Bureau of the Census. (1993). *Current population survey: March, 1993* (Machine-readable data file). Washington, DC: Bureau of the Census.

Van Nostrand, J. F. (1993). Common beliefs about the rural elderly: What do national data tell us? *Vital Health Statistics, 3*(28). Washington, DC: National Center for Health Statistics.

CHAPTER 8

Gay Men in Later Life

George S. Getzel, D.S.W.

The notion of an aged gay man presents a collision of commonly held societal stereotypes and beliefs. Many persons think that being aged and sexual are mutually exclusive attributes. Old people are too old to have sex and if they are sexually active, they should cease and desist. Being sexually active or having sexual interest in late life is identified as an embarrassing symptom of senility or depraved conduct.

Adding to our ageist-induced confusion is the notion of an elderly gay man. Our imaginations and patchwork of societal prejudices are sorely taxed: if the aged are not sexual, how can they be homosexual? While examples of older homosexual men are not as readily available as heterosexual ones, they do exist. In part, they are modeled on the parody of the bawdy old man in pursuit of a young woman. Homosexual men are perceived as unhappy predators of young boys. Thomas Mann (1930), in his novella *A Death in Venice*, depicts Gustave Aschenbach as a voyeur of an adolescent boy at the beach. Given the negative stereotype, Aschenbach's death gives moral closure to a pitiable late life.

Unfortunately, ideas about gay men are strongly influenced by the stigma attached to homosexuality and widespread ignorance about homosexuals. For example, heterosexual males and females in high school in the 1940s and 1950s might not have been able to identify a peer who engaged in homosexual activities at that time. This was due, in part, to the denial of homosexuality during that period, which was abetted by homosexuals' justified concerns about the social and legal consequences of revealing their behaviors and interests. Many gay men and lesbians growing up then are presently in their 60s and 70s (Nardi, Sanders, & Marmor, 1994).

Various stereotypes of older gay men still prevail. Homosexual males are perceived as subversive of the norms of society and dangerous influences over young people. Homosexuality is still popularly labeled as pathological, despite changes in psychiatric taxonomies. Homosexual males are seen as "tortured souls" incapable of close social relationships. Research on older gay men challenges these stereotypes and adds useful insights to gerontological theory and practice.

OBJECTIVES

This chapter will review the literature on older gay men and examine the core issues surrounding the study of sexuality in late life. The characteristics of older gay men will be discussed, as well as their attitudes and outlook on the aging process. Special attention will be given to the informal supports available to older gay men and their health concerns. Social service delivery will be discussed through the analysis of a case illustration.

The beginning of gay and lesbian scholarship occurred in the wake of the Stonewall Rebellion and the beginning of the Gay Rights Movement in 1969. While homosexual behaviors were noted in ancient times, aging gay men have only recently been acknowledged in the social science and human service literature (Berger & Kelly, 1986; Kimmel, 1993).

CORE ISSUES

A discussion of homosexuality should begin with an examination of general attitudes toward sex. In his historical analysis of discourses on sexuality in Western society, Foucault (1978) stated that notions of sexual repression are not adequate to explain a society's difficulties in addressing sexuality. Sex is denied in human affairs or approached in a veiled, clandestine fashion by different groups of people during different historical periods. A more fruitful inquiry lies in answering the questions: Why is the discussion or lack of discussion of sexuality so important to the operation of a society? How are sexual behaviors discussed during a historical period? What power is generated by the manner in which sexuality is discussed? What is the content of varying discourses on sexuality in a society? How are different groups in society affected by the knowledge they have of sex? What power do different groups have to act on what they know?

The research on gay men in late life entails new discourses that challenge prevailing ideas about human sexuality. Language is a central element in the construction of open and hidden discourses on the topic. For example, homosexual men, an oppressed group, may develop a dissembling stance toward the revealing of their sexual behaviors and a hidden discourse to justify their situation in the private sphere of peer interaction. Similarly, heterosexual men may have open and hidden discourses on how sexual impulses, attitudes, and behaviors are addressed. Specific language or labels are of central importance to the analysis of all human sexuality.

Labels are important in looking at aging and homosexuality. Self-labeling is related to the norms of the social network in which individuals participate. For example, younger homosexual men may prefer to be called "gay." Older men may refer to themselves as "homosexuals." With the aging of younger historical cohorts, it is likely more individuals will refer to themselves as "gay"—a term with varying sociocultural and political meanings.

In this chapter, "homosexual" refers to sexual behaviors with persons of the same gender. The term "gay" is generally used to refer to lifestyle, and "homoerotic" used in reference to male/male attraction. While sexual behaviors are learned, sexual preferences have a complex origin in the biology and the social environment of individuals. Finally, while gender identification among gay men is usually male, transgender identifications are also possible.

Determining the number of aging gay men in the population is inextricably tied to the difficulties of labeling and self-identification. Self-disclosure of homosexual behaviors, or a gay lifestyle, remains an emotionally charged and politically significant decision with serious consequences for an individual's economic and social well-being (Martin & Dean, 1990). The accuracy of information volunteered about homosexual behaviors remains suspect, particularly if there are criminal laws prohibiting homosexuality. For example, the debate about the percentage of the population that engages in homosexual behavior, or identifies itself as "gay," has recently assumed a renewed intensity (Barringer, 1993; "Homosexual attraction," 1994; Schmaltz, 1991).

Despite methodological controversies and debates about findings, the limited number of exploratory studies of gay men reveal important data about the conditions and outlook of a growing number of self-identified older gay men. After an exhaustive search of the literature, these important yet preliminary studies serve as the basis of discussion in this chapter.

CHARACTERISTICS OF OLDER GAY MEN

Kelly (1977) undertook one of the earliest studies of older gay men (in Southern California). His findings challenged stereotypes of older gay men. For example, the representative older gay man in his sample was not lonely or isolated. Gay men had a high rate of association with other gay men, regardless of their age. The youngest and the oldest gay men were less likely to associate with other gay men, which for the former may be related to their "coming-out" process and in the latter due to health issues and deaths in their generational age cohort. Among men 65 or older, 30% indicated low participation in activities within the gay community and 22% indicated moderate participation. No respondent was totally disengaged from activities in the gay community. Association with heterosexual friends tended to decrease significantly with age.

Berger (1984), in his research with older gay men, noted that homosexual arousal, homosexual behavior, the reactions of others, and self-concept were factors for gay men from adolescence through old age. Generally, men experience the "coming-out" process earlier than women. By the age of 27, all his respondents realized that they were homoerotically aroused by a particular person or situation. With the recognition of homoerotic feelings, they began to interact with gay and lesbian peers in adolescence or early adulthood, except in the cases of married men and women with children. Married persons, in some cases, abandoned their spouses and assumed a homosexual identity in their 40s.

Despite efforts to engage persons of color, Berger's sample was all white, affluent, and well-educated. They were recruited from gay organizations and were not representative of most gay persons, who are not members of gay organizations. Berger (1984) found that most respondents were able to maintain bonds with their families (parents, siblings, children, and others). These ties existed, in some cases, whether the respondent revealed his sexual identity or it was assumed but unspoken by family members. A minority of respondents had serious interpersonal conflicts with family members when their homosexuality was discovered. Berger found that older gay men tended to socialize less in bars, clubs or sexually oriented establishments and more in their own homes—safe places insulated from the prejudices of the general community and younger gay men. Domestic life provided legitimation to older gay men that was not otherwise available.

Changes of sexual preference in late life require sophisticated longitudinal studies. Generational discourses about "variety" in sexual preferences and behaviors influence self-descriptions of sexuality. It might be that older generations of gay men (preStonewall Rebellion adults) view their choices as only between homosexual and heterosexual, with little room for sexual variety.

Homosexual men who had married may reflect a generational condition of living before the Gay Rights Movement. For the older generation, marriage may have served as a stable social environment, given the precariousness of a public homosexual identity fraught with a stigma. Although it is unlikely that a homosexual man currently needs marriage for legitimation and stable supports, as in the past, some gay men continue to navigate the demands of a family with a separate gay identity.

Research is sorely lacking on older gay men from different socioeconomic backgrounds and of different racial and ethnic backgrounds. Gay men living in suburban and rural areas have not been studied. Research in these areas present serious challenges because of the seeming "invisibility" of these cohorts. Researchers must be ethically sensitive to the privacy and human rights concerns of gay men who do not have the protection of larger gay communities.

Attitudes to Aging

Older gay men give evidence of good psychological adjustment, despite research suggesting that younger gay men see themselves as more attractive than older men (Adelman, 1991; Lee, 1987b). While a youthful appearance may be seen as a point of superiority among younger gay men, it does not seem to seriously diminish older men's sense of self-worth. Berger (1984) indicated that age was not correlated with measures of self-acceptance, life satisfaction, anxiety about homosexuality, or fear of aging and death. Older respondents were significantly less depressed and less concerned about psychosomatic symptoms. These findings suggest that older gay man have strengths in late life.

Informal Supports

Little research has been undertaken on the range of informal social supports available to gay men. The AIDS pandemic has stimulated interest in the sources of support available in the community for growing numbers of persons requiring long-term care (Hart, Fitzpatrick, McLean, Dawson, & Boulton, 1994). The gay community has been influential in developing services to people with AIDS, using the assistance of kin, friends, neighbors, and trained volunteers. In the last 20 years, gay men and lesbians have formed voluntary associations to provide human rights protection, social services, and health programs.

Less visible to the outside observer are the informal friendship networks of gay men: vital resources for this population. Several studies point to the existence of rich informal social support for gay men throughout adult development (Berger & Kelly, 1986; Friend, 1990; Kimmel, 1993). These friendship networks serve as family-equivalents or additions to the extant kinship connections of siblings, parents, children, and other relatives. As one older gay man put it, "I have a family and I have close friends, *my family of choice.*"

A recent study of older gay men and lesbians matched with heterosexual men and women between 60 and 93 years old living in Southern and Central California found that heterosexual and homosexual men and women did not differ in depression scores after controlling for age, educational level, partner status, and gender (Dorfman et al., 1995). The presence of large social networks was associated with lower geriatric depression scores. A standard measurement of the quantity and quality of informal support was statistically insignificant between heterosexual and homosexual respondents—both generally had high levels of informal social support. Older gay men and lesbians were more apt to have more friends as supports than heterosexual men or women. Older gay men had significantly fewer kin identified as supports than older lesbians, heterosexual men, or heterosexual women. Although sexual orientation did not predict the number of friends used as social supports, older gay men tended to have friends in the absence of kin supports. The overall strength of the informal social supports of older gay men did not differ significantly from those of their lesbian and heterosexual male and female counterparts.

For gay men, friends are important resources to ward off loneliness. Socialization with members of one's generational cohort appears to be a vital component for emotional stability and social integration of older gay men. This group of men seem to have the capacity to maintain informal supports, despite fewer kinship ties or the absence of kinship supports.

Giving secondary importance to friendship networks, in studies of gay men, undervalues a core source of familial-equivalent influence. For gay men, the distinction between friends and kin may be difficult to make. Are lovers to be considered friends or kin? There are legal and cultural issues related to the legitimacy of gay relationships. Some jurisdictions permit the registration of gay and lesbian domestic partners living in the same households; some health care insurance policies allow coverage of domestic partners.

Older couples surviving into late old age have major stresses, as one or both partners become seriously ill. In the beginning phase of a health crisis, ill older partners generally depend on each other before seeking support from available kin. Older gay men, if they survive as couples, may not have children or other available kin to call on for long-term care planning and provision. Thus, as their age cohort may be severely desolated, they may be forced to turn to formal community organizations.

HEALTH ISSUES

Kimmel (1993) stated that the study of older gay men must take into consideration their unique historical experiences, including when they became aware of their sexuality; how they handled their stigmatized identities; and what developmental demands they encounter in the aging process.

Little systematic knowledge is available about the health and mental health needs of older gay men. In addition, social agencies for older gay men and lesbians have only been started in the last 20 years, and not without considerable difficulties (Dawson, 1982; Lee, 1987a). In 1995, the first mental health program specifically designed for gay men and lesbians was established in New York City with federal funds for AIDS services under the Ryan White Act (Goldstein, Goodman, & Landsberg, 1995).

The needs of older persons with HIV infection and AIDS bear special attention. Despite the early pattern of 10% of all cases of persons diagnosed with AIDS being 50 years or older, little attention has been given to this age group (Riley, 1991). There is evidence that gay men, regardless of age, benefit from HIV prevention education; yet there has been little effort made in such education directed to older persons (Blakelee, 1994). Gay men, 50 years or older, are the largest subpopulation of HIV-infected older adults. Many older men engaging in homosexual behaviors are apt to be "closeted" and not readily reachable through traditional, gay-oriented AIDS organizations. Broad-scope educational outreach to all older persons is the most effective way to reach older gay men.

Older gay men who are infected by HIV, or clinically symptomatic, require services that are sensitive to their aging concerns. Older and younger gay men do not share the same cohort histories. Younger men's "coming-out" experiences are postStonewall and occurred after the start of the HIV/AIDS pandemic. Support groups should be homogeneously composed of older persons with AIDS, in that older gay men (compared to younger men) have longer work histories and different life experiences (including marriages and children). Older gay men benefit from sharing these distinctive commonalities in the group.

There is evidence of a greater frequency of alcoholism and polydrug use among gay men (Ratner, 1993). Clinicians should be mindful of the possibility of these problems when working with older gay men. Substance abuse is also associated with an increase in high-risk sexual behaviors related to HIV infection and sexually transmitted disease (Mulry, Kalichman, & Kelly, 1994). Alcoholics Anonymous and other recovery programs can provide useful social supports for older gay men as well as intergenerational contacts with younger gay men.

SOCIAL SERVICES

Gay-specific services for older gays and lesbians are emerging in cities with large gay populations. Initially, it may be difficult for older gay men and lesbians, who have been secretive with neighbors and in the workplace for all their adult lives, to join a gay-identified program or agency. Yet, they may feel uncomfortable in mainstream (heterosexual-oriented) community centers and social agencies where they may encounter homophobic reactions from other clients and service providers.

Founded in 1977, Senior Aging in a Gay Environment (SAGE) in New York City was the first social service program for gay men and lesbians in the United States (Dawson, 1982). SAGE has grown in size and serves gay men and lesbians of diverse backgrounds from different sections of New York City. Services provided include social activities, counseling, support groups, HIV prevention service, case management to the homebound, information, and referral to long-term care and other programs. SAGE provides technical assistance to nongay service providers to sensitize staff to the particular needs of aging gay and lesbian clients.

Outreach to traditional service providers in the aging network will grow important as these providers identify more older openly gay men needing their services. If there is bias toward gay consumers of services, legal advocacy and other forms of political pressure will be needed.

Awareness of the lifestyles of older gay persons should be seen within the context of multicultural education and sensitivity training. The religious auspices of some facilities present special obstacles for gay older persons. There may be a need for long-term care facilities and assisted living residences specifically for older gay men and lesbians, if sectarianism blocks access to services. The Gay Rights Movement had faced and continues to face obstacles at all levels of government to guarantee civil rights on the basis of sexual orientation. The service needs of the elderly gay should not be overlooked in the areas of bias, neglect, and abuse by providers. The expansion of the rights of gay men and lesbians has important implications for Social Security eligibility and coverage under private health plans.

CASE ILLUSTRATION

The following case points to some of the concerns that may face an older gay couple recently seen by a social worker over the past year and a half:

Allan and Martin are 54 and 68 years old respectively. They have lived together as lovers in the same household since meeting 29 years ago. They celebrate their anniversary together each New Years. Their relationship has been stormy at various times, but has solidified substantially over the last 10 years.

Allan has found substantial peace of mind since his recovery from alcoholism and success as a book illustrator. Although considering himself in semi-retirement, Martin continues to work as a lawyer 3 days a week, which provides needed money. Allan has been recently diagnosed with AIDS. Martin initially came for counseling because of depression and his worries about being left alone after Allan dies. Additionally, Martin was worried about predeceasing Allan. Martin was being treated for high blood pressure and an arthritic condition that he feared would prevent him from working. Allan was not able to obtain affordable health insurance after he was diagnosed with AIDS.

The social worker discovered that Allan had not pursued getting health insurance, in part, because of a belief that if he took care of himself his HIV infection would not turn into an AIDS diagnosis. Although privately skeptical, Martin joined Allan in the faith that together they could overcome the progression of the virus by living in an unpressured and healthy manner. Both Allan and Martin entered a period of crisis when Allan's T-cell count fell below 200, a clinical basis for an AIDS diagnosis.

This crisis period was a fruitful time for professional work with the couple. A number of current and historic problems became evident. Martin had a good deal of submerged anger at Allan for his infidelity 10 years ago, which Martin assumed to be the source of HIV, since Martin recently tested HIV-negative. It took awhile for Martin to get retested. He said to the social worker that he secretly wished to be HIV-positive: his fantasy was that he and Allan would die together—a romantic but an unlikely scenario. Sheepishly, Martin indicated that if he was dead he would be spared all the tragedy and pathos. Martin did not avail himself of health insurance that Allan needed. Martin was very anxious about revealing his homosexual status implied in Allan's enrollment as a domestic partner. During his entire work history, Martin's sexual orientation was undisclosed in the work place.

Discussion

The social worker assisted the couple in discussing their historical relationship. They reviewed the peaks and valleys in their relationship, and the strong bond that endured. Allan expressed unhappiness with Martin's closeted life that reflected generational differences about "coming-out." The worker helped them discuss their differences, which resulted in Martin sharing his anger and fears about Allan's sexual indiscretions. Allan expressed his mixed feelings about Martin's HIV-negative status—relief and jealousy that his lover was uninfected. Subsequently, Martin came out as a gay man at work, even introducing Allan to fellow employees at a Christmas party. They also decided to register at City Hall as domestic partners.

As Allan's health status declined, Martin joined a care givers group at the gay community-based organization in the neighborhood. The social worker assisted the couple to complete advanced directives and wills, which has greatly reduced their anxiety. Martin explored affiliation with a group for aging gay men. He noted that he was more socially isolated than he previously recognized.

Allan is currently struggling with the issue of disclosing his AIDS diagnosis to his older sister and brother-in-law, who have accepted his relationship with Martin for years. Allan's difficulty is related to his guilt about "cheating" on Martin and burdening his family with worries. Since Allan has discussed his AIDS diagnosis with his niece, he has suspicions that his sister might know. There may a conspiracy of silence between them.

This case describes some of the problems that face contemporary older gay men. Culturally sensitive practice is vital in meeting the needs of gay men as they encounter the normative crises of aging and the special issues of being gay in an inhospitable society. An array of social and health services that provide positive accessibility must be developed to maintain the highest quality of life possible. AIDS has become an inextricable part of the service needs of older gay men whose friendship networks have been seriously depleted. Work with kin and friends is a necessity.

CONCLUSION

Continued research and programmatic innovation should focus on older gay men in all their diversity. Many societal obstacles interfere with a sympathetic and disinterested examination of gay men's lifestyles and psychosocial problems. The expansion of human rights is a necessary precondition for deepening the understanding of homosexuality in gerontological theory and practice in the closing years of this century.

REFERENCES

Adelman, M. (1991). Stigma, gay lifestyles and adjustment to aging: A study of late-life gay men and lesbians. *Journal of Homosexuality, 20,* 7–32.

Barringer, F. (1993, April 15). Sex survey of American men finds 1% are gay. *New York Times,* pp. 1, 18.

Berger, R. (1984). The realities of gay and lesbian aging. *Social Work, 29,* 57–62.

Berger, R., & Kelly, J. (1986). Working with homosexuals in the older population. *Social Casework, 67,* 203–210.

Blakelee, S. (1994, January 10). People over the age of 50 disregard safeguards against AIDS. *New York Times,* p. 8.

Dawson, K. (1982). Serving the older gay community. *Siecus Report,* 5–6.

Dorfman, R., Walters, K., Burke, P., Hardin, L., Karanik, T., Raphael, J., & Silverstein, E. (1995). Old, sad and alone: The myth of the aging homosexual. *Journal of Gerontological Social Work, 23,* 29–43.

Foucault, Michel. (1978). *The history of sexuality: An introduction.* New York: Vintage Books.

Friend, R. A. (1990). Older lesbian and gay people: Responding to homophobia. *Marriage and Family Review, 14,* 242–263.

Goldstein, P. G., Goodman, H., & Landsberg, G. (1995). Mental health services for HIV affected populations in New York City: A program perspective. New York: The Coalition of Voluntary Health Agencies.

Hart, G., Fitzpatrick, R., McLean, J., Dawson, J., & Boulton, M. (1990). Gay men, social support, HIV disease: A study of social integration of the gay community. *AIDS Care, 2,* 163–170.

Homosexual attraction is found in 1 of 5. (1994, September 6). *New York Times,* p. 14.

Kelly, J. (1977). The aging male homosexual: Myth or reality? *Gerontologist, 17,* 328–332.

Kimmel, D. C. (1993). Adult development and aging: A gay perspective. In L. D. Garnets & D. C. Kimmel (Eds.), *Psychological perspectives on lesbian and gay male experiences* (pp. 517–534). New York: Columbia University Press.

Lee, J. A. (1987b). What do homosexual aging studies contribute to theories of aging. *Journal of Homosexuality, 13,* 43–71.

Lee, J. A. (1987a). Invisible men: Canada's aging homosexuals: Can they be assimilated into Canada's "liberated" gay communities? *Canadian Journal on Aging, 8,* 79–97.

Mann, T. (1930/1963). *Death in Venice and seven other stories.* New York: Vintage. (Original work published 1930).

Martin, J . L., & Dean, L. (1990). Developing a community sample of gay men for an epidemiologic study of AIDS. *American Behavioral Scientist, 33,* 546–561.

Mulry, G., Kalichman, S. C., & Kelly, J. A. (1994). Substance use and unsafe sex among gay men: Global versus situational use of substances. *Journal of Sex Education and Therapy, 20,* 175–184.

Nardi, P. M., Sanders, D., & Marmor, J. (1994). Growing up before Stonewall: Life histories of some gay men. London: Routledge.

Ratner, E. F. (1993). Treatment issues for chemical dependent lesbians and gay men. In L. D. Garnets & D. C. Kimmel (Eds.), *Psychological perspectives on lesbian and gay male experiences* (pp. 567–558). New York: Columbia University Press.

Riley, M. W.(1991). AIDS & older people: The overlooked segment of the population. In Riley, M. W., Ory, M. G., & Zabloty, D. (Eds.), *AIDS in an aging society: What we need know* (pp. 3–27). New York: Springer Publishing.

Schmalz, J. (1993, April 16). Survey stirs debate on the number of gay men in the U.S. *New York Times,* p. 20.

CHAPTER 9

The Transition to Retirement

Abraham Monk, Ph.D.

Individuals differ in how they anticipate, decide, prepare, and ultimately adjust to retirement. There is no single or simple path to insure a positive retirement experience. Some people enjoy it immensely and may even regret not having started it earlier. Others regard retirement as a major trauma and dread every minute of it. Furthermore, there is no instant adaptation to this stage in a person's life. It should not be surprising that after spending 3 or 4 decades in the workforce; that is, a person's entire adult life, such an adjustment could require a protracted and, at times, painful process.

Retirement has historically been a dominant male experience simply because both the rate of men's labor force participation, and the duration of such participation, far exceeded that of women. At the beginning of the century, 69% of men but only 13% of women were working full-time, outside the home. Furthermore, men averaged 32.1 years of such employment over their lifetime, as contrasted to 6.3 years for women. The gap, however, narrowed steadily, and by 1980 men's overall employment rate declined to 55%, while that of women rose to 38%, almost three times their 1900 rate (Best, 1981; U.S. Department of Labor, 1986; U.S. Senate, Special Committee on Aging, 1991).

When focusing on individuals between the ages of 62 and 64 years, it appears that men and women traversed different, almost opposite, employment and retirement paths between 1965 and 1993. The employment of men in that age group declined from a 73.2% rate in 1965 to

46.1% in 1993. This constituted a reduction of almost 40% in less than 30 years. Women of similar ages actually experienced a slight increase in their rate of employment during the same period, from 29.5% to 31.8% (U.S. House of Representatives, Committee on Ways and Means, 1994). True, women in this age group started out with a much lower participation rate—less than half that of men in 1965—but they gradually affirmed their presence in the labor force, while men underwent a pronounced withdrawal in what amounts to a massive exodus from full-time employment. Once they reached the 65 years of age threshold, 84% of men and 92% of women were no longer in the workforce in 1993 (U.S. House of Representatives, Committee on Ways and Means, 1994).

The trend to retire early among men can be partially attributed to the better prospects of financial security, which resulted, in turn, from improved Social Security and private pension benefits. It may have also been the consequence of negative circumstances, such as later life unemployment caused by technological and occupational obsolescence and the massive layoffs that usually follow corporate mergers, downsizings, and plant shutoffs. In other instances it may be the correlate of mandatory policies, or sheer—albeit veiled—discrimination against older workers. Quinn and Burkhauser (1994) noted that the tendency toward earlier retirement among men is prevalent in almost all developed countries, and they largely attribute it, at least in the United States, to strong policy and economic incentives. These inducements may, however, be reversed in the future, if eventual labor force shortages prompt employers to try to retain older workers longer on their jobs.

The present reality remains, however, characterized by the intensification of retirement among men. This chapter examines how the actual transition into retirement occurs, focusing primarily on the different modes of individual adaptation to the post-retirement stage of life.

THE TRANSITION TO RETIREMENT

The formal entry into retirement constitutes, in most instances, a one-time event. People cease to work on a given day and receive a ceremonial tribute from relatives, colleagues, and friends. The retirement transition transcends, however, those few discrete episodes in a person's life. It involves, instead, a succession of stages of varying duration.

Atchley (1994) identified no less than eight such stages or phases, although he warned that they do not constitute a uniform, fixed sequence applicable to all retirees.

The *first* is the "preretirement" phase, when people become aware of their impending separation from employment and begin anticipating what the future holds for them. The *second* is the "honeymoon" that follows the formal retirement event. It is a joyful period, especially for those who can afford it, of trying out new things and fulfilling old wishes. Some retirees may embark on a *third* stage, which Atchley labels the "immediate retirement routine," should they have already cultivated an assortment of interests, and be able to organize their lives into consistent and enduring patterns of activities. Others may find refuge instead in the *fourth* stage, one of "rest and relaxation." Such rest may constitute, however, only a temporary respite. Once boredom and uneasiness set in, these retirees may seek to reinitiate a semblance at least of their previous occupational lives.

The following are another four stages identified by Atchley (1994):

1. *Disenchantment.* In its more extreme forms, this may end up in feelings of depression.
2. *Reorientation.* To overcome the preceding disenchantment, some retirees will embark in a renewed search for more realistic and appropriate life choices.
3. *Routines.* The selection and subsequent commitment to a new set of alternatives may lead to a new personal equilibrium. The retiree has then found a new and a more satisfying pattern of activities.
4. *Termination.* In this late stage, people may finally reach a point where retirement no longer plays a critical role in their lives. They either reentered the workforce in a full or limited capacity, or are deeply involved with new interests and pursuits. In the worst of circumstances, poor health and chronic functional impairments may preclude their capacity to lead independent lives.

THE RETIREMENT TRANSITION AMONG EXECUTIVES

Atchley's detailed sequence of phases evolved from a series of empirical studies that began in the mid-1960s and stretched to the 1980s. A more succinct analysis of the transition into retirement, as applied to executive males, identifies four stages (Leedy & Wynbrandt, 1987). During the first, the *realization* phase, men deal with their imminent retirement not just as a general idea, but in concrete terms with practical day-to-day implications. The next stage of *acceptance* implies that the process of planning one's life is being set in motion, together with the intent to resolve the emotional conflicts produced by the separation from work and career. The third stage is one of *disengagement*, when people cut off the emotional bonds that keep them dependent on their lifelong career. This is the necessary prelude to the fourth and last stage of *separation*, when the male retiree forges a new post-career lifestyle.

Some interpretations perceive retirement adaptation as a predominantly negative sequence of phases. Most corporate executives, according to Sonnenfeld (1988), anticipate such a negative adjustment and even associate the idea of retirement with death. He further suggests that the process follows the same stages as those identified by Kübler-Ross (1969) in the adjustment of terminally ill patients to the awareness of their imminent demise. Corporate leaders thus start out with *denial*, refusing to accept that their careers are about to reach a terminal point. Next comes a stage of *anger*, followed by a third one of *bargaining*, when they try to lessen the blow and hope to negotiate a postponement (perhaps a part-time assignment or a consultative relationship that would salvage some of the symbolic trappings of their current position). The fourth stage is one of *depression*, when they succumb to the realization that retirement is inevitable and that they are powerless to counter it. Finally, the stage of *acceptance* represents a coming to terms, either in defeat or in mature contentment, with their new life condition.

IS THE RETIREMENT TRANSITION A POSITIVE OR A NEGATIVE PROCESS?

The analogy with the five stages outlined by Kübler-Ross (1969) may constitute an extreme interpretation, applicable only to a small proportion of retirees in the executive and professional suites. Stage models, in general, are useful auxiliary frameworks, but they lack universal validity. They simply cannot predict a course of entry into retirement that applies to all potential retirees.

Empirical studies have been of little help in this regard, as researchers have not so far agreed whether the retirement transition ends up as a predominantly positive or negative process. Some investigators have concluded that the retirement experience deteriorates and becomes more negative over time. Ekerdt, Bossé, and Levhoff (1985) found that there is greater optimism and future orientation in the first year of retirement, but that it is followed by a possible letdown and lower sense of life satisfaction in the second year. Beck (1982) obtained just the opposite results, and found that the retirement experience is far more difficult and negative in the first year, and that there is no evidence that an initial "honeymoon" phase, as identified by Atchley (1994), actually takes place.

These conflicting findings may, however, reflect differences in research design. The studies were done over a wide span of time, and the populations targeted for inquiry may not have had the same socioeconomic characteristics. It must also be borne in mind that retirement is affected by concurrent historical events. People may thus dread the prospects of retirement during inflationary periods; conversely, they may feel more confident about it under stable economic conditions. Retirement outcomes also depend on whether people leave the workforce of their own volition or whether they are forced to depart. Similarly, it matters whether they started out with a favorable attitudinal disposition and consciously prepared for it. The transition, in sum, could lead to either a relatively easy adjustment or to a stressful personal crisis.

RETIREMENT AS A PERSONAL CRISIS

Whether or not retirement constitutes a major source of stress, experienced by most retirees as a painful personal transition, is still debated among researchers, counselors and retirees alike. Back (1969) alluded to the "ambiguity" of retirement, because on the one hand it constitutes an achievement (the completion of a lifelong enterprise), but on the other it is feared as a disturbing crisis. To the extent that retirement may be experienced by some men as a crisis, what are some of the causes for a negative experience?

One interpretation argues that retirement represents a loss of power—the giving up of a prized position of control and authority (Cowgill, 1972; Foner, 1984). It does not matter that most employed men never achieve a real position of power. What counts, according to Gerzon (1981), is the "illusion" of such power, seemingly associated with work. It may be pertinent to introduce here a gender qualifier and relate retirement to a series of male sex-role expectations in our culture, such as the drive to success, self-reliance, independence, and performance (Doyle, 1983).

Another explanation similarly defines retirement as the loss of the work role without having it replaced with a new role which is commensurate in power or prestige to the one relinquished. It then follows that retirement constitutes a demotion to an anomalous "roleless" condition, a sort of limbo where men no longer know what is expected of them, or whether they still fit in a world within which they used to be familiar and comfortable (Rosow, 1967).

A third interpretation centers around the fact that for some men, their jobs constitute the source of their personal validation. They experience the "I am my career" syndrome (Leedy & Wynbrandt, 1987, p. 252), and once separated from their jobs, they feel stripped of their personal identity. They have great difficulty adjusting to their new status because they mourn what Werwoerdt (1976) calls their "lost paradise."

Some researchers of the retirement process do not give much credence, however, to single-cause theories such as those enunciated above. Palmore, Fillenbaum, and George (1984) pointed out that the work role is not as central in the lives of most people as it has been led to believe. For these authors, single-cause interpretations that underscore the work role or the continuity of personal identity factors overlook other potential stressors, such as the drop in income and standard of living, and—most specially—the loss of health.

It is to be expected that both the prospects and the reality of retirement may cause stress and anxiety to some retirees, but there is also substantial research evidence that the majority of men interviewed are generally satisfied with retirement. Friedmann and Orbach (1974) stated over a quarter of a century ago that retirement is being increasingly accepted as a normal life event which contributes to enrichment and positive gains in certain areas of life, such as social and affective relationships. People, they affirmed, tend to retire into more intensive family relations, and they become closer to kin and relatives. Barfield and Morgan (1978) studied a national sample of retirees and found that only one in five expressed strong negative feelings about their retirement. Streib and Schneider (1971) reported finding that most people experienced retirement as a more pleasant reality than they had previously anticipated. Only 5% considered retirement worse than they expected, and one-third stated it was even better than they anticipated.

What factors may then predict who will end up with either a positive or a stressful retirement outcome? A more recent study of a sample of over 1,500 male retirees by Bossé, Aldwin, Levenson, and Workman-Daniels (1991) found that retirement was rated as almost the least stressful, actually the 30th, on a list of 31 potential life events. The three most stressful, in rank order were "death of spouse," "death of son or daughter," and "institutionalization of spouse." Only a handful of retirees found retirement to be stressful. Bossé and associates found that the best predictors of such retirement stress were poor health and financial hardship.

Financial difficulties may be a valid predictor of stressful adaptation to retirement, but it does not necessarily follow that all low-income retirees end up with such negative experiences. A study of retired union members (Charner, Fox, & Trachtman, 1990) established that most were living on tight budgets, with the bulk of their monthly income earmarked for basic necessities. There was very little left for discretionary expenses or emergencies, and they felt very threatened by even minor inflationary variations in prices. They were particularly concerned about health care coverage gaps. Most had already purchased a private health insurance plan to supplement Medicare, but they were keenly aware that many essentials remained uncovered, such as prescription drugs, dental care, and eye examinations.

Notwithstanding these concerns, most respondents claimed to be quite satisfied with their retirement. They also stated that they did not wish to return to work, and that they considered themselves to be "active." They spent most of their time watching television, listening to the radio, reading, socializing, and doing physical fitness exercises. They were coping quite well and found intrinsic rewards in retirement, despite the adverse financial circumstances.

GENDER DIFFERENCES IN RETIREMENT STRESS

Most studies on post-retirement stress and retirement satisfaction have focused on retired men. There is a dearth of studies that compare gender differences and, again, due to differences in research design and methodology, their results cannot easily be pooled. George, Fillenbaum, and

Palmore (1984) analyzed data from the Retirement History Study and the Duke Second Longitudinal Survey and concluded that men experience a greater drop in life satisfaction rates than women, but that both sexes equally report an increase in psychosomatic symptoms during retirement. When controlling for health, income, and occupational status, Jaslow (1976) found that women were more seriously impacted by poor health and lower incomes than men.

It is conceivable that working women may be far more vulnerable in retirement than men: they earned consistently less, even in comparable occupations; they received less pension coverage and may have worked for smaller companies that offered no pension benefits. Their work histories were more often discontinuous; that is, they may have entered and left the workforce several times, having accumulated at the end fewer credits in both Social Security and private pension plans. A study by Seccombe and Lee (1986) reveals that women express lower levels of retirement satisfaction than men, but the difference turned out to be rather minimal, and is attributed to the fact that women had, on the average, lower incomes. The study confirms, however, that the determinants of retirement satisfaction (for married persons as well as higher-status and better-paid workers) are substantially the same for both sexes. For the more affluent, positive feelings stem from the fact that they enjoy a higher standard of living and better health.

MODALITIES OF RETIREMENT ADJUSTMENT

Most retirees are basically satisfied with their retirement, once they have completed the corresponding transition from their former work-related status. They have reached this point in their lives by developing their own retirement lifestyles. These lifestyles reflect, in turn, differences in personal background, as well as in ways of coping and adjusting to novel life situations. Three such frequently mentioned lifestyles or modalities of retirement adjustment are identified here: withdrawal, compensation, and accommodation.

Withdrawal

Some people opt for reducing their level of activities and prefer to focus on a few selective routines. They are not eager to learn new things and consequently rely on past knowledge. They shun assuming new responsibilities or making major commitments; nor are they seeking to make new friends. Their success rests, then, on having reached a satisfying equilibrium through a voluntary form of disengagement. Yet, despite this reduction of outward energy investment, they may remain actively involved with their own thoughts and reminiscences. Retirement is, then, a time for turning inward and for personal stock-taking. These men may figuratively adopt a "rocking chair" posture in order to meditate, ponder about meanings, and relive memories. Some will put those thoughts in writing, in the form of diaries, autobiographies, poetry, or philosophical musings.

Far from finding their withdrawal to be emotionally confining or intellectually depressing, those who follow its path extol its liberating virtues. Retirement, in the form of disengagement, represents for many men the opportunity to shake off the rat race with its oppressive sequel of schedules, obligations, and constraints. It gives them a chance to unwind, take a respite, and perhaps even concentrate on just a few specialized interests, but without deadlines or stipulated performance expectations. They are free to do as much as they wish and whenever they feel like doing it. They abhor long-range planning and would rather take each day one at a time.

Such an unstructured approach to life constitutes for some an interlude of decompression, especially after retirement from a very regimented job, but others gladly adopt it as their permanent lifestyle. There are those who need to get away from everything for just a while as a form of stress management. There are also those who would go fishing, or paint on a hilltop, day in and day out, almost indefinitely.

Compensation

A second pattern of adjustment seeks to actively compensate and replace what has been lost in the transition to retirement. It entails an exploratory stance and an active interest in learning new things. These are the people Neugarten, Havighurst, and Tobin (1968) characterized as "reorganizers." They are endowed with an "openness to experience," a personality trait that—according to Costa and McRae (1980)—facilitates a positive adjustment.

It is typical of these individuals to engage in creative pursuits, start a new career, or learn new skills in order to catch up with their grandchildren and the fast-changing world around them. They want to participate in activities by whatever means. Consequently, they volunteer their skills and expertise for service to other people, they mentor the young, and they take on new causes.

This "openness to experience" stance may go hand-in-hand with a need to both maintain a high level of activity and hold on to former pursuits and routines. It is not uncommon for these men, therefore, to seek to retain a sense of continuity with whatever they did prior to retiring. Three compensatory patterns may be noted here:

1. There are individuals wishing to maintain continuity at all cost. Their stubborn determination may well lead to disappointment and even depression, when they realize that they no longer have the stamina to meet their unrealistic objectives.
2. There are also those who have developed a flexible capacity to substitute, for past activities, new ones properly scaled down and offering similar functional and/or symbolic gratifications.
3. There are, finally, men who overcompensate by doing too much to replace retirement-related losses. Instead of their former 9-to-5 job, they may start their own business (i.e., a "bed and breakfast" hotel) and put all their energies into the effort. They may also take on challenges conventionally sanctioned as "unthinkable" for their age, such as parachuting or learning to pilot planes.

Regardless whether retired men do it for its narcissistic shock value, or because they simply need to prove themselves by testing the limits of their abilities and endurance, many of the stresses that these proactive men face in retirement are self-induced. The main thing for them is to keep busy and live as intensely as ever. They are convinced that once they slow down there will be nothing left to look forward to but death. In essence, these men like to surprise themselves by tackling one challenge after another. There is the risk, however, that as possibilities to compensate dwindle or narrow down, they may find themselves immobilized by fear and dejection, unable to cope with their future.

Accommodation

The third mode of retirement adjustment was defined as "accommodation" by Shanas (1972) to characterize a new distribution of personal energies and resources into nonworking roles, rather than a search for substitutions and compensations.

Essential to this mode is the initial realization by retirees that their life conditions (including health, income, and even their own sense of self) are bound to change. As a consequence, they must forge a personal compromise with retirement as their new reality. Second, as their overall personal resources diminish, the retirees must reexamine and redefine their life priorities and maximize the investment of their personal resources—health, functional abilities, income, social relations, etc.—in areas or goals to which they assign greater personal meaning and importance.

Accommodation is often confounded with adjustment, but it actually implies a critical review and restructuring of a person's life. It means that each retiree has to affirm what is essential for his life for it to have meaning. This does not happen by chance, nor is it the result of a sudden inspiration. It requires instead a discipline of critical reflection which may ultimately lead to "transformative learning" (Mezirow & Associates, 1990). In this form of learning, people examine all the assumptions on which their beliefs are grounded, they seek and analyze alternative ways of looking at things, forge a new perspective, and act upon it.

This would appear as a normal discursive act of thinking which every older person should be capable of routinely performing. Many retired men may need help, however, to identify their subjective premises and beliefs, and then to interpret and understand them. Moreover, they need encouragement, in the form of adult education, group therapy, support groups, individual counseling, or retirement preparation programs, to eventually act upon those new self-images or understandings of self. "Transformative learning," according to Mezirow and Associates (1990) is not ". . . a private affair . . . it is interactive and intersubjective from start to finish" (p. 364).

The Therapeutic Learning Program, outlined by Gould (1990), includes a problem resolution process very similar to Mezirow's "transformative learning." It begins with a three-question sequence which a retiree may ask himself:

1. What is my problem in retirement? What can I do about it, and what prevents me from doing it?
2. What is the best and less risky course of action?
3. What are the fears and doubts that inhibit me from starting to act?

This apparently simple sequence has the potential of inaugurating a reconfiguration process that could lead, in turn, to a more realistic personal accommodation. Yet, in order to succeed, transformative learning must be continuous, because accommodation itself continues through life. Whatever adjustments a man made in his retirement at 65 may no longer apply at 70 or 75. Retirement may be conceived, in this sense, as a life career of repeated reformulations of personal priorities, and successive reassessments of personal circumstances and resources. There are different gains and losses at different points in a person's retirement. Accommodation ultimately consists in capitalizing on the gains side of the balance sheet, no matter how few and dwindling, while accepting—with fortitude, rather than with resignation—that some or many of the losses are irreversible.

CONCLUSION

The three patterns of retirement described in this chapter—withdrawal, compensation and accommodation—are not to be taken as normative prescriptions, nor do they exhaust the range of adaptations. All three may be equally conducive to a successful retirement, depending on how well an older man prepared for it. The patterns constitute alternative approaches to life many men follow once completing their transition to retirement. Their choice is not necessarily a conscious one, and depends upon their personal idiosyncrasies, interests, interpersonal circumstances, and overall attitude vis-á-vis retirement itself. Again, these three patterns are cursory representations extrapolated from a myriad of styles of adaptation; consequently, they are not mutually exclusive absolutes. Men may incorporate characteristics of all three patterns, even if one becomes the more dominant, or they may waver from one pattern to another at different points in their life. Thus, a person may adopt a more compensatory approach to retirement at 65, but then switch to a withdrawal or accommodation lifestyle a decade later.

It should be reiterated that, notwithstanding the strong orientation to work in industrial societies like the United States, most retired men are capable of finding satisfaction and deriving pleasure from their retirement. This applies to both blue-collar workers and executives. Of course, the extent to which men positively adjust to retirement is contingent not only on subjective factors (such as coping modalities, attitudinal orientation, and personality characteristics), but it is also affected by the type of job they held and its location in the labor market. Calasanti (1996) calls attention to several related considerations when contemplating retirement: pay levels, the degree of stability, opportunities for promotion enjoyed while employed, and the anticipated economic loss.

Finally, it is obvious that most people retire when they are old or middle-aged, not when they are young. Retirement is, therefore, juxtaposed and confounded with the developmental features of the later stages of the life cycle. Consequently, many of the stresses and changes, both positive and negative, attributed to retirement are bound to occur, regardless whether the older man continues to work or not.

REFERENCES

Atchley, R. C. (1994). *Social forces and aging* (7th ed.). Belmont, CA: Wadsworth.

Back, K. W. (1969). The ambiguity of retirement. In E. W. Busse & E. Pfeiffer (Eds.), *Behavior and adaptation in late life.* Boston: Little, Brown.

Barfield, R. E., & Morgan, J. N. (1978). Trends in satisfaction with retirement. *The Gerontologist, 18*, 19–23.

Beck, S. H. (1982). Adjustment to and satisfaction with retirement. *Journal of Gerontology, 37*, 616–624.

Best, F. (1981). *Work sharing: Issues, policy options, and prospects.* Kalamazoo, MI: Upjohn Institute for Employment Research.

Bossé, R., Aldwin, C. M., Levenson, M. R., & Workman-Daniels, K. (1991). How stressful is retirement? Findings from the normative aging study. *Journal of Gerontology, 46*, 9–14.

Calasanti, T. M. (1996). Gender and life satisfaction in retirement: An assessment of the male model. *Journal of Gerontology: Social Sciences, 51B*, S18–S29.

Charner, I., Fox, S. R., & Trachtman, L. N. (1990). *Union retirees: Enriching their lives, enhancing their contribution*: Vol. 1. Washington, DC: Academy for Educational Development, National Institute for Work and Learning.

Costa, P. T., & McRae, R. R. (1980). Influence of extroversion and neuroticism on subjective well-being: Happy and unhappy people. *Journal of Personality and Social Psychology, 38*, 668–678.

Cowgill, D. O. (1972). A theory of aging in cross-cultural perspective. In D. O. Cowgill & L. D. Holmes (Eds.), *Aging and modernization*. New York: Appleton-Century-Crofts.

Doyle, J. A. (1983). *The male experience*. Dubuque, IA: William C. Brown.

Ekerdt, D. J., Bossé, R., & Levkoff, S. (1985). An empirical test for phases of retirement: Findings from the normative aging study. *Journal of Gerontology, 40*, 95–101.

Foner, N. (1984). *Ages in conflict*. New York: Columbia University Press.

Friedmann, E. A., & Orbach, H. L. (1974). Adjustment to retirement. In S. Arieti (Ed.), *American handbook of psychiatry* (pp. 609–645). New York: Basic Books.

George, L., Fillenbaum, G., & Palmore, E. (1984). Sex differences in the antecedents and consequences at retirement. *Journal of Gerontology, 39*, 364, 371.

Gerzon, M. (1981). *A choice of heroes*. Boston, MA: Houghton-Mifflin.

Gould, R. L. (1990). The therapeutic learning program. In J. Mezirow & Associates (Eds.), *Fostering critical reflection in adulthood: A guide to transformative and emancipatory learning*. San Francisco: Jossey-Bass.

Jaslow, P. (1976). Employment, retirement and morale among older women. *Journal of Gerontology, 31*, 212–218.

Kübler-Ross, E. (1969). *On death and dying*. New York: Macmillan.

Leedy, J. J., & Wynbrandt, J. (1987). *Executive retirement management*. New York: Facts on File.

Mezirow, J., & Associates (1990). *Fostering critical reflection in adulthood: A guide to transformative and emancipatory learning*. San Francisco: Jossey-Bass.

Neugarten, B. L., Havighurst, R. J., & Tobin, S. S. (1968). Personality and patterns of aging. In B. L. Neugarten (Ed.), *Middle age and aging*. Chicago, IL: The University of Chicago Press.

Palmore, E., Fillenbaum, G., & George, L. (1984). Consequences of retirement. *Journal of Gerontology, 39*, 109–116.

Quinn, J. F., & Burkhauser, R. V. (1994). Retirement and labor force participation of the elderly. In L. G. Martin & H. P. Samuel (Eds.), *Demography of aging* (pp. 50–101). Washington, DC: National Academy Press.

Rosow, I. (1967). *Social integration of the aged*. New York: Free Press.

Seccombe, K., & Lee, G. R. (1986). Gender differences in retirement satisfaction and its antecedents. *Research on Aging, 8,* 426–440.

Shanas, E. (1972). Adjustment to retirement: Substitution or accommodation? In F. M. Carp (Ed.), *Retirement* (pp. 219–243). New York: Behavioral Publications, Inc.

Sonnenfeld, J. (1988). *The hero's farewell: What happens when CEOs retire.* New York, NY: Oxford University Press.

Streib, G. F., & Schneider, C. J. (1971). *Retirement in American society: Impact and process.* Ithaca, NY: Cornell University Press.

U.S. Department of Labor, Bureau of Labor Statistics. (1986, February). *Worklife estimates: Effects of race and education* (Bulletin 2254). Washington, DC: Author.

U.S. House of Representatives, Committee on Ways and Means. (1994). *Where your money goes: America's entitlements* (p. 856). Washington, DC: Brassey's.

U.S. Senate, Special Committee on Aging. (1991). *Aging America: Trends and projections* (DHHS Publication No. FCoA 91–28001). Washington, DC: U.S. Government Printing Office.

Werwoerdt, A. (1976). *Clinical geropsychiatry.* Baltimore, MD: Williams and Wilkins.

D. Special Problems

The Physical Health of Older Men: The Significance of the Social and Physical Environment

William A. Satariano, Ph.D., M.P.H.

INTRODUCTION

It would be difficult to consider the physical health of older men without including some reference to the physical health of older women. Although men are less likely than women to survive to the age of 85, those who do survive seem to have fewer chronic conditions and disabilities than women of the same age (Ory & Warner, 1990). There is evidence, in fact, that older men have a better active life expectancy than older women; that is, a greater likelihood that their senior years will be spent in independence and mobility (Katz, et al., 1983).

Although older men have fewer health conditions than older women, it is important to note that older men are still at greater risk than women of the same age for two serious chronic conditions: heart disease and lung cancer. Based on data from the National Health Interview Survey, Verbrugge and Patrick (1995) report that the prevalence rate of ischemic heart disease for men ages 45 to 64 is 87.3 per 1,000 men, compared to only 43.0 per 1,000 for women of the same age. The prevalence rate refers to the rate of current cases; that is, the rate of those alive with the condition per 1,000 people in the reference population.

While the difference in the prevalence rates is reduced between men and women aged 65, the rate is still greater in older men (179.0 vs. 120.7). Risk factors for ischemic heart disease include cigarette smoking, high blood pressure, and elevated serum cholesterol. There is also evidence that older men experience a greater level of activity limitation associated with ischemic heart disease than do women of the same age (Verbrugge & Patrick, 1995).

Lung cancer is the leading cause of cancer death among men and women in the United States (Miller et al., 1993). These data are usually expressed as a cancer mortality rate. A cancer mortality rate is the number of deaths with cancer as the underlying cause of death occurring in a specified population during a year. It is reported as the number of deaths due to cancer per 100,000 people. The average, annual age-adjusted mortality rate for lung cancer among men aged 65 and older between 1973 and 1990 was 469.3 per 100,000 men. In contrast, among women in that age group, the age-adjusted mortality rate was 160.6 per 100,000 women. The incidence rate for lung cancer is second only to prostate cancer among men and second only to breast cancer among women. A cancer incidence rate is the number of new cases of cancer of a specific site or type occurring in a specified population during a year, reported as the number of cancers per 100,000 people.

As is true of most forms of cancer, the incidence rates for men and women increase with age. The average, annual age-adjusted incidence rate for lung cancer among men under the age of 65 between 1973 and 1990 was 36.7 per 100,000 men in that age group. For men age 65 and older, the age-adjusted rate was 501.5 per 100,000. Among women under the age of 65, the rate was 21.3, compared to a rate of 203.7 for women ages 65 and older. The leading cause of lung cancer is cigarette smoking. It is estimated that 85% of all cases can be attributed to tobacco consumption (Lubin et al., 1984). In fact, the elevated risk of lung cancer in older men is usually attributed to the prevalence of cigarette smoking in that age cohort of men. Likewise, the increase in the rate of lung cancer among women is explained in terms of the increase in the popularity of cigarette smoking among women, especially after World War II and, in particular, after the Korean War.

In addition to heart disease and lung cancer, prostate cancer is of particular concern to older men. As noted previously, prostate cancer is the most frequently occurring cancer among men in the United States (Miller et al., 1993). It is clearly the cancer of older men. The age-adjusted incidence rate in men under the age of 65 is only 22.7 per 100,000, compared to 884.1 per 100,000 in men ages 65 and older. Prostate cancer is also the second leading cause of cancer death among older men. While the age-adjusted mortality rate in men under the age of 65 is only 2.9 per 100,000, it increases to a rate of 227.1 per 100,000 for men ages 65 and older. Relatively little is known about the etiology of the disease. Dietary fat and elevated levels of male hormones (especially testosterone) have been implicated.

A COMMON THEME

In considering the physical health of older men, there are two important questions: Why do some older men develop specific health conditions, while others of the same age do not? Of those men who develop health problems, why do some survive longer or better than others? Addressing these questions are central to gerontological research, and should ultimately lead to better public health interventions to enhance the health of older men.

The key is to look across different health conditions and find common themes as a way of understanding differences in the risk of disease, disability, and death in older men. Consider socioeconomic status. There is a substantial body of evidence indicating that men of lower socioeconomic status are not just at elevated risk for a few health conditions; rather, they are at risk for a wide variety of conditions, including diabetes, heart disease, and chronic obstructive pulmonary disease, as well as leading forms of cancer (including cancers of the lung and prostate) (Adler et al., 1993; Susser, 1985). These conditions are also more likely to appear at younger ages, be diagnosed at a more advanced stage, and occur concurrently with other health conditions (House, Kessler, & Herog. 1990). Finally, men in a lower socioeconomic position are more likely to be disabled and die prematurely from those conditions.

What is it about lower socioeconomic status that elevates the risk of disease, disability, and death? A poor diet, lack of exercise, cigarette smoking, and poor access to health services have all been associated. Recent research suggests, however, that the health effects of socioeconomic status involve much more. Haan, Kaplan and Camacho (1987) have investigated the reasons for the association between socioeconomic status and poor health by studying 9-year mortality in a random sample of residents aged 35 and over in Oakland, California. They found that residents of a federally designated poverty area experienced higher age-, race-, and sex-adjusted mortality, compared to residents of non-poverty areas. Most important, the relationship between place of residence and mortality persisted, even after adjusting for characteristics of the individual residents. These factors included baseline health status, race, income, employment status, access to medical care, health insurance coverage, smoking, and alcohol consumption. The authors conclude that the risk of ill health for residents of poverty areas may be due more to the environmental demands facing residents than to the characteristics of the individual residents themselves. Along these lines, MacIntyre, MacIver, and Sooman (1993) indicate that these demands may be associated with the availability of decent housing, transportation, affordable and nutritious food, and safe and healthy recreation, as well as access to social and health services.

Examining the intersection between the individual and the environment offers a promising strategy for developing a more parsimonious approach for understanding and enhancing the physical health of older men. This approach enables the examination of factors associated with the risk of disease, access to prevention, treatment, and rehabilitation services, as well as the duration and quality of survival. This approach is also in keeping with the ecological model of aging, originally proposed by Lawton and Nahemov (1973). The primary concept behind the ecological model of aging is that behavior is a function of the competencies of the individual person, the demands of the environment, and the interaction or adaptation of the person to the environment. In many ways, a focus on the social and physical environment helps to fulfill the promise of public health, supplying a piece to the health puzzle that is not supplied by clinical medicine with its focus on the individual patient.

THE HOUSEHOLD

The household may be one of the best entrees for studying the environment of older men. By entering the home, one may examine both living arrangements of older men and the physical structure of the dwelling itself. Both factors are associated with health outcomes.

Living Arrangements of the Household

Older men are more likely to be married and, as a result, have a better chance of being cared for in the home if they suffer from health problems or disabilities. Women, on the other hand, are more likely to live alone and be institutionalized if they cannot care for themselves. In 1993, 77% of men aged 65 and older were married, compared to 42% of women of that age. Only 18% of older men live alone, compared to 43% of older women (Barer, 1994).

Although men are less likely to live alone, those men who do live alone seem to be at elevated risk for a variety of health conditions. Davis, Neuhaus, Moritz, and Segal (1992) examined the association of living arrangements and survival among 7,651 adults, aged 45 to 74 years, in the National Health and Nutrition Examination Survey (NHANES 1, 1971–1975). Men who lived alone or with someone other than a spouse had significantly shorter survival times compared with those living with a spouse. The reasons for this elevated risk of death were not completely clear. Adjusting for the number of chronic conditions did not reduce the association of living arrangements with survival. Diet may play a role. In a separate study, Davis, Murphy, Neuhaus, and Lein (1990) examined the dietary practices of 4,402 people aged 55 and over enrolled in the Nationwide Food Consumption Survey. Dietary quality was based on percent of recommended dietary allowances for 3-day intakes of nine nutrients. In general, those who lived alone were more likely to eat fewer meals and, in general, consume a less healthful diet. This was especially the case for men.

Research on the health effects of bereavement also suggests that older men who live alone are at elevated risk of death. A committee of the National Academy of Sciences reviewed the research on bereavement and reported several findings (Klerman & Clayton, 1984) which are summarized below:

After the death of a spouse, there is a statistically significant increase in mortality for men under the age of 75. The risk is particularly elevated during the first year and remains elevated for up to 6 years among those men who do not remarry. For women, there is no elevated risk of death in the first year. It is unclear whether there is a higher mortality rate in subsequent years. There is also evidence that the suicide rates increase during the first year is elevated among widowers. There is only a modest increase in suicide among widows. In contrast to widows, widowers are at elevated risk of death from accidents, cardiovascular disease, and some infectious diseases.

Barer (1994) suggests that older men may not be as well equipped as older women to deal with the loss of a spouse, and notes that "widows are better able than widowers to develop and sustain intimate relationships. They tend to form confidant relationships with other widowed women, whereas widowed men, who had relied on their wives for their emotional needs, are left with no one" (p. 30). It was also noted that when a man is widowed, other men his age are most likely to still be married. It is not surprising, therefore, that widowers are more likely than widows to remarry. Of course, given differences in life expectancy and customs about "appropriate" differences in age between married men and women, older men have a larger pool of eligible mates.

Even though older men are more likely than women to be married, women are more likely to serve as caregivers for an ill spouse. Most research on caregiving, in fact, has focused on women (Wright, Clipp, & George, 1993). It is important to realize, however, that regardless of gender, spousal caregivers report poorer health than those of the same age in the general population. Stone, Cafferata, and Sangl (1986) report that 44% of caregivers report their health as "fair" or "poor," compared to 30% of people of the same age in the general population. Despite the focus on female caregivers, several studies have reported on the health problems of male caregivers, including elevated blood pressure and reports of poorer health found for husbands of cognitively impaired wives (Moritz et al., 1989). The characteristics of the living arrangements of older men are clearly associated with their level of health and functioning.

Physical Structure of the Household

There is also a growing body of research examining the effects of the physical design of housing on the health and functioning of older people (Regnier & Pynoos, 1987). The results suggest that the functional capacity of older people can be either enhanced or impaired by physical design (Christenson & Taira, 1990). Physical design also affects the extent to which older people are able to satisfy everyday needs, such as bathing and cooking (Christenson & Taira, 1990).

Special attention has been given to the physical environment and the risk of falls (Berg & Cassells, 1992). It is estimated that approximately one-quarter of persons aged 65 to 74, and one-third or more of those aged 75 and older, report a fall in the previous year. Falls result in a variety of injuries, including fractures of the hip, wrist, humerus, and pelvis as well as hematoma, joint dislocation, severe laceration, sprain, and other disabling soft tissue injury. Falls also represent the leading cause of accidental death among people aged 65 and older, with older men being more likely than older women to suffer a fatal fall.

Although falls are often thought to be a marker of frailty, environmental factors are reported to play a primary role in the risk of falls in healthy people. It is reported (Berg & Cassells, 1992) that environmental hazards potentially include the poor design and disrepair of stairways, inadequate lighting, clutter, slippery floors, unsecured mats and rugs, and lack of nonskid surfaces in bathtubs, among many others. Environmental factors are reported to be implicated in one-third to one-half of falls. Unfortunately, studies have yet to assess hazards outside the home or quantify exposure to hazards (in terms of frequency, duration, and intensity) to develop a true estimate of risk (Berg & Cassells, 1992). Most studies simply report the presence or absence of a hazard. In addition, definitions of environmental hazards and methods of assessment have not been well standardized.

THE AUTOMOBILE

The automobile, and the use of other modes of transportation, also represents a convenient point of entry for studying the physical health of older men. Transportation is important for several reasons. First, it represents the means by which an older person is able to get to places beyond walking distance to obtain goods and services and to maintain contact with friends and relatives. Second, transportation (in particular, the use of the automobile) represents one of the few settings that requires the coordination and execution of a variety of functional capacities, including cognition, vision, and upper- and lower-body strength. Third, automobile crashes represent one of the leading causes of accidental death in the elderly, especially among older men. There is evidence indicating that driving performance and crashes in older people are associated with a variety of factors, including the number and type of symptoms, level of physical and visual function, and cognitive performance (National Highway Traffic Safety Administration, 1989).

Most older people, especially men, rely on the automobile to get to places beyond walking distance. With increased age, the frequency of driving decreases. Although the effects of various chronic conditions on driving performance have been hypothesized, no consistent association is reported. In a recent study, the odds of driving less than 5,000 miles per year were associated with level of functional status (e.g., difficulty climbing stairs and performing heavy household tasks), rather than particular diagnosed conditions (Marttoli et al., 1993). Functional status, as a more direct behavioral measure, may be a more sensitive indicator of driving performance than information about diagnosis of one or more chronic conditions. Results also suggest that older people involved in more outside activities, e.g., employment and participation in social activities, are more likely to drive (Marttoli et al., 1993).

Research on the risk of crashes suggests that older men are at elevated risk for being in a crash. This may be due to the fact that older men are more likely to drive than older women (National Highway Safety Traffic Administration, 1989). Research on the role of cognitive health problems and functional status on the risk of crashes is somewhat inconsistent. For example, cognitive impairment, as measured by the Mini-Mental test, was shown to be associated with crashes in one study, but unrelated in another (Foley, Wallace & Eberhard, 1995; Stewart, Moore, Marks, May, & Hale, 1993). There is also no consistent association with medication use. Symptoms associated with the odds of crashes were found to include feeling cold in feet and hands, an irregular heartbeat, and having a history of back pain (Stewart et al., 1993). In this study, only bursitis has been identified as a chronic condition associated with the risk of being in a crash. Others have identified diabetes and cardiovascular disease as elevating the odds of an injury-producing crash (Decina & Stalin, 1993). A recent study of visual assessment found that those with low contrast sensitivity were at elevated risk of such accidents (Koepsell et al., 1994). Interestingly, there is relatively little research examining the association between automobile and highway design and the risk of injuries.

CHALLENGES AND NEW DIRECTIONS

An examination of the intersection between the individual and the environment presents some unique challenges.

Most research in public health focuses on the exposures, behaviors, and health outcomes of individuals. Although the research objective may be to examine the health of families and the community, the unit of analysis is almost exclusively the individual (Marshall, Matthews, & Rosenthal, 1993). For example, sampling strategies are designed to randomly select individuals, not families or other aspects of the social environment. Once families are identified, it is not completely clear how information about family health should be obtained, perhaps by interviewing individual family members, or by developing techniques which combine ethnographic techniques with survey sampling. It is only by developing different strategies of sampling and field interviewing and observation that there can be a greater understanding of the health effects of living arrangements for older men. How does caregiving affect the health of the caregiver? Indeed, how does the health of one family member influence the health of another, in this case, the older man?

The household and automobile (and other modes of transportation) should be used as a context or setting for studying the intersection between the individual and the environment. It is also necessary that investigations identify how those places intersect with the broader social, political, and economic environment. Research in this area is especially important, given that older men are at elevated risk for both suffering a fatal fall and being involved in an automobile crash.

Studies in ethnically diverse populations are needed. Men of color are at elevated risk for a variety of health conditions (Manton, Patrick, & Johnson, 1989). Research indicates that the extended family plays an important role in different ethnic groups (Chatters, Taylor, & Neighbors, 1989). If measures of the social environment do not include the kin network, there may be an incomplete picture of family supports.

More sophisticated indicators of the physical and technological environment need to be developed. Presently, as Carp (1987) notes, the environment is typically measured in terms of individual perceptions. Subjects are asked about their reactions to the environment. Direct measures of the environment are not included. Carp (1987) outlines strategies for direct assessments of the environment (e.g., assessments of the number of floors, number of rooms, and level of lighting). Other indicators may include the availability of particular goods and services, highway design, and traffic volume.

Longitudinal studies should be established, on the basis of data from a variety of sources, including interviews, health records, and environmental indicators.

New research teams need to be established. In addition to researchers in gerontology and public health, it will be necessary to include individuals with expertise in human factors research, architecture, engineering, and environmental psychology.

THE SPPARCS STUDY: AN EXAMPLE

The Study of Physical Performance and Age-Related Changes in Sonoma (SPPARCS), funded by a grant from the National Institute on Aging, is designed to investigate the epidemiology of aging and physical performance in a sample of 2,096 male and female residents of Sonoma, California aged 55 and over. One of the key objectives of this 5-year longitudinal study is to examine the extent to which living arrangements and the physical environment either enhance or impede an older person's capacity to complete everyday activities and recuperate following illness. It provides an example of one way to address the intersection between the individual and the environment. It also affords an opportunity to highlight the special health problems facing older men, in particular, the risk of falls and the risk of automobile crash injury.

The city of Sonoma is approximately 40 miles to the northeast of San Francisco, California at the southern end of the wine-growing region of the Sonoma Valley. The city and its unincorporated surrounds contain considerable numbers of retirees. Based on the 1990 census, the city had a population of 8,121 of whom 39.5% were ages 55 and over and 30.5% were 65 and over.

The Sample

The sampling frame was the entire city and selected immediately contiguous neighborhoods outside of the boundaries of the city. The contiguous areas included a retirement community adjacent to the city (63% aged 65 and over in the 1990 census; area 0.7 square miles) and several other neighborhoods that were more general population sites.

Recruitment was based on a design that was used to recruit subjects in the Alameda County Health Study (Berkman & Breslow, 1983). A community-wide survey (census) of all households in the target area was conducted to enumerate the number of potentially eligible subjects. All residents aged 55 and over were eligible for the study. The 2,386 households for which complete census data were available produced 3,509 age-eligible individuals. Of these, only 3,057 actually were available to be enrolled. Of these 3,057 individuals, 2,092 (68.4%) were successfully enrolled and completed the baseline interview. By sampling households rather than individuals, approximately 800 pairs of spouses aged 55 and over were enrolled.

Sources of Information

In addition to medical records and laboratory assessments of pulmonary and cardiovascular function, the main source of information in the SPPARCS study is the home interview. The interview addresses a comprehensive set of topics, including questions on level of moderate and vigorous physical activities, the number and types of chronic conditions and symptoms, physical and cognitive function, falls and injuries, depression, medication use, health behavior, and demographic and socioeconomic factors. In addition, the interview includes questions on marriage, living arrangements, and social networks, as well as driving performance and the use of alternative means of transportation.

The Household

The number, age, and relationship of each household member is recorded. The participant is also asked about whether any member of the household is ill or in poor health and whether the participant assists anyone in the household in the completion of daily activities (such as dressing, grooming, bathing, or feeding). Questions about caregiving responsibilities for other relatives and friends are also included.

In addition to living arrangements, respondents are also asked about the physical characteristics of the household and neighborhood. Included are questions about whether they have difficulty getting in or out of a tub or shower, reaching for items on top shelves, using a stepstool, turning door knobs or faucets, and getting up or down stairs. Respondents are also asked whether their home includes particular items, such as a seat in the shower or bath and grab bars or railings in any room. Questions are also included about the immediate neighborhood. Respondents are asked whether any of the following represented problems in their neighborhood: Heavy traffic, speeding cars, excessive noise, vandalism, crime in general, no sidewalks or poorly maintained sidewalks, and inadequate lighting at night.

The social and physical characteristics of the household figure prominently in assessing differences in health and functioning. For example, respondents are asked about whether they fell in the previous 6 months and the circumstances of the fall; for example, whether it was due to a trip, slip, bump (i.e., an environmental or extrinsic cause) or fainting or a sudden drop (an intrinsic cause). In terms of the completion of instrumental activities of daily living, such as meal preparation, housekeeping, and grocery shopping, respondents are asked to identify all the people in the household who perform the task and then to name the person who is most likely to perform the task. Questions also are included on the type and frequency of vigorous and moderate physical activities. In addition, respondents are asked whether they presently limit or avoid physical exercise for any reasons. Included in a list of reasons are problems with eyesight, concern about falling or injury, any other health problem, ailment or disability, as well as the lack of someone to exercise with, and concern about crime or violence when outside.

The Automobile

Special attention is being given to driving and use of alternative types of transportation among older residents in Sonoma. The interview includes questions about the license status (current, past, or never held), the timing of driving, and the average number of miles they drive each week. Participants are also asked whether they have limited or avoided driving for any reason, including health problems, ailments, or disabilities, as well as the lack of someone to drive with, concern about crime, and concern about getting lost. Finally, participants also are asked about their level of difficulty in getting to places beyond walking distance.

In addition to asking participants questions about driving, driving records are obtained from the California Department of Motor Vehicles to identify the number and type of citations and crashes experienced by respondents both before and after the baseline interview. With this information, it will be possible to identify the health and social factors associated with an elevated risk of crashes in the elderly. This will be particularly important for understanding the physical health of older men, given that the risk of crashes, in general, and fatal crashes, in particular, are elevated in older men.

Analytic Plan

One of the major objectives of the SPPARCS study is to examine the association between functional capacity (e.g., pulmonary function) and functional performance (e.g., frequency and type of physical exercise). It is hypothesized that characteristics of the social and physical environment will either enhance or impede the association between capacity and performance. For example, given a particular level of pulmonary function, married men living in a well-lighted neighborhood with well-paved sidewalks are more likely to engage in physical exercise than older men of the same age and level of pulmonary function who live alone in less accommodating neighborhoods. In this study, which is currently in the field, special attention will be given to comparing the association between functional capacity and performance between men and women.

There is also evidence to suggest that spouses tend to share a similar level of health. The reasons for this concordance between spouses is not completely clear. As noted previously, the SPPARCS sample consists of 800 spouse pairs. One of the objectives of this study is to examine the degree of concordance between spouses for a number of indicators of health and functioning, including the prevalence of particular health conditions, exercise capacity, and pulmonary function. There will also be a determination of the extent to which the strength of concordance varies by the number of years the spouses have been together. This will provide an excellent opportunity to examine the effect of living arrangements and marital status on the health of older men. Although older men in Sonoma are not necessarily representative of older men in other regions of the United States, the protocol for the SPPARCS project could be employed in other areas to better characterize the health and functional status of older men.

CONCLUSION

It was contended that it would be difficult to consider the physical health of older men without at least a passing reference to the physical health of older women. Indeed, it is believed fair to suggest that it is impossible to assess the health of any group without a consideration of others. Older men do not exist in a vacuum. They interact with others in a social and physical environment. With this in mind, future researchers face two significant challenges. First, it will be necessary to develop strategies to identify and study the group, rather than the individual, as the unit of investigation and analysis. Second, it will be critical to include indicators of the physical environment (e.g., characteristics of the house and highway) that can be assessed independently of the individual. By addressing these challenges, there will be a better understanding of (and ability to enhance) the health, functioning, and mobility of older men.

REFERENCES

Adler, N., Boyce, W. T., Chesney, M., Cohen, S., Folkman, S., Kahn, R. L., & Syme, S. L. (1994). Socioeconomic status and health: The challenge of the gradient. *American Psychologist, 49*, 15–24.

Barer, B. (1994). Men and women aging differently. *The International Journal of Aging and Development, 48*, 29–39.

Berg, R. L., & Cassells, J. S. (Eds.). (1992). *The second fifty years: Promoting health and preventing disability.* Washington, DC: National Academy Press.

Berkman, L. F., & Breslow, L. (1983). *Health and ways of living: The Alameda County Study.* New York: Oxford University Press.

Carp, F. M. (1987). Environment and aging. In D. Stokols & I. Altoman (Eds.), *Handbook of environmental psychology* (pp. 329–360). New York: John Wiley.

Chatters, L. M., Taylor, R. J., & Neighbors, H. W. (1989). Size of the informal helper network mobilized during a serious personal problem among black Americans. *Journal of Marriage and the Family, 51*, 667–676.

Christenson, M. A., & Taira, E. D. (1990). *Aging in the design environment.* New York: The Haworth Press.

Conference on research and development needed to improve safety and mobility of older drivers (1990). Lister Hill Conference Center, National Library of Medicine, April 23–24, 1989. Washington, DC: National Highway Traffic Safety Administration, U.S. Department of Transportation, PB-90-258567.

Davis, M. A., Murphy, S. B., Neuhaus, J. M., & Lein, D. (1990). Living arrangements and dietary quality of older U.S. adults. *Journal of the American Dietetic Association, 90,* 1667–1672.

Davis, M. A., Neuhaus, J. M., Moritz, D. J., & Segal, M. (1992). Living arrangements and survival among older middle-aged and older adults in the NHANES I Epidemiologic Follow-up Study. *American Journal of Public Health, 82,* 401–406.

Decina, L. E., & Stalin, L. (1993). Retrospective evaluation of alternative vision screening criteria for older and younger drivers. *Accident Analysis and Prevention, 25,* 267–275.

Foley, D. J., Wallace, R. B., & Eberhard, J. (1995). Risk factors for motor vehicle crashes among older drivers in a rural community. *Journal of the American Geriatrics Society, 48,* 776–781.

Haan, M., Kaplan, G. A., & Camacho, T. (1987). Poverty and health: Prospective evidence from the Alameda County Study. *American Journal of Epidemiology, 125,* 989–999.

House, J. S., Kessler, R. C., & Herog, A. R. (1990). Age, socioeconomic status, and health. *The Milbank Quarterly, 68,* 383–411.

Koepsell, T. D., Wolf, M. E., McCloskey, L., Buckner, D. M., Louie, D., Wagner, E. H., & Thompson, R. S. (1994). Medical conditions and motor vehicle collision injuries in older adults. *Journal of the American Geriatrics Society, 42,* 695–700.

Katz, S., Branch, L. G., Branson, M. H., Papsidero, J. A., Beck, J. C., & Greer, D. S. (1983). Active life expectancy. *The New England Journal of Medicine, 309,* 1218–1224.

Klerman, G. L., & Clayton, P. (1984). Epidemiological perspectives on the health consequences of bereavement. In F. Solomon & M. Green (Eds.), *Bereavement: Reactions, consequences, and care* (pp. 15–44). Washington, DC: National Academy Press.

Lawton, M. P., & Nahemov, L. (1973). Ecology and the aging process. In C. Eisdorfer & M. P. Lawton (Eds.), *The psychology of adult development and aging* (pp. 619–674). Washington, DC: American Psychological Association.

Lubin, J. H., Blott, W. J., Berrino, F., Flamant, R., Gillis, C. R., Kunze, M., Schmahl, D., & Visco, G. (1984). Modifying the risk of developing lung cancer by changing habits of cigarette smoking. *British Medical Journal, 288,* 1953–1956.

MacIntyre, S., MacIver, S., & Sooman, A. (1993). Area, class, and health: Should we be focusing on places or people? *Journal of Social Policy, 22,* 213–234.

Manton, K. G., Patrick, C. H., & Johnson, K. W. (1989). Health differentials between blacks and whites: Recent trends in mortality and morbidity. In D. P. Willis (Ed.), *Black Americans and health policies* (pp. 129–199). New York: Transaction Books.

Marshall, V. M., Matthews, S. H., & Rosenthal, C. J. (1993). Elusiveness of family life: A challenge for the sociology of aging. *Annual Review of Gerontology and Geriatrics, 13*, 39–72.

Miller, B. A., Ries, L. A. G., Hankey, B. F., Kosary, C. L., Harras, A., Devesa, S. S., & Edwards, B. K. (1993). *SEER Cancer Statistics Review 1973–90* (NIH Publication No. 93–2789). Bethesda, MD: National Cancer Institute.

Moritz, D. J., Kasl, S. V., & Berkman, L. F. (1989). The health impact of living with a cognitively impaired spouse: Depressive symptoms and social functioning. *Journal of Gerontology, 44*, S17–S27.

Martolli, R. A., Ostfeld, A. M., Merrill, S. S., Perlman, G. D., Foley, D. J., & Cooney, L. M. (1993). Driving cessation and changes in mileage driven among elderly individuals. *Journal of Gerontology: Medical Sciences, 48*, MS255–260.

Ory, M. G., & Warner, H. R. (1990). *Gender, health, and longevity.* New York: Springer.

Regnier, V., & Pynoos, J. (1987). *Housing the aged: Design directives and policy considerations.* New York: Elsevier.

Stewart, R. B., Moore, M. T., Marks, R. G., May, F. E., & Hale, W. E. (1993). *Driving cessation and accidents in the elderly: An analysis of symptoms, diseases, cognitive dysfunction and medications.* Washington, DC: AAA Foundation for Traffic Safety.

Stone, R., Cafferata, G., & Sangl, J. (1986). *Caregivers of the frail elderly: A national profile.* Washington, DC: U.S. Department of Health and Human Services.

Susser, M. (1985). Social class and disorders of health. In M. Susser (Ed.), *Sociology in medicine* (pp. 213–274). New York: Oxford University Press.

Verbrugge, L. M., & Patrick, D. L. (1995). Seven chronic conditions: Their impact on U. S. adults' activity levels and use of medical services. *American Journal of Public Health, 85*, 173–182.

Wright, L. K., Clipp, E. C., & George, L. K. (1993). Health consequences of caregiver stress. *Medical Exercise, Nutrition, and Health, 2*, 181–195.

CHAPTER 11

Recognizing and Treating Alcohol Abuse and Alcohol Dependence in Elderly Men

Kathleen J. Farkas, Ph.D.
& Lenore A. Kola, Ph.D.

As many clinicians have learned, there is no age limit for substance abuse problems. People of all ages use alcohol and other drugs, but substance abuse is rarely raised in discussions of the problems of later life. Substance abuse symptoms in an elderly person are more likely to be misdiagnosed or ignored than they would be in a younger person, due to a lack of information about the signs and symptoms of substance abuse, lack of training in substance abuse treatment, and the social stigma which still can accompany a substance abuse diagnosis. In fact, family and friends may even encourage use in elderly relatives to increase socialization, improve appetite, and to help with sleeping problems.

Several interrelated health and social factors put the elderly at risk for substance abuse problems; problems resulting from the use of legal drugs (i.e., alcohol and prescription drug use) and illegal drugs (i.e., street drugs). Health-risk factors include the incidence of chronic conditions and mental disorders, and age-related pharmacodynamics. Most people over age 65 have at least one chronic condition, and it is common to have several ailments which can be painful and limit mobility. Alcohol and other prescription and nonprescription drugs can be used to soothe pain. The elderly may use alcohol to counteract depression and anxiety.

While younger people also use alcohol for mood management, it is noteworthy that a significant number of elderly people are seriously depressed. Age-related pharmacodynamics refers to how alcohol and other drugs work in an elderly person's body. In general, physical changes which accompany age, such as decreases in cellular fluids and increases in proportions of body fat, serve to increase a person's sensitivity to the effects of alcohol. Elderly people may experience increased effects of alcohol, such as dizziness and/or drowsiness, without increasing the amount they consume. Many people decrease the amount of alcohol they drink in later life because of such experiences.

In terms of social-risk factors, many elderly persons experience an increase in unstructured time and may not have as many job and family responsibilities as they did earlier in life. The loss of a spouse is seen as an especially stressful event, and newly widowed men are vulnerable to maladaptive coping strategies, such as increased alcohol use. For some men, the death of a wife may not only mean the end of married life, but also may mean the end of a social life which was centered around the wife's activities and social relationships. This loss of a social network can bring loneliness and isolation, which can serve as additional risks for increased drinking. The multiple losses and the ensuing grief processes of later life constitute particular risk factors for the elderly.

An increase in unstructured time may mean more time to socialize and to increase the amount of alcohol consumption per week. An elderly man who settles in a retirement community which has an emphasis on social interaction and social events may find that, for the first time in his life, he has the time and the opportunity to have a cocktail before dinner, and finds he is drinking more than he did when he was younger. On the other hand, an elderly man may find that the same amount of alcohol he once consumed with no problem may result in clinical symptoms, such as slurred speech, instability, falls, and confusion (Gambert, 1992). This retirement scenario may be especially risky for an elderly man if he does not have family, friends, or colleagues nearby to recognize a change in his drinking behavior or to spot problems which might be related to alcohol use. Later life also brings changes in social roles which may have an impact upon social status, self-perception, and the use of alcohol.

For some men, late life may serve to enhance social standing, in that only the strong survive and some groups revere the elderly for their experience and knowledge. For other men, late life may bring a step down in social status, and the lack of power and recognition may precipitate feelings of rejection and depression. Since alcohol can be used to either celebrate or to console, social loss factors alone usually do not predict alcohol abuse problems.

Over the past 30 years, it has been learned that substance abuse among the elderly can include prescription drugs, over-the-counter medications, alcohol, tobacco and illicit drugs, such as heroin or amphetamines. Alcohol, however, has remained the drug of choice for people over 60, and currently is the drug most often abused by this age group. While recognizing that these other substances can present serious problems for elderly people, the scope of this chapter will be limited to alcohol abuse and dependence.

Elderly people tend to use alcohol less often than the general population, but a significant subset of elderly people, elderly men in particular, experience alcohol-related problems. Elderly men are more likely to drink alcohol and to experience more problems related to alcohol abuse and alcohol dependence than are elderly women. In fact, contrary to many aspects of gerontology, alcohol abuse and dependence may be one area in which we know more about men that we do about women (Friedman, Fleming, Roberts, & Hyman, 1996). While it is true that initial diagnosis and treatment efforts in alcohol abuse and dependence focused on men, van Wormer (1995) argues that the literature is virtually silent on male-gender issues in diagnosis and treatment, while the needs of females have been well documented, since women are often treated as a special population in alcohol and other drug abuse publications.

PREVALENCE OF ALCOHOL ABUSE AND DEPENDENCE IN ELDERLY MEN

Earlier theorists explained the lack of alcoholism among elderly people as an issue of survivorship; that is, the majority of alcoholics died early in life and only a few were fortunate to reach old age (Drew, 1968). While alcohol abuse and alcohol dependence among the elderly is still not a widely researched topic, there is an emerging body of knowledge on the prevalence, diagnosis, and treatment of alcohol abuse and dependence among elderly people (Farkas, 1992). Liberto, Oslin, and Ruskin

(1992) conducted a review of the literature on alcoholism among older persons and found that the rates of alcohol use, alcohol abuse, and alcohol dependence vary depending upon the type of sample, the type of questions, and the time frame of the study. These authors illuminated the distinctions between prevalence rates in community samples and prevalence rates in hospital and outpatient populations, and differences in cross-sectional versus longitudinal information about alcohol use.

Community-based studies typically use a cross-sectional approach, and indicate that between 10% and 22% of people older than 60 drink alcohol daily. Questions about daily drinking, or even about heavy drinking, do not necessarily indicate alcohol abuse or dependence, and community-based studies often lack clinically significant indicators of alcohol abuse and dependence. As reported in Liberto et al. (1992), the Epidemiologic Catchment Area Study (using an accurate and clinically significant measurement tool) found a 1-year prevalence rate for alcohol abuse and dependence of 3.1% for elderly men and .46% for elderly women. In another community survey, Jinks and Raschko (1990) found that 2.2% of all elderly people met the Diagnostic Interview Schedule criteria for alcohol abuse and dependence, used by the Epidemiologic Catchment Area Survey, and that 9.6% of elderly men fell into the abuse and dependence category. While the findings on difference in alcohol use between African-American and white elderly are mixed, Herd (1990) found that white men over age 60 had higher rates of drinking than African-American men, controlling for income level. In contrast to the stereotype of the skid row drinker, several studies have shown that it is the higher-income elderly who are more likely to drink alcohol and less likely to abstain in comparison to lower-income elderly (Borgatta, Montgomery & Borgatta, 1982; Dunham, 1981; Goodwin Sanchez, Thomas, Hunt, Garry, & Goodwin, 1987). This finding makes sense when one considers the financial burden of alcoholic beverages for elderly persons on a limited income.

The scope of alcohol problems among the elderly becomes much larger when studies of alcohol abuse and dependence focus upon elderly people in the hospital. Liberto et al. (1992) summarized the prevalence rates for hospital studies as between 20% to 50% "with even higher rates for men" (p. 977). These rates are tempered by studies of outpatient settings. Buchsbaum, Buchanan, & Lawton (1991) found a 5% prevalence rate in a primary care medical care setting using the DSM-III criteria. Liberto et al. (1992) cite evidence that 6% of men in a veteran's screening clinic were drinking more than 50 grams of alcohol per day. Of all institutional settings, nursing homes have the highest rates of alcohol abuse problems, and up to 40% of nursing home patients are reported to have alcohol abuse problems (Buchsbaum et al., 1991). While not all nursing home patients are elderly, the high rates of alcohol abuse problems among this population present an area of concern for prevention and treatment efforts.

The Diagnostic and Statistical Manual (DSM) of the American Psychiatric Association includes a useful typology of issues and behaviors related to alcohol use. The most recent edition is DSM IV which replaces the previous edition, DSM III-R. The DSM criteria for diagnosis are widely used in the social work, medical, and nursing professions and present useful concepts important in the diagnosis of alcohol problems among the elderly.

What is known about the stability of alcohol use patterns over the life span? How do people change their drinking habits over the life course? If they do, what is the importance of these changes in detecting and treating alcohol abuse and dependence in later life? One way to approach the answers to these questions is to examine the age of onset of alcohol abuse and dependence problems.

Researchers and clinicians use three patterns to discuss onset: early onset, late onset, and intermittent patterns (Liberto et al., 1992). Early onset is when a person begins drinking alcohol excessively in his 20s or 30s and continues this pattern of abuse and dependence into later life. Friedman et al. (1996) have labeled the early onset group as "survivors" and characterize them as more often having alcohol-related problems, such as cirrhosis, pancreatitis, hypertension, or diabetes. Late onset is when a person begins an excessive drinking pattern at an older age, typically in response to a psychosocial stressor. An intermittent pattern is characterized by a history of excessive drinking in earlier life, but includes either abstinence and/or lighter drinking for long periods of time before a return to excessive drinking in late life. Without considering the lifetime pattern of alcohol use, the intermittent pattern is often mistaken for the late onset pattern.

Studies of onset patterns have consistently shown that approximately one-third to one-half of elderly alcohol abusers fall into the late onset pattern and that more men than women fall into the early onset or the intermittent onset groups.

SCREENING OF ALCOHOL ABUSE
AND DEPENDENCE

Screening and assessment are the building blocks of prevention and treatment efforts. Screening questions should be brief and lead to information about the need to know more about an individual's use of alcohol and other drugs. All professionals who work with elderly people in health care or social service settings should develop a screening strategy for alcohol problems and routinely use this screening strategy with all elderly, not only those who appear to have problems. Too often, professionals skim over issues which they think might be embarrassing to their patients or clients. Since the elderly may experience more social stigma regarding alcohol problems than younger people, it is especially important that universal screening questions be worded nonjudgmentally and be asked in a supportive and respectful manner.

Fortunately, there exist several useful screening tools for alcohol problems, and at least two of them have been developed specifically for the elderly. These screening tools are known by their acronyms. A popular tool is the CAGE, which has been used in a variety of settings and with a variety of age groups (Mayfield, McLeod, & Hall, 1974). The CAGE questions are:

1. Have you ever felt you should cut down on your drinking?
2. Have people annoyed you by criticizing your drinking?
3. Have you ever felt guilty about your drinking? and
4. Have you ever had a drink first thing in the morning (an eye-opener) to steady your nerves or to get rid of a hangover?

The CAGE questions are direct and may offer elderly men an opportunity to talk about their concern regarding alcohol use. The CAGE questions, however, may be too direct and present a stereotypical image of an alcoholic. For some elderly men, the CAGE questions may be too threatening. The CAGE has been criticized as lacking sensitivity in older populations, especially if elderly women are included in the screening group along with elderly men.

The HEAT, a variation of the CAGE, is another four-point screening option (Willinbring & Spring, 1988). The HEAT questions are:

1. *How* do you use alcohol?
2. Have you ever thought you used to *excess*?
3. Has *anyone else* ever thought you used too much?
4. Have you ever had any *trouble* resulting from your use?

These questions are more open-ended, and the response to the first question, about how alcohol is used, provides the opportunity to discuss drinking patterns and reasons for drinking with the elderly client. As with the CAGE questions, any affirmative response warrants additional questions and discussion. It may be useful to ask screening questions in relation to various periods in the person's life. For example, one could ask the screening questions using a 6-month time frame (e.g., "Within the past 6 months, how have you used alcohol?"). The clinician might then repeat questions using a 1-year interval and then a lifetime perspective. By comparing the responses for different time periods in the person's life, the clinician will be able to elicit information about onset and other life stressors important in the diagnostic process.

The CHARM (Friedman et al., 1996) builds upon the HEAT and the CAGE and provides a flow of questions for use with elderly people. The first questions are general ones about stresses in a person's life and the ways the person copes with these stresses. The clinician then asks if the person has drunk any alcohol in the past year. If the response is negative, the following questions include: Did you have a problem with alcohol in the past? If so, how long ago? If the answer to the alcohol use question is in the affirmative, then the CHARM questions follow:

1. Have you ever thought about cutting down?
2. How? Do you have rules about drinking? Has your drinking pattern changed lately?
3. Has anyone expressed concern about your drinking?
4. What role does alcohol play in your life?
5. Have you ever used alcohol more than you intended? and
6. Have you ever had a problem with your medications?

The advantage of the CHARM protocol is that it offers additional questions to introduce the issues of stress and coping, and includes the area of medication problems, which can provide another avenue in the exploration of alcohol abuse.

ASSESSMENT AND DIAGNOSIS

Assessment and diagnosis efforts abound in the field of alcohol and other drug abuse, and clinicians will differ in their interpretations and in their use of the various tools in their work with elderly people. Graham (1986) has argued that the current methods to identify and measure alcohol abuse among the elderly are misleading. Her suggestions include revised measures which take into account the three onset patterns and the special health and social aspects of later life.

As mentioned on page 179, the DSM IV criteria has been commonly used by professionals for diagnosing the existence of alcohol problems in older populations. Using this criteria, substance abuse is defined as a maladaptive pattern of substance use leading to clinically significant impairment or distress. One of the four criteria for substance abuse is the failure to fulfill social roles, such as obligations at home, school, or work. The reliance on the criteria of social roles and on the social changes inherent in late life can impede an accurate diagnosis with elderly men. For example, "failure to fulfill major role obligations" may be meaningless in the case of an elderly man whose role obligations have been reduced through widowhood, retirement, and the geographic separation from children and grandchildren. Driving a car is an activity which might provide an opportunity to talk about alcohol use, but not always. Many elderly restrict their driving to daytime hours or to short neighborhood trips, and they may not use the car to drive to social occasions where alcohol is served, or do not drink alcohol outside of the home. An alcohol-related traffic violation, or an arrest for DWI, may not be a particularly useful indicator of substance abuse among the elderly.

The issue of intentional versus unintentional substance abuse is pertinent in working with the elderly and is important for interpreting information about substance abuse. It is possible that some elderly people may not make the connection between ingestion of alcohol and changes in mood states and/or impairment in cognitive and motor functions. Especially for elderly people who do not have a history of problem drinking, it is important to talk about the possible effects that even a small amount of alcohol may have on an older person. Some sensitivity is warranted in helping people to understand the differences between experiencing an alcohol-related problem and continued use after alcohol's role has been recognized. Using the DSM-IV criteria for substance abuse, alone, may result in missed opportunities to diagnosis current problems with alcohol and alcohol use patterns which put elderly men at risk of developing future problems with alcohol.

Two key issues are raised in the assessment of substance dependence: tolerance and withdrawal. Tolerance, in younger populations, is indicated by the need to use more of the substance in order to achieve the desired effects. In an elderly group, however, the changes in body mass and in metabolic processes may allow the elderly person to keep his intake stable or even, in some cases, to decrease it slightly with the same intoxicating results. Clinicians must be able to rule out general medical conditions and other mental disorders before making the diagnosis of withdrawal. Since the symptoms of alcohol withdrawal can mirror a number of other physical conditions which the elderly experience, the clinician who has not done a careful screening for alcohol problems, or who assumes that alcohol is not a problem of the elderly, can be often misled.

The clinical approach one takes in screening, assessment and diagnosis of alcohol problems is especially important in dealing with the elderly. In the general population, the idea that alcoholism is a disease has become common, thus reducing the stigma and shame for many people who experience alcohol-related problems themselves or in their families. However, the elderly may be one group which still may cling to previous ideas that alcohol problems are caused by moral weakness or personal deficits. Growing up in the shadow of temperance and Prohibition, some of today's elderly may still experience the stigma which was formerly associated with alcohol problems and alcoholism.

Men, in particular, may be vulnerable to feelings of decreased self-worth and powerlessness associated with growing older, and the additional burden of a diagnosis of alcohol abuse or dependence must be handled with sensitivity and professionalism. Physicians, social workers, and nurses may serve as potential gatekeepers in alcohol treatment for the elderly, since they routinely see many older persons and work with them and their families over time. Since alcohol-related problems are often mistaken for other health and social problems experienced by the elderly, it is important that all professionals working with older people be able to provide adequate screening and referral services.

TREATMENT OPTIONS

The options in alcohol and other drug treatment for all age groups are expanding. No longer is there the belief that twelve-step groups, such as Alcoholics Anonymous (AA), provide the only therapeutic avenues for success. While AA continues to be a viable treatment for many people, and has specific advantages for elderly men, there are other treatments which provide important clinical options for the elderly, their families, and their health care providers.

Several general issues relevant to the treatment of alcohol abuse in the elderly have been discussed by Hester and Miller (1995), who have outlined the most often used approaches in the treatment of alcohol abuse and dependence. While the twelve-step approach, and its philosophy, undergirds the most frequently used treatment in alcohol and other drug abuse, the field is moving toward incorporating additional treatment options. These options can include psychosocial treatment techniques that utilize supportive and problem-solving groups, cognitive behavioral approaches, social skills training, anxiety and stress management, and/or medication. Relatively few studies have examined treatment effectiveness with groups of elderly and, to date, no particular treatment approach has been shown to be more effective than others in working with elderly men.

Several general issues about alcohol abuse treatment for the elderly are worth discussing before focusing upon specific treatment approaches. These general issues include age-specific treatment, inpatient versus outpatient treatment, and treatment effectiveness.

Proponents of age-specific treatment models argue that the elderly are more likely to benefit from alcohol treatment groups which are formed only with other elderly people, who are likely to share similar alcohol-related problems and similar life experiences. In an age-segregated group, an elderly person may feel less isolated and more likely to participate. Kofoed, Tolson, Atkinson, Toth, and Turner (1987) found that the elderly in an age-specific treatment setting had higher rates of treatment completion than those in mixed-age settings. However, the smaller numbers of elderly relative to younger people seeking treatment limits the availability of elder-specific treatment programs in many areas of the country.

Cost considerations and changes in reimbursement mechanisms have slowed the growth of inpatient models of alcohol treatment. Outpatient treatment programs typically offer a series of sessions over a period of several weeks. For many elderly men, there is no reason to argue that inpatient treatment has any advantage over outpatient models. However, for some, who may have become physically vulnerable after a period of heavy alcohol use and poor nutrition, inpatient treatment models offer the secondary benefits of regular nutritionally balanced meals and sustained periods of abstinence and rest. Lack of transportation is another area which may present barriers for elderly men to attend outpatient treatment. While getting to the treatment setting every day is often portrayed as part of the life-training skills needed for recovery, it may be that the effort an elderly person has to spend to get there each day may not be worth the perceived benefit. A careful assessment of transportation and physical barriers can make the difference between treatment failure and success in an elderly population.

Outreach programs, which provide assessment and services at home, are standard components of many social service programs for the elderly. However, outreach is just beginning to be included in most alcohol treatment systems. Outreach may be a necessary part of the assessment process for many elderly people. The home setting offers many opportunities to evaluate social and medical problems, and provides the clinician with indicators for a further investigation of drinking patterns. Many home assessments of drinking have been initiated, for example, after a visiting social worker or nurse notes a trash can full of empty beer cans or liquor bottles. The capability to make home visits may allow the clinician to gently, but persistently, influence the elderly person to seek treatment. By making routine home visits, the clinician can increase the client's exposure to treatment options, rather than waiting until the client comes to the office for an appointment or is forced into treatment during a crisis. Home-based treatment may be the only type available to elderly people who are cognitively impaired and still living at home.

Advanced age has been used as a screening mechanism to exclude people from a variety of health, mental health, and social services. Age has also been used as a reason to exclude people from alcohol treatment, with the rationale that older people do not have many reasons to quit drinking, that they will not benefit from treatment, and that they should be left to enjoy drinking as a last pleasure in life. Elderly people, when provided access to treatment, are active participants and benefit from the services. Graham and associates (1995) found that, similar to studies of younger people in treatment, elderly "clients who remain in treatment longer are more likely to show improvement, and tend to be more open and cooperative during treatment" (p. 186). The Graham team also found that demographic variables or personality characteristics were not useful to predict which of their older clients would be successful in treatment; again, mirroring the experiences of clinicians working with younger people in treatment.

The goal of screening and assessment efforts is not only to detect problems, but also to provide motivation for the individual to take actions which will reduce the problems and promote healthy behaviors. In a controlled study of treatment protocols among younger people with alcohol problems, Miller and Rollnick (1991) found that the single best predictor of treatment failure, regardless of treatment type, was client resistance. Graham et al. (1995) came to a similar conclusion with a sample of elderly in treatment and stated that "clients who are more open and concerned about their problems and more cooperative tend to show better outcomes from treatment" (p. 184). A skilled practitioner will develop a systematic screening protocol to assess alcohol use and abuse in all elderly people. Such efforts will maximize the levels of support and reassurance in the assessment process in order to increase the chances that the client will be able to accept the diagnosis and be willing to move forward on a therapeutic path.

TREATMENT APPROACHES

Two treatment approaches—Motivational Enhancement Therapy and twelve-step groups—are especially well suited to clinical work with elderly men and are discussed below. The concepts used in these treatment approaches, if not the treatment techniques themselves, should be considered in any work with the elderly, as they emphasize personal responsibility and choice which can only enhance the diminished self-esteem felt by many elderly men with alcohol problems.

Motivational Enhancement Therapy

One area of recent research and treatment, Motivational Enhancement Therapy (MET), may be especially useful to the practitioner working with the elderly. MET presents a clinical stance and sets forth a process between the client and the clinician which enables the client to make choices in his or her life (Miller & Rollnick, 1991). MET proposes six core elements important to change in drinking behaviors. These core elements include the following:

1. Feedback of personal risk or impairment;
2. Emphasis on personal responsibility for change;
3. Clear advice to change;
4. A menu of alternative change options;
5. Therapist empathy; and
6. Facilitation of client self-efficacy or optimism.

There are two major phases of MET: building motivation for change and strengthening commitment to change. The focus of the clinical work is to enable the client to decrease his ambivalence about changing his drinking behaviors and to increase his motivation to initiate changes in his life. Using MET, the clinician uses empathy freely and listens and presents feedback concerning the client's views on his drinking patterns, the problems associated with drinking, and the opinions of friends and family members. The clinician tries to present personal risk factors for impairment due to drinking as well as advice on change strategies.

One of the areas where MET differs from other counseling strategies which have been used by alcohol and other drug abuse treatment counselors is that MET avoids any discussion of labeling of problems or diagnosis. The clinician using MET will not give a diagnosis, even if the client asks the direct question, "Do you think I am an alcoholic?" Below is an example of a MET therapeutic transcript illustrating the response to a labeling question.

> *Client*: Do you think I am an alcoholic?
> *Clinician*: That's a word that means many things to different people. I don't want you to worry about what to call yourself. What matters, really, is that we take a good close look at what's going on here. I can see why you're concerned, and I'd like to help you find out what risk you might be facing, and what—if anything—you could do about it (Miller & Rollnick, 1991, p. 144).

Using this approach, the therapist avoids a confrontation and an argument around labeling and shifts the focus to the drinking behaviors and their consequences, while at the same time affirming personal responsibility and choice.

For men, who may experience a great deal of loss of self-esteem and control in later life, MET offers some clear advantages. The emphasis of personal responsibility for change and the lack of argumentation should facilitate a collaborative approach to problem solving. If an older man is not pushed into a corner by having to admit that he is an alcoholic, then he may be more willing and able to make changes. MET can be conducted in short sessions and can be done in a home setting. This method is gentle, but it does not overlook or ignore problem areas.

The technique requires time and experience to master, and clinicians using MET should participate in a training session to ensure that they are using techniques properly. Clinicians will need to develop a menu of change strategies to discuss with men who are interested in making changes in their lives. These strategies can range from a dramatic step, such as entering a treatment facility and beginning abstinence, to a less dramatic one, such as removing the throw rugs in the house to diminish the risk of falls after drinking. Clinicians may need to assess their levels of tolerance for risk-taking, since building motivation for change may take place over an extended time period and treatment may take place as the client continues to use alcohol.

Twelve-Step Groups

Alcoholics Anonymous groups, and the twelve-step approach, can provide a particularly useful atmosphere for elderly men's recovery. The founder of AA, Bill Wilson, developed the initial approach based upon his own alcohol problems and recovery. These may be similar to the experiences of elderly men, especially those who have had problems with alcohol all of their lives or intermittently as they moved through adulthood. AA offers a peer support model built on acceptance of self and acceptance of others. This peer support can increase low levels of self-esteem and provide hope to older men who have lost other areas of social interaction. The potential of AA to increase social interactions and social support networks is of special note for men with late onset problems, and contacts made through AA can be the beginning of new friendships. AA participation requires that the elderly person be physically able to attend the meetings and be mentally able to benefit from the experience of the group. AA is not a treatment option for those elderly persons who are housebound or who are cognitively impaired to the extend that they cannot sit through a meeting or understand the information given.

Using a step-by-step practical approach to recovery, AA is abstinence-based and affords participants the opportunity to hear other stories of recovery and struggle. Twelve-step approaches offer an inexpensive form of treatment in that there is no charge to attend any AA meeting. The AA philosophy, and the twelve steps, are available in many AA books and pamphlets, but the group format and the use of "leads" and speakers make AA principles and ideas available to those elderly whose literacy skills are low or whose eyesight may preclude much reading.

Potential barriers for elderly men may lie in the effort it takes to attend the first meeting and in finding a group which feels comfortable. AA does not accept referrals, but will accept anyone who is willing to come to the meetings and listen. Clinicians should remember that it takes a great deal of courage for most people to admit they have a problem and to make the initial effort to attend an AA group meeting. It is useful for the clinician to keep a supply of current AA schedules, to understand the differences in types of meetings, and to be able to explain the basic format of an AA meeting. Helping people develop reasonable expectations about what they might experience at AA meetings is a valuable first step in the process of recovery. For clinicians who are not in recovery, or who have never had experience with AA, attending several open meetings is very valuable to understand the format and the feelings which go along with first-time attendance.

Some AA groups do not differentiate between members, and some are designated for women or men only. Few, if any, AA meetings are officially designated for elderly people. However, there may be some groups which, for a variety of reasons, may be attended by a majority of elderly people. Some elderly men may feel more comfortable in a group of age peers. Sometimes the location and the timing of an AA group may indicate that the majority of members will be over 60. For example, a meeting held at a senior citizen apartment in the middle of the day may be a good place to start. It is important to note that it may take several visits to a particular group, or it may take a series of visits to different groups, before finding one which offers a level of comfort for an elderly person. Twelve-step approaches are also available to spouses and other family members of elderly persons with drinking problems. Alanon, for example, holds group meetings for family members whose elderly relatives have a life-time of alcohol-related problems or are struggling with alcohol for the first time.

CONCLUSION

The next several years will bring many changes to the understanding and treatment of all age groups of alcohol abusers. Future changes in how alcohol problems are viewed will stem from research on treatment matching, which is intended to maximize therapeutic benefits by matching specific treatment protocols with particular types of alcohol problems or particular patient characteristics. Instead of using the same service package for all patients, treatment professionals will be more likely to tailor specific treatment plans to meet individual needs.

Other changes in treatment will come from the administrative and political changes in health care services. Alcohol and other drug abuse resources will feel the impact of managed care and accountability efforts, as health care and social services systems continue to struggle with financial and social reform initiatives.

While the numbers of elderly people who abuse alcohol are small in comparison to the numbers of younger abusing people, there are compelling reasons to develop further research and treatment models specific to elderly people. Census figures on the growth of the elderly population during the next 20 or 30 years indicate that 52 million people, or 18% of the population, will be 65 years of age or older (Spencer, 1989). As future cohorts age, it is reasonable to expect that their drinking patterns will differ from those of the present cohort of elderly. This will necessitate future innovations in assessment and treatment and greater awareness of differences between elderly men and women who abuse alcohol.

REFERENCES

American Psychiatric Association. (1987). *Diagnostic and statistical manual of mental disorders* (3rd ed. rev.). Washington, DC: Author.

American Psychiatric Association. (1994). *Diagnostic and statistical manual of mental disorders* (4th ed.). Washington, DC: Author.

Borgatta, E. F., Montgomery, R. J. V., & Borgatta, M. L. (1982). Alcohol use and abuse, life crisis events, and the elderly. *Residential Aging, 4*, 378–405.

Buchsbaum, D. G., Buchanan, R. G., & Lawton, M. J. (1991). Alcohol consumption patterns in a primary care population. *Alcohol and Alcoholism, 26*, 215–220.

Drew, L. R. H. (1968). Alcohol as a self-limiting disease. *Quarterly Journal of Alcohol Studies, 29*, 956–976.

Dunham, R. G. (1981). Aging and changing patterns of alcohol use. *Journal of Psychoactive Drugs, 13*, 143–151.

Farkas, K. J. (1991). Alcohol and elderly people. In F. J. Turner (Ed.), *Mental health and the elderly* (pp. 328–354). New York: The Free Press.

Friedman, L., Fleming, N. F., Roberts, D. H., & Hyman, S. E. (Eds.). (1996). *Source book of substance abuse and addiction.* Baltimore: Williams and Wilkins.

Gambert, S. R. (1992). Substance abuse in the elderly. In J. H. Lowinson, P. Ruiz, R. B. Millman, & J. G. Langrod (Eds.), *Substance abuse: A comprehensive textbook* (pp. 843–851). Baltimore: Williams & Wilkins.

Goodwin, J. S., Sanchez, C. J., Thomas, P., Hunt, C., Garry, P., & Goodwin, J. (1987). Alcohol intake in a healthy elderly population. *American Journal of Public Health, 77*, 173–177.

Graham, K. (1986). Identifying and measuring alcohol abuse among the elderly: Serious problems with existing instrumentation. *Journal of Studies on Alcohol, 47*, 322–326.

Graham, K., Saunders, S. J., Flower, M., Timney, C. B., White-Campbell, M., & Pietropaolo, A. Z. (1995). *Addictions treatment for older adults: Evaluation of an innovative client-centered approach.* New York: The Haworth Press.

Herd, D. (1990). Subgroup differences in drinking patterns among black and white men: Results from a national survey. *Journal of Studies on Alcohol, 51*, 221–232.

Hester, R. K., & Miller, W. R. (1995). *Handbook of alcoholism treatment approaches: Effective alternatives* (2nd ed.). Boston: Allyn and Bacon.

Jinks, J. J., & Raschko, R. R. (1990). A profile of alcohol and prescription drug abuse in a high risk community-based population. *DICP: Annals of Pharmocotherapy, 24*, 378–405.

Kofoed, L. L., Tolson, R. L., Atkinson, R. M., Toth, R. L., & Turner, J. A. (1987). Treatment compliance of older alcoholics: An elder-specific approach is superior to "mainstreaming." *Journal of Studies on Alcohol, 48*, 47–51.

Liberto, J. G., Oslin, D. W., & Ruskin, P. E. (1992). Alcoholism in older persons: A review of the literature. *Hospital and Community Psychiatry, 43*, 975–984.

Mayfield, D., McLeod, G., & Hall, P. (1974). The CAGE questionnaire: Validation of a new alcoholism screening instrument. *American Journal of Psychiatry, 131*, 1121–1123.

Miller, W. R., & Rollnick, S. (1991). *Motivational interviewing: Preparing people to change addictive behavior.* New York: Guilford Press.

Spencer, G. (1989). *Projections of the populations of the United States, by age, sex and race: 1988 to 2080* (Series P–25, no. 1018). Washington, DC: U.S. Department of Commerce.

van Wormer, K. (1995). *Alcoholism treatment: A social work perspective.* Chicago: Nelson-Hall.

Willenbring, M., & Spring, W. D. (1988). Evaluating alcohol use in elders. *Generations, 12*(4), 27–31.

CHAPTER 12

Mental Disorders of Elderly Men

John L. McIntosh, Ph.D.,
Jane L. Pearson, Ph.D.,
& Barry D. Lebowitz, Ph.D.

Although the overall prevalence of mental disorders in the United States is the same for males and females, the prevalence rates for specific mental disorders vary by gender and age. Reviewed here are the most prevalent disorders among older adults, with attention to those that exhibit gender differences in prevalence rates; specifically, sleep disorders, dementia, anxiety, depression, and suicide. Gender differences in depression and suicide are considered at length, with a focus on elderly men.

SLEEP DISORDERS

Between 30 and 50% of the elderly have some sort of sleep disturbance, and persons who sleep on average less than 7 hours per night have a 1.5 times greater mortality rate than those sleeping 8 hours (Kripke, Simons, Garfinkel, & Mammond, 1979). Relative to younger age groups, the elderly report frequent night wakening, early morning wakening, excess "fragile" sleep, and more frequent use of sleeping pills. About one of every three older women complains about sleep problems, and this is about two times the rate of complaints by older men (e.g., Campbell, Gillin, Kripke, Erikson, & Clopton, 1989). Yet, on objective measures of sleep, such as circadian temperature rhythm (Campbell et al., 1989) and particular sleep disorders (e.g., apnea), men outnumber women in disturbed sleep patterns (Hoch, Buysse, Monk, & Reynolds, 1992).

Sleep problems can result from normal aging (e.g., disturbances in circadian sleep-wake rhythm, increased sleep fragmentation), and as a condition secondary to medical illness (especially pain-related disorders, and respiratory and neurologic diseases) and psychiatric illness (depression, dementia, anxiety). Like other comorbid conditions, sleep disorders can contribute to the further deterioration of medical and psychiatric problems (Hoch et al., 1992).

Sleep research, which documents predictable sequences of physiologic processes, includes electroencephalographic (EEG) study, temperature monitoring, and (more recently) changes in hormonal systems. Because these systems and their interactions are just becoming documented in the elderly, theories regarding possible gender differences in sleep disorders are lacking. Investigations of the effects of steroidal hormones on circadian period and sleep consolidation are needed (see Bremner, Vitiello, & Prinz, 1983, for an example of aging effects on testosterone). In addition, many sleep researchers are pointing to the importance of individual variation within gender, where longitudinal research is necessary to document age-related changes in individual sleep patterns (including hormonal cycles and EEG patterns).

DEMENTIA

The fourth edition of the *Diagnostic and Statistical Manual of Mental Disorders* (DSM-IV; American Psychiatric Association, 1994) identifies over nine different etiologies for dementia. The most prevalent of these are Alzheimer's Disease (AD), followed by vascular or multi-infarct vascular dementia (MID); AD has been estimated to account for about half of all dementias, MID for an additional 10%, and mixed AD and MID for about 20% more. Risk for AD increases with age; for persons age 65 and older, the prevalence rate ranges up to 12% (Evans et al., 1989). Persons age 85 and above have about a one-in-four chance of having dementia (Jorm, Korten, & Henderson, 1987).

Although age is the most consistently cited risk factor for nonfamilial-type Alzheimer's Disease, recent reports examining the oldest old have suggested that the risk for AD may level off at age 95 (Ritchie & Kildea, 1995). Thus, AD may be best conceptualized as an aging-related disorder, rather than simply an age-related one.

Because the etiology and definite diagnosis of dementia cannot be determined until autopsy, the rates of AD and MID cited here are based on assessments of cognitive impairment (as is the case for many community surveys), or clinical assessments (typically conducted in clinical settings). Therefore, variation in case definition, samples, and level of clinical assessment contributes to the wide range of prevalence estimates. These methodological issues represent even greater problems when possible gender differences in prevalence rates for dementias of various etiologies must be estimated, especially when level of education or cardiovascular disease are considered significant risk factors as well.

Prevalence rates of dementia have either been considered equivalent for men compared to women—as in the case of Epidemiological Catchment Area-based (ECA) measures of cognitive impairment (George, Landerman, Blazer, & Anthony, 1991)—or higher for women, particularly when the criteria of clinically diagnosed AD is applied (Rocca et al., 1991). In terms of incidence rates, however, there are no significant gender differences in AD (e.g., Paykel et al., 1994). Investigations that detect small differences show women's rates prevailing (e.g., Rocca et al., 1991). The nearly equal incidence of dementia by gender may reflect several factors: there may be a slower progression in women, women with dementia survive longer than do men, and/or men's higher general mortality rates may mean that men with dementia die of other causes.

Among the biological risk factors for AD, apolipoprotein E (ApoE) has received significant attention as a possible marker in genetic testing (e.g., ACMG/ASHG Working Group, 1995). As a plasma protein involved in the transport of cholesterol, certain forms of ApoE have been linked not only with AD, but also with cholesterol metabolism and coronary heart disease. Little information exists to indicate whether there are gender differences in the prevalence of various harmful or protective forms of ApoE.

ANXIETY

The National Institute of Mental Health Epidemiological Catchment Area studies (Robins & Regier, 1991), based on DSM–III criteria, are the primary source of prevalence rates for most mental disorders. With regard to anxiety, the ECA assessed panic, phobic disorders, and obsessive-compulsive disorders; generalized anxiety disorder was considered in three sites in the second wave of the survey (Blazer, Hughes, George, Swartz, & Boyer, 1991). In terms of age and gender effects, older persons (age 65+) were found to have lower rates than the general population, and older women had higher rates than older men. For example, the elderly had the lowest rates of generalized anxiety disorder (using no other diagnostic exclusions) with a prevalence of 2.22% compared to 3.76% for all age groups (Blazer, Hughes, et al., 1991). For panic disorder, rates among the elderly were 0.04% for males and 0.41% for females; for phobic disorder the figures were 4.90% and 8.84%, respectively (Eaton, Dryman, & Weissman, 1991). Blazer, George, and Hughes (1991), reporting on the North Carolina ECA site, provided prevalence rates of generalized anxiety disorder among persons age 65 and older by gender and ethnicity. Their findings indicated that white males had a rate of 1.0%, with African-American males at 0.3%, white females 2.9%, and African-American females 3.7%.

Cohort effects may be influencing the age effects found in the prevalence of anxiety disorders in the elderly, such that persons born earlier have benefited from some protective effect. Another hypothesis involves concomitant cardiovascular disturbances, especially with panic disorder, that may raise mortality at younger ages, so that fewer persons with panic disorders reach older adulthood (Eaton et al., 1991).

Women's higher anxiety rates in later life may be related to longer survival. Because older women, as they age, have an increased likelihood of medical conditions, higher rates of visits to primary health care providers, and more frequent prescription of psychotropic medications than men, another area of inquiry is the degree to which the somatic symptoms of anxiety disorders reflect or interact with physical illness or medication side effects (Cohen, 1991).

DEPRESSION

The 1–year prevalence for major depression in men and women age 65 and older was found to be about 1% (Weissman, Bruce, Leaf, Florio, & Holzer, 1991). The comparable rate for persons age 45 to 64 was 2.3%.

When the diagnostic criteria of major depression were used, there were no gender differences in the rate of late life depression. This is in contrast to findings in young and middle adulthood, where rates of depression are markedly higher for women.

Different age and gender patterns appear, however, if the threshold for depression is lowered, or if criteria are broadened to include other affective disorders such as adjustment, bipolar, or dysthymic disorders. A number of survey studies, relying on self-report responses to checklists, such as the Center for Epidemiologic Studies Depression Scale (CES–D), report either no age effects, or increased numbers of symptoms with age (e.g., Blazer, 1994). A consistent finding across these CES–D studies is that women report more symptoms than men across all age groups.

When the definition of depression is broadened to include all affective disorders, as was done in the Eastern Baltimore reappraisal study (an investigation springing from the ECA), rates of all depressions combined were observed to increase with age (Romanoski et al., 1992). Again, females displayed higher rates across all age groups. For persons age 75, women had a prevalence rate of about 9%, and men had a rate of 3.5%. A similar pattern of depressive symptoms increasing among older women was found in a North London community (Livingston, Hawkins, Graham, Blizard, & Mann, 1990) and a New York City sample (Kennedy et al., 1989).

Rates of depression in the elderly are much higher among those who have more physical problems. For example, among nursing home residents, prevalence rates for depression range from 15 to 25%, with about 10% annual incidence of new episodes of major depression (see NIH Consensus Development Panel on Depression in Late Life, 1992). Comorbid depression is also common among older medical inpatients. For example, Koenig and his associates (Koenig, O'Connor, Guarisco, Zabel, & Ford, 1993) reported a prevalence rate of 13% for major depressive disorder. Among the elderly with comorbid psychiatric illness and chronic physical illness, women outnumber men (Verbrugge, 1990).

There is strong evidence that major depression in the elderly increases risk for disability and mortality, including suicide (e.g., Koenig & Blazer, 1992). Subthreshold symptoms, such as those assessed by the CES–D, are also significantly detrimental, increasing risk for lowered daily functioning and disability related to physical illness (Blazer, 1994; NIH Consensus Development Panel, 1992).

As will be discussed below, death by suicide is primarily a male phenomenon. Why are older women more likely to report depressive symptoms compared to men, but older men more likely to take their own lives? Given the contradictory findings for age and gender trends in depression prevalence rates, it is not surprising that there are few well-formulated hypotheses that have been tested to explain either age or gender differences in depression. Nonetheless, there are a number of interesting questions being posed to explain some intriguing age and gender patterns.

Blazer (1994), among others, has suggested that older respondents with major depression may have been undercounted in the ECA estimates because they are less likely to endorse dysphoric mood as part of their symptom clusters. Lyness and colleagues have also reported that older patients in inpatient psychiatric services often underreport their depressive symptoms (Lyness et al., 1995). With regard to gender differences, a few recent studies have suggested that older men are more likely to underreport depressive symptoms (e.g., Allen-Burge, Storandt, Kinscherf, & Rubin, 1994).

Because prevalence rates are influenced by case definition (which symptoms, for how long), incidence, and duration of disorder, theories that address gender or age differences in depression prevalence must consider how these influences are affected by gender and age. Nolen-Hoeksema's theory of gender differences in interpersonal style and cognition (see Nolen-Hoeksema, Morrow, & Fredrickson, 1993) is an example of how a psychosocial theory of depression could address these three factors. Rumination, a cognitive style more common among women, may prolong depressive episodes (Nolen-Hoeksema et al., 1993), whereas men tend to distract themselves—for example, with other activities. Although this gender-typed style may contribute to prolonged depressive episodes among women, it may also protect them from acting on suicidal thoughts. Men, on the other hand, may successfully distract themselves and alleviate their depression and its causes or prevent ruminating about them. To date, no one has examined how ruminative cognitive style or interpersonal sensitivity influences onset or duration of depression in older women. This may be especially important in studies of bereavement. The significant overlap between depressive and anxiety symptoms in depressive diagnoses in late life (Koenig & Blazer, 1992) would also suggest this may be a reasonable avenue to explore.

SUICIDE

Epidemiology: Current Levels of Gender and Age Differentials

Unlike depression, death by suicide is predominantly a male phenomenon. Rates of suicide consistently show men's risk at levels four times those of women. For example, in 1992 (the most recent data available; all 1992 data are derived from S. Murphy, personal communication, April and May, 1995; figures to be published later in the 1992 annual volume of National Center for Health Statistics, *Vital Statistics of the United States*) men committed suicide at a rate of 19.6 per 100,000 population compared to 4.6 for women (and 24,457 suicides vs. 6,027, respectively). On the other hand, men are far less likely to make a nonfatal suicide attempt than are women. Research typically indicates that women attempt three times more often than men (e.g., Bille-Brahe, 1993). Therefore, when men make an attempt on their lives, the event is much more likely to end fatally.

Suicide risk, however, is portrayed better when considering both sex and age simultaneously. Men and women not only demonstrate substantially different overall rates of suicide, but also show distinct patterns by age. While women's rates are lower than those for men at all ages, rates for women increase with age, peaking during middle adulthood, and decline slightly thereafter in late life. Men's rates increase throughout the life span, peaking in older adulthood, with highest levels for the oldest group (i.e., 85 years of age and above). Among men, all age groups beyond 65 years evidence higher suicide risk than any younger age grouping. The greatest risks for suicide, therefore, are elderly men. For example, in 1992 women age 65 and over had a rate of 6.0 per 100,000 population, while aged men had a rate over six times higher at 38.5. In fact, this risk differential between the sexes is greater than at any other life period. From among the average of 17 elderly suicides each day in 1992, 14 were men. In addition, suicide is dramatically overrepresented among elderly men. More specifically, elderly men in 1992 were 5.1% of the population but accounted for 16.4% of the suicides (comparable figures for elderly women are 7.5% and 3.8%, respectively). In other words, one of every six suicides of all ages is an elderly man.

When the demographic variable of race is included, suicide risk is further clarified, with the highest level observed for elderly white males.

The rates for the elderly groups (age 65 and above) in 1992 were 2.6 for nonwhite women, 6.4 for white women, 14.5 for nonwhite men, and 41.1 for white men. White men, therefore, exhibited a risk for suicide that was more than twice that of the elderly as a whole and nearly three times that for the nearest other age-sex-race grouping.

U.S. epidemiological research for age and attempted suicide shows that men are at lower risk for nonfatal attempts throughout the life span when compared to women, with the highest rates seen in the young and lowest rates in old age for both sexes (e.g., Bille-Brahe, 1993). As noted already, men's attempts are more often fatal, and this is particularly true in late life.

Epidemiology: Trends Over Time by Age and Gender

As noted elsewhere (see McIntosh, Santos, Hubbard, & Overholser, 1994), elderly suicide rates over time are best characterized by long-term declines, with rates in the 1990s approximately one-half to one-third those observed during the 1930s. Although a consideration of suicide rates from the 1980s to the present would yield an analysis that elderly suicide rates have increased ("Suicide among older persons," 1996), the long-term trends do not support this conclusion. Despite a brief tendency toward increases in the 1980s, the long-term trends remain in a downward direction and have continued from the late 1980s. This decline has almost exclusively been produced by the decreases in rates for elderly men, whereas women's rates have changed little or declined slightly. Despite the differential trends, men's rates remain markedly higher than those for women.

A number of potential factors have been advanced to account for the declines in suicide rates for the elderly as a whole (i.e., both sexes combined), including the development and availability of antidepressants, increases in health care access and economic programs for older adults, political and social activism for and by the elderly, improved elder social service programs, and changing attitudes toward retirement (McIntosh et al., 1994). Among the factors associated with the declining rates, investigations (see McIntosh et al., 1994, for a review) have observed significant correlations between the rate changes and increases in economic measures for the old, particularly for elderly white males. The differential impact of these factors, other than economic ones on older males compared to older females, has not been studied.

The decreased risk observed for the elderly from the 1930s to the early 1990s is not representative of the predictions advanced by some prognosticators (for a review, see McIntosh et al., 1994). These authors predict considerably higher future rates of elderly suicide associated with the arrival of the baby boomer generation to age 65 and above from approximately 2010 to 2030. These rate levels are based on the size of the baby boom generation and the resultant effects that large numbers of individuals in a population group have on its social and psychological well-being.

On the other hand, McIntosh (McIntosh et al., 1994) has contended that future levels of suicide, as a measure of the well-being of the elderly, are not inevitably destined to be high. McIntosh argues that the large size of the boomer generation may actually produce greater attention to issues of late life and the allocation of greater resources to meet the needs of this large group in old age. In addition, many other factors not considered in earlier predictions could significantly influence suicide rates in late life, including advances in health care and pain management, economic conditions, and treatments for mental health problems and particularly depression. In other words, the size of a cohort alone does not necessarily determine its mental health. It is likely that factors affecting the quality and nature of life in old age, as well as the years of late middle age, will be crucial in producing the specific groups' adaptation and failures in coping in the future. McIntosh concluded that even in the event that late life suicide risk does not change from that of current older adults, increases in elderly individuals in the population of the future insure that a large number of elder suicides would result and require significant attention by mental health professionals.

In any event, successive cohorts of elderly to the present have been increasingly lower risks for suicide when compared to generations of elderly in the past. Although current elders are at lower risk than their predecessors to late life, it should be emphasized that they remain the highest-risk age group for suicide in the population, and among this group, the subgroup at substantially highest risk is men.

Motivations in Elderly Suicide and Depression

The obvious concentration of suicides among elderly men implies that reasons for suicide in late life are largely those found among men. Suicidal motivations for the elderly, compared to the young, are more often intrapersonal or social in nature (for a review of these issues see McIntosh et al., 1994). Suicidal etiology in the old is likely to involve the interaction and combination of several factors rather than any single one. Suicides by older adults most often seem to be responses to their entire life circumstances. The multifactorial nature of suicide is true for all ages but is particularly relevant among the elderly. The occurrence of any single factor alone among those noted below is unlikely to produce suicide in an older adult.

Put another way, through a lifetime, older adults have accumulated coping methods, social supports, and other resources that have usually permitted them to adapt to single factors or problems that arise, and probably even the combination of some factors. It is likely that a breakdown or failure of these resources would occur only with the existence of several conditions simultaneously that finally overwhelm or exhaust one's ability to cope adequately. Tolerance levels for psychological and other pain, special vulnerabilities to particular problems, and social resources are highly individual, however. Therefore, conditions that will produce intolerable levels of pain and stress will not be exceeded for some older adults at high levels of pain, whereas for others the threshold may be reached with many fewer stressors. Clark (1993) hypothesized that elderly suicides possess a character flaw that has existed throughout their lives but remained hidden until problems and stressors of late life revealed them, producing their suicide.

Motivations to depression and suicide in the aged derive from biopsychosocial factors. That is, psychological, physiological, and social realms, both individually and in combination, produce the cognitive and other circumstances that are associated with or lead to depression and suicide among older adults. Among psychological aspects of suicide, depression is one of the most important contributing factors in the elderly (as well as for other age groups). From psychological autopsy studies, a strong relationship exists between suicide and unipolar, late-onset depression, particularly for older adults. Research findings suggest that depression underlies two-thirds or more of the suicides of late life (e.g., Conwell & Brent, 1995). Other factors that psychologists and gerontologists have suggested that might contribute to suicidal ideation in old age include negative evaluations of one's life (especially as a part of "life review," e.g., Butler, 1963), issues regarding the control of the time of death, and society's negative attitudes toward aging and older adulthood.

Biological factors experienced in old age which may lead to suicide include depression associated with physical decline and illnesses, as well as incurable illness accompanied by pain (e.g., Conwell, Rotenberg, & Caine, 1990). Although the majority of all those who commit suicide do not have health problems, physical illness has repeatedly been observed as a factor in elderly suicides and suicide attempts more often than for other age groups, especially among the old-old (McIntosh et al., 1994). Health problems have tremendous implications for changing and disrupting the individual's social and psychological worlds as well. Another interaction issue occurs with respect to depression. The strong relation between depression and physical health may be interpreted as representing situations in which depression may have resulted from illness, but depression may also have been a preexisting condition worsened by the presence of health problems, or even a comorbid disorder that developed along with illness. In any event, physical conditions emerge as a common aspect of many elderly suicides. In addition, the presence of pain may increase the strength and intensity of the individual's feelings of hopelessness and helplessness, particularly when the pain is chronic in nature or has proven (or is interpreted) to be intractable.

Social explanations of elderly suicide have emphasized the lessened societal involvement and integration of older adults (e.g., Durkheim, 1897/1951). Lower levels of integration derive from the loss of loved ones and general interpersonal restriction, as well as from disengagement that often accompanies older adulthood such as in retirement (with its resultant changes in income, status, roles, and independence). These losses and changes, of course, do not invariably mean that suicide will occur. Durkheim (1897/1951) also emphasized the lack of clear norms (i.e., anomie) in suicide and this has often been utilized to understand suicide in the context of changing roles in older adulthood.

Two social factors that represent special suicide risk in late life are the often related factors of social isolation and marital disruption (McIntosh et al., 1994). Suicide rates are consistently higher among the widowed and divorced, with high rates for all unmarried groups (including the never-married) in late life. The loss of people in the lives of older adults derives from several sources other than the death or loss of a spouse, however. Social isolation is also associated with high risk for suicide attempt and completion, and older adults are the population group most likely to be living alone and feeling isolated. The presence of either of these factors does not assure that suicide will occur, of course, and the strength of the individual's entire relational system is an important dimension to consider.

It is clear that older adulthood is associated with many of the more prominent forces toward suicide and depression. Almost necessarily, an older adult will possess several high-risk conditions associated with elevated depressive and suicide risk. Much remains to be learned regarding predictive variables with respect to geriatric suicides (and among other age groups as well). Accurate prediction of individuals who will attempt suicide, and under which specific combination of factors, has proven to be more elusive than the elaboration of the factors associated with risk. Certainly the individual's personality and lifelong coping style, experience dealing with traumas and stresses, and the availability of a supportive network, along with previous losses and problems, are salient factors.

Issues Regarding Motivations to Suicide and Depression Among Elderly Men

As noted above, elderly males' high suicide risk, and their large contribution to late-life suicide, means that any discussion of motives that produce thoughts of suicide, as well as overt suicidal actions, in old age will largely focus on the forces that produce such behavior in older men. However, there are several special factors that may contribute to depression, and in some cases suicide, that deserve to be highlighted because they are particularly prominent among elderly men.

Obvious group differences between men and women in late life today involve their work histories and the accompanying issue of retirement from work roles. In the current generation of elders, men have engaged in lifelong careers in much larger numbers (a difference that will diminish with subsequent generations). American society has emphasized and valued productivity and work, and men in our culture have often identified with their occupation and work. Loss of the work role through retirement, then, potentially has major ramifications for the elderly man. Retirement may produce perceptions of the loss of status, role, control, and direction in life, useful and meaningful activity in which to engage, and power in society, as well as the loss of income and the independence that it affords. Additionally, the loss of the work role also lessens the involvement of the individual with others in the workplace, a situation that increases suicide risk, according to Durkheim's (1897/1951) sociological theory of suicide. Many investigations have demonstrated the increased vulnerability to suicide among retired men (McIntosh et al., 1994; Osgood & McIntosh, 1986). Durkheim's other explanation that applies in this context is that the loss of work through retirement may thrust the elderly man into a situation of uncertainty about appropriate actions and behaviors. Durkheim referred to this situation as a state of *anomie*, or normlessness, that increases suicide risk and is often observed concomitantly with lessened integration or involvement.

Particularly important in any discussion of retirement and suicide is a consideration of white males, the highest risk for suicide. Compared to African-American males and females, as well as white females, aged white males in American society have traditionally suffered the most severe loss of social status and position, power, and money with retirement and late life. Many authors have related their high suicide rates to the severe losses noted above that were formerly obtained through participation in work (Osgood & McIntosh, 1986). Women and minority males, by comparison, are two groups with traditionally lower status/ positions in society. By this reasoning, these groups lose less upon retirement and are not forced to adapt as much as white males, and thus tend to display lower rates of suicide. As another factor, these groups may also have generally found status and value in other social realms that have less often been true for white males.

Another loss in late life that impacts greatly on involvement in social interactions is the loss of spouse through death or divorce. Although death of spouse more typically befalls the elderly woman, men who become widowed in late life have received special attention with respect to suicide, even though their numbers are small when compared to women. Research on widowhood has often concluded that it takes an especially greater toll upon widowers (i.e., men), which includes the more extreme reaction of suicidal behaviors (Stroebe & Stroebe, 1983). Divorced men, as noted above, have dramatically higher rates of suicide in late life than do divorced elderly women or the divorced of younger ages. Once again, Durkheim (1897/1951) predicted high suicide risk in the case of both widowhood and divorce, and—as for retirement—the common issues are those of social involvement and normlessness.

The loss of a marriage relationship, however, has great implications beyond simply social factors per se. The loss of one's spouse, in many cases following decades of marriage, represents the loss of a major social role as a husband/wife and roles within the family unit, but it also entails the loss of a companion, friend, confidant, and sexual partner. The psychological impact is typically extreme and may be quite long-lived, often producing sadness, loneliness, feelings of meaninglessness and emptiness, and sometimes clinical levels of depression and even suicidal behavior.

Durkheim and other sociologists (see McIntosh et al., 1994; Osgood & McIntosh, 1986) have suggested that men derive more benefits from marriage than do women. In American society, the wife often assumes the primary responsibility for social contacts with the larger family and maintains the social contacts with friends and relatives over the years of marriage. When the wife dies in late life, the bereaved widower may feel as though he has been left totally alone, since he is unaccustomed to maintaining these ties. Feelings of social isolation may result, particularly if involvement with community organizations (and work) is not present.

A primary example of the multifactorial aspects of suicide in late life, and the interactions and combinations of potent factors, occurs with the existence of retirement and/or widowhood in the context of the other major changes and losses of late life. One explanation of men's high suicide rates in old age (compared to women) involves the suffering of double losses by widowers. Bereaved men lose not only their roles in the family and with their spouse, but also their role in the occupational realm as well. Blau (1956), for instance, referred to these specific multiple social losses as cumulative role loss. That is, several roles are lost, and the greater their number, the larger the negative impact. Similar conclusions arise from the psychological literature on stressors and adaptation. For instance, prior to retirement, a man may rely greatly on his occupation and fellow workers for identity and status, both personally and socially. Following retirement, he may rely more heavily on his wife to derive personal social status and worth. Her death, therefore, takes on personal and social importance, under such circumstances, that exceeds the losses of either retirement or widowhood alone.

Another special aspect that may increase suicide risk among aged men arises from the biological realm. As indicated, physical health problems represent an important factor in suicide and depression in late life. Physical illness has more often been identified as a contributing factor in the suicides of the older men than for older women (McIntosh et al., 1994). Significant health problems threaten continued employment and may well prompt or force retirement (with all of its other effects), as well as limiting or altering mobility and social contacts that may produce greater isolation and loneliness. Illness may also reduce independence and control for the individual. Again, the combinations and interactions of changes and losses in late life seem most potentially devastating for the old and, in many circumstances, may more often impact the lives of elderly men than women.

A final issue in late-life suicide that obviously affects the risk of a fatal outcome in suicidal actions is the differential choice of methods for the sexes. Although men of all ages often use firearms (the most lethal method) in their suicidal actions, and especially their suicide completions, elderly men employ firearms in their suicides in even higher proportions than men as a whole. For instance, in 1992 males of all ages killed themselves with guns in 64.7% of the cases (compared to 39.3% for women), whereas men aged 65 and above employed firearms in 76.5% of their deaths by suicide (35.0% for elderly women). The choice of firearms is influenced by many factors, such as knowledge and familiarity with guns, availability, perception of method gender-appropriateness by the individual and society, and even seriousness of intent. The selection of firearms, however, has great impact on the likelihood of a fatal outcome. Unlike many other methods, the use of guns permits little or no time for a change of mind, rescue, or intervention by others. In addition, the damage inflicted is likely to be more life-threatening, and often there is less that can be done to save the person's life.

Prevention of Elderly Men's Suicide

Recognition that white elderly men are at substantially higher suicide risk than any other age-sex-race grouping prompted the United States Department of Health and Human Services to include a mental health initiative regarding this group in its *Healthy People 2000: National Health Promotion and Disease Prevention Objectives*. The statement of objective is to reduce the rate of suicide for this group, from the 1987 baseline level of 46.7 per 100,000 population, to a rate no greater than 39.2 by the year 2000 (National Center for Health Statistics, 1993). The 1992 rate of 41.1, and the downward trends noted above, offer promise that this mental health objective will be reached. To insure that this goal is met, or even exceeded, there are several aspects related to prevention of suicide and a number of measures that might be implemented.

Suicide prevention among the aged, and elderly men in particular, is complicated by a number of facts. While the suicide literature suggests that the overwhelming majority of suicidal individuals of all ages communicate their intent to others, some research (Osgood & McIntosh, 1986) shows that—compared to younger individuals—elders less frequently give clues to their suicidal thoughts, and they seem more intent on dying as the result of their actions (as opposed to gaining attention or "crying for help"). One of the primary clues to future suicidal behavior is a past suicide attempt. However, research on the topic (McIntosh et al., 1994) has shown that the elderly of both sexes are less likely to have made a previous attempt compared to younger individuals. A final issue related to communication and recognition of the depressed and suicidal older adult arises because the old often present physical, rather than direct mental health, symptoms and these are most often communicated to medical rather than mental health professionals (with only the latter trained to intervene with depression and suicide).

Another complication in elderly suicide prevention is created by the almost total dearth of suicide prevention programs designed for older adults, and none specifically to address the most suicidal group of all: elderly males (McIntosh et al., 1994). Related to this lack of programs is the tendency of the old, and men especially, to rarely contact suicide prevention or crisis intervention centers, mental health, or social services agencies that are often utilized by other groups experiencing depression and suicidal ideation (McIntosh et al., 1994). While many factors contribute to this underutilization of prevention schemes by the elderly, an additional aspect that lessens the likelihood of communicating warning signs and turning to others for help results from their socialization as men in our society. Particularly among the current cohorts of elderly, men learned to believe that they should not display their feelings or seek the assistance of others, but rather should solve their own problems and take personal control of the situation. When solutions do not result, and feelings of helplessness and hopelessness are heightened, the choice of suicide to take control may become more attractive for the aged male.

Although prevention of suicide among older men may be more difficult as a result of the factors above, there are many steps that may be taken to prevent their needless deaths, both as individuals and as a group. The most important, and potentially effective, element of prevention involves obtaining professional mental health intervention for the older man. As noted, the suicidal man is most likely depressed, with the cognitive components that are most often associated with suicide probably present: hopelessness, helplessness, and the perception of his psychological pain at intolerable levels. As at other ages, the old are good candidates for individual, family, and group psychotherapies to treat depression, and they respond well to antidepressants and other psychotropic medication, as well as electroconvulsive therapy in the case of severe depression with suicidal ideation.

The major problem, of course, with obtaining therapy for older men is their general reluctance to seek such assistance on their own and the low likelihood that they will be readily identified by others as being depressed. Therefore, a primary and essential aspect of suicide prevention in elderly men involves identification by others of their depression and suicidal intent. One source of identification would involve health professionals who are likely to be visited by the suicidal man, but with physical, not mental, complaints. Training doctors and other health professionals to recognize depression and seek appropriate intervention is an important need in this regard. Other gatekeepers (e.g., EMTs, law enforcement, firefighters, nursing home and senior center staff, social service personnel, funeral directors, etc.) who come into frequent contact with older adults and who might, therefore, be able to recognize the symptoms of depression and suicidal warning signs are also prime targets of specialized training. In addition to these groups, there remains the need for more professionals trained in gerontologic specialties, and for a greater priority to older adults in the mental health service delivery system.

A particularly crucial aspect of case identification and referral with older adults, and even more so with men in late life, is the development of new methods to find and help the depressed and suicidal elderly. Whatever form these methods take, from buddy systems of phone calls and visits, to programs designed specifically for older adults or elderly males, one element should be included: an active outreach component as an integral part of any such service program. This outreach may involve going to community locations elder males frequent (for focused identification and referral), providing transportation to services, or even delivering mental health services in community locations, outside the clinic or therapist's office.

Other measures to prevent suicide and depression among older men follow directly from the reasons and special factors already identified with respect to this group. Physical health problems (including reports of pain), with their common appearance in late-life suicide, especially for males, should be taken seriously, detected, and treated as early as possible to lessen or prevent more serious problems that may result if symptoms are dismissed, unrecognized, or untreated. Certainly, encouraging regular exercise and good nutritional practices can benefit older adults and improve their overall physical health. In addition, the availability and affordability of good medical services are important, as is the encouragement of regular routine medical care and examinations.

The loss of people in the life of the old, particularly those older men who may be more prone to social isolation and loneliness, must be addressed to lower the likelihood and severity of depression and suicide. Any efforts to maintain existing social relationships and community involvement, as well as efforts to develop new relations and contacts, should help to lessen isolation and loneliness. In the special case of spousal loss through death or divorce, as already noted, even greater efforts are likely to be necessary to assist the bereaved elderly man with the multidimensional ramifications that accompany this major life change and stressor. Referrals to bereavement support and therapy resources may also be appropriate, though this may require special efforts, since men are generally underrepresented in their utilization of such resources.

The importance of retirement as a source of stress and adjustment problems for elderly men demands that this issue be addressed to prevent depression and suicide. These efforts would include such measures as encouraging and supporting continued work involvement, rather than retirement, when desired by the older man, and assisting with the development of second careers or finding new roles or settings from which the retiree may derive feelings of worth, importance, and self-esteem. Emotional and economic planning, and preparation for retirement, may lessen adjustment problems and disillusionment. Other economic changes associated with aging, and their potential psychological burdens, can be alleviated or diminished with careful financial planning and savings programs as well as the availability of affordable long-term care or catastrophic health care insurance.

The use of firearms in such high proportions by elderly males suggests that efforts to address this issue afford promise and should be included in any broad-scale prevention efforts. Lowering the availability of such a highly lethal method of suicide would likely reduce the number of suicides among older adult men. Although some men would undoubtedly seek other methods to effect their deaths, some suicides would likely be averted if the additional time and effort were required to consider and obtain alternative methods. It is also possible that the other methods chosen would be less lethal and permit more time and opportunity for intervention and rescue than do firearms. Although men do not utilize medications and other drugs in their suicides as often as women, responsible and careful prescription and dispensing of medications would likely prevent some men's suicide attempts and deaths as well.

Finally, the multifactorial nature of elderly suicide has implications for prevention. The almost certain existence of multiple factors in the production of depression, suicidal thoughts, or suicidal actions dictates that the problem be confronted on several fronts and not just a single one. In order to prevent a suicide among an elderly male in the long term, it will likely be necessary that problems in biological, psychological, and social realms be addressed simultaneously or successively, and actions taken to alleviate the factors that are present. On the other hand, from the standpoint of immediate intervention, and prevention of imminent behavior or active suicidal contemplation, the theoretical work of Shneidman (McIntosh et al., 1994) and its clinical implications are especially relevant. Shneidman (1993) adamantly contends that suicide is produced by the perception of intolerable psychological pain (i.e., "psychache"). His clinical prescription, for what he perceives as the causative agent in suicide, is to lessen the pain. If the pain is diminished, even slightly in some cases, the individual may well still be unhappy and in pain, but the pain may be perceived as within tolerable levels. In other words, the individual would choose to live rather than die. In the context of the multifactorial etiology of men's suicide in late life, this suggests that for crisis intervention purposes, the selection and lessening of one or two factors producing suicidal ideation may dramatically lower the immediate risk of suicide. This is not to imply that the larger set of issues are left unaddressed. Rather, it emphasizes the short-term and long-term goals of suicide prevention efforts with older adults.

CONCLUSION

For far too long, the highest risk group for suicide has been ignored. Elderly men are the most likely group to die by their own hand. Many of these needless deaths could be prevented, as could the suffering associated with depression. Effective prevention and treatment measures are possible if their central design confronts the somewhat unique factors and circumstances of older men that lead to depression, suicide, and other mental health problems. The need for such expenditure of energy and resources is important now and will be even more true when the number of older adults, including men, increases substantially in the early decades of the next century. Immediate and ongoing efforts have the potential to enhance the lives, lessen the emotional toll of various mental health problems, and prevent the premature and unnecessary deaths of elderly men of today and tomorrow.

REFERENCES

Allen-Burge, R., Storandt, M., Kinscherf, D. A., & Rubin, E. H. (1994). Sex differences in the sensitivity of two self-report depression scales in older depressed inpatients. *Psychology and Aging, 9*, 443–445.

American College of Medical Genetics/American Society of Human Genetics Working Group (ACMG/ASHG) on ApoE and Alzheimer Disease. (1995). Statement on the use of apolipoprotein E testing for Alzheimer Disease. *Journal of the American Medical Association, 274*, 1627–1629.

American Psychiatric Association (1994). *Diagnostic and Statistical Manual of Mental Disorders* (4th ed.). Washington, DC: American Psychiatric Association.

Bille-Brahe, U. (1993). The role of sex and age in suicidal behavior. *Acta Psychiatrica Scandinavica, 87*(Suppl. No. 371), 21–27.

Blau, Z. S. (1956). Changes in status and age identification. *American Sociological Review, 21*, 198–203.

Blazer, D. G. (1994). Epidemiology of late-life depression. In L. S. Schneider, C. F. Reynolds, B. D. Lebowitz, & A. J. Friedhoff (Eds.), *Diagnosis and treatment of depression in late life* (pp. 9–19). Washington, DC: American Psychiatric Association.

Blazer, D. G., George, L. K., & Hughes, D. (1991). The epidemiology of anxiety disorders: An age comparison. In C. Salzman & B. D. Lebowitz (Eds.),

Anxiety in the elderly: Treatment and research (pp. 17–30). New York: Springer.

Blazer, D. G., Hughes, D., George, L. K., Swartz, M., & Boyer, R. (1991). Generalized anxiety disorder. In L. N. Robbins & D. A. Regier (Eds.). *Psychiatric disorders in America* (pp. 180–203). New York: Free Press.

Bremner, W. J., Vitiello, M. V., & Prinz, P. N. (1983). Loss of circadian rhythmicity in blood testosterone levels with aging in normal men. *Journal of Clinical Endocrinology and Metabolism, 56,* 1278–1281.

Butler, R. N. (1963). The life review: An interpretation of reminiscence in the aged. *Psychiatry, 26,* 65–76.

Campbell, S. S., Gillin, J. C., Kripke, D. F., Erikson, P., & Clopton, P. (1989). Gender differences in the circadian temperature rhythms of healthy elderly subjects: Relationships to sleep quality. *Sleep, 12,* 529–536.

Chia, B. H. (1979). Suicide and the generation gap. *Life-Threatening Behavior, 2,* 194–208.

Clark, D. C. (1993). Narcissistic crises of aging and suicidal despair. *Suicide and Life-Threatening Behavior, 23,* 21–26.

Cohen, G. D. (1991). Anxiety and general medical disorders. In C. Salzman & B. D. Lebowitz (Eds.), *Anxiety in the elderly: Treatment and research* (pp. 47–62). New York: Springer.

Conwell, Y., & Brent, D. (1995). Suicide and aging I: Patterns of psychiatric diagnosis. *International Psychogeriatrics, 7,* 149–164.

Conwell, Y., Rotenberg, M., & Caine, E. D. (1990). Completed suicide at age 50 and over. *Journal of the American Geriatrics Society, 38,* 640–644.

Durkheim, E. (1951). *Suicide: A study in sociology* (J. A. Spaulding & G. Simpson, Trans.). New York: Free Press. (Original work published 1897).

Eaton, W., & Kessler, R. (1981). Rates of symptoms of depression in a national sample. *American Journal of Epidemiology, 114,* 428–538.

Eaton, W. W., Dryman, A., & Weissman, M. M. (1991). Panic and phobia. In L. N. Robbins & D. A. Regier (Eds.), *Psychiatric disorders in America* (pp. 155–179). New York: The Free Press.

Evans, D. A., Funkenstien, H. H., Albert, M. S., Scherr, P. A., Cook, N. R., Chown, M. J., Hubert, L. E., Hennekens, Ch. H., & Taylor, J. D. (1989). Prevalence of Alzheimer's disease in a community population of older persons: Higher than previously reported. *Journal of the American Medical Association, 262,* 2551–2556.

George, L. K., Landerman, R., Blazer, D. G., & Anthony, J. C. (1991). Cognitive impairment. In L. N. Robbins & D. A. Regier (Eds.), *Psychiatric disorders in America* (pp. 291–327). New York: Free Press.

Hoch, C. C., Buysse, D. J., Monk, T. H., & Reynolds, C. F., III (1992). Sleep disorders and aging. In J. E. Birren, R. B. Sloane, & G. D. Cohen (Eds.),

Handbook of mental health and aging (2nd ed.) (pp. 558–581). New York: Academic Press.

Jorm, A. F., Korten, A. E., & Henderson, A. S. (1987). The prevalence of dementia: A quantitative integration of the literature. *Acta Psychiatrica Scandinavica, 76,* 456–479.

Kennedy, G. J., Kelman, H. R., Thomas, C., Wisniewski, W., Metz, H., & Bijur, P.E. (1989). Hierarchy of characteristics associated with depressive symptoms in an urban elderly sample. *American Journal of Psychiatry, 146,* 220–225.

Kessler, R. C., Foster, C., Webster, P. S., & House, J. S. (1992). The relationship between age and depressive symptoms in two national surveys. *Psychology and Aging, 7,* 119–126.

Koenig, H. G., & Blazer, D. G. (1992). Mood disorders and suicide. In J. E. Birren, R. B. Sloane, & G. D. Cohen (Eds.), *Handbook of mental health and aging* (2nd ed.) (pp. 379–407). San Diego: Academic Press.

Koenig, H. G., O'Connor, C., Guarisco, S., Zabel, M., & Ford, S. (1993). Depressive disorder in elderly inpatients admitted to general medicine and cardiology at a private hospital. *American Journal of Geriatric Psychiatry, 1,* 197–210.

Kripke, D., Simons, R., Garfinkel, M., & Mammond, C. (1979). Short and long sleep and sleep pills. *Archives of General Psychiatric, 36,* 103–116.

Livingston, G., Hawkins, A., Graham, N., Blizard, R., & Mann, A. H. (1990). The Gospel Oak Study: Prevalence rates of dementia, depression and activity limitations among elderly residents in inner London. *Psychological Medicine, 20,* 137–146.

Lyness, J. M., Cox, C., Curry, J., Conwell, Y., King, D. A., & Caine, E. D. (1995). Older age and the underreporting of depressive symptoms. *Journal of the American Geriatrics Society, 43,* 216–221.

McIntosh, J. L., Santos, J. F., Hubbard, R. W., & Overholser, J. C. (1994). *Elder suicide: Research, theory and treatment.* Washington, DC: American Psychological Association.

National Center for Health Statistics. (1993). *Healthy people 2000 review, 1992* (DHHS Publication No. (PHS) 93–1232–1). Washington, DC: U.S. Government Printing Office.

NIH Consensus Development Panel on Depression in Late Life. (1992). Diagnosis and treatment of depression in late life. *Journal of the American Medical Association, 268,* 1018–1024.

Nolen-Hoeksema, S., Morrow, J., & Fredrickson, B. L. (1993). Response styles and the duration of episodes of depressed mood. *Journal of Abnormal Psychology, 102,* 20–28.

Osgood, N. J., & McIntosh, J. L. (1986). *Suicide and the elderly: An annotated bibliography and review.* Westport, CT: Greenwood Press.

Paykel, E. S., Brayne, C., Huppert, F. A., Gill, C., Barkley, C., Gehlhaar, E., Beardsall, L., Girling, D. M., Pollitt, P., & O'Connor, D. (1994). Incidence of dementia in a population older than 75 years in the United Kingdom. *Archives of General Psychiatry, 51,* 325–332.

Ritchie, K., & Kildea, D. (1995). Is senile dementia age-related or ageing-related? Evidence from meta-analysis of dementia prevalence in the oldest old. *The Lancet, 346,* 931–934.

Robins, L. N., & Regier, D. A. (Eds.). (1991). *Psychiatric disorders in America: The epidemiologic catchment area study.* New York: Free Press.

Rocca, W. A., Hofman, A., Brayne, C., Breteler, M. M. B., Clarke, M., Copeland, J. R. M., Dartigues, J., Engedal, K., Hagnell, O., Heeren, T. J., Jonker, C., Lindesay, J., Lobo, A., Mann, A. H., Molsa, A., Morgan, K., O'Connor, D. W., da Silva Droux, A., Sulkava, R., Kay, D. W. K., & Amaducci, L. (1991). Frequency and distribution of Alzheimer's disease in Europe: A collaborative study of 1980–1990 prevalence findings. *Annals of Neurology, 30,* 381–390.

Romanoski, A. J., Folstein, M. F., Nestadt, G., Chahal, R., Merchant, A., Brown, C. H., Gruenberg, E. M., & McHugh, P. R. (1992). The epidemiology of psychiatrist-ascertained depression and DSM-III depressive disorders. *Psychological Medicine, 22,* 629–655.

Schmid, C. F., & Van Arsdol, M. D., Jr. (1955). Completed and attempted suicides: A comparative analysis. *American Sociological Review, 20,* 273–283.

Shneidman, E. S. (1993). *Suicide as psychache: A clinical approach to self-destructive behavior.* Northvale, NJ: Jason Aronson.

Stroebe, M. S., & Stroebe, W. (1983). Who suffers more? Sex differences in health risks of the widowed. *Psychological Bulletin, 93,* 279–301.

Suicide among older persons: United States, 1980–1992. (1996, January 12). *Morbidity and Mortality Weekly Report, 45,* 3–6.

Verbrugge, L. M. (1990). Pathways of health and death. In R. D. Apple (Ed.), *Women, health and medicine in America: A historical handbook* (pp. 41–79). New York: Garland Press.

Weissman, M. M., Bruce, M. L., Leaf, P. J., Florio, L. P., & Holzer, C. E. (1991). Affective disorders. In L. N. Robbins & D. A. Regier (Eds.), *Psychiatric disorders in America* (pp. 53–80). New York: Free Press.

CHAPTER 13

The Victimization of Elderly Men

Jordan I. Kosberg, Ph.D.
& Stan L. Bowie, Ph.D.

This chapter focuses upon the victimization of elderly men. Such victimization includes crime on the street and within the home by strangers, abuse and maltreatment within the community by members of the informal support system (e.g., family, friends, and neighbors) and by formal caregivers (e.g., home care workers, professionals), and abuse and maltreatment within institutional settings.

In addition to the actual victimization of the elderly, in general, and elderly men, in particular, this chapter will also discuss the fear of older men of being victims of crime which can, in turn, adversely affect the quality of their lives. This chapter begins with an overview of issues pertaining to the victimization of the elderly, in general, and then focuses specifically upon elderly men.

INTRODUCTION

Official crime statistics (U.S. Department of Justice, 1994) suggest that the elderly, as a group, are not victimized as frequently as are younger individuals. It can be concluded that crime against the elderly is, thus, not a serious problem. Yet, methodological problems in the survey reports need to be considered. Further, though victimization of the elderly is relatively lower than for younger groups, there are important considerations not included in the statistics which pertain to all elderly, but which—in many instances—are especially applicable to elderly men.

First of all, as disclosed in any survey of crime reports or literature review, it is rather uncommon for victimization statistics to be differentiated by chronological age. The result is that it may be virtually impossible to come to any definitive conclusions regarding the prevalence or incidence of crime against the elderly. Relatedly, when and where there are studies which focus upon the elderly, or findings are controlled by age, often these studies on crime or abuse against the elderly fail to differentiate by gender (thus precluding comparative analyses).

There are those who question the validity of crime statistics in general. Fattah and Sacco (1989) refer to the prevalence of differing definitions of crime and of abuse in research findings and report statistics, and suggest that such diversity makes it impossible (and questionable) to merge findings from different studies. Additionally, these authors suggest that a large proportion of studies which focus upon crime against the elderly take place within urban areas, and do not accurately reflect victimization within suburban or rural areas of the country.

Fattah and Sacco (1989) further suggest that there are certain subpopulations which are understudied and their victimization underreported: the homeless, the poor, and those living within "skid-row areas." Relatedly, they point out that the use of phones for the identification of subjects (telephone sampling procedures), and as the means for collecting data, discriminate against those without phones. It is suspected that elderly men comprise a large proportion of such subpopulations who are somewhat "invisible" populations (Keigher, 1991).

There are many elderly victims—like victims of any age—who fail to report their adversities for different reasons. Butler, Lewis, and Sunderland (1991) have discussed the underreporting of crime against the elderly due to elderly victims being "too feeble or too fearful to contact authorities" (p. 25). They may be embarrassed at being a victim of a crime, particularly those crimes resulting from fraudulent "get-rich-quick" schemes or "quick solutions" to health problems. They may fail to report their abuse because the abuser may be a relative, because they see themselves to be the cause of the problem, or because they fear that one of the perceived solutions to the problem (i.e., institutionalization) will be worse than the problem itself (Kosberg, 1988). Finally, the elderly victim may not be familiar with how (or to whom) to report the problem.

It is a sad fact that the fear of crime—which is not considered in crime statistics—adversely affects elderly persons' quality of life. Indeed, such older populations have been measured to be more fearful than younger populations, and this influences when and where they go and/or influences whether or not they leave their dwelling (out of fear of crime on the street or fearing that their home will be broken into, should they leave it). Wan, Odell, and Lewis (1982) have pointed out the paradox that while the elderly are less often victims of crime (particularly violent crimes), they are more fearful. Stated differently: because the elderly are more fearful (and stay out of harm's way), they are less likely to become victims.

While the elderly have been found to have the lowest victimization rates of any age group in the U.S., "In a number of respects, however, crimes committed against the elderly are often more serious than crimes against younger people" (Whitaker, 1987, p. 1). There is some suggestion that the elderly are more likely to be repeatedly victimized (often by the same offender) and that the commission of a crime often results in greater adverse consequences (i.e., hospitalization, injury, and losses that cannot be replaced due to limited income). Research by the U.S. Department of Justice (Bachman, 1992) found that the injuries of elderly victims of violent crime are likely to be more serious than those of younger victims, and that they are more likely to face assailants who are strangers and are more likely to be victimized or assaulted at or near their home. These findings, plus the prevalence of fear of victimization (whether in the home, on the street, or within an institutional facility) make the problem of victimization of the elderly a significant one, indeed.

Elderly men are an extremely diverse group. Those few surveys and research studies focusing upon the victimization of elderly by gender tend not to consider such important variables as racial and ethnic background, socioeconomic status, urban and rural location, or marital status, nor differentiate between the young-old (those 65 to 74) and old-old (those 75 and older). Thus, information included in this chapter on the victimization of elderly men—when not based upon specific empirical findings—may result from the authors' extrapolation of general findings or from their speculations about what might be true. Needless to suggest, both extrapolations and speculations necessitate empirical verification in the future.

The vulnerability of elderly persons to victimization is inversely related to the perception of their value in society (seen differently by each individual). Kosberg (1988) has suggested that the combination of ageism (perceiving the elderly to be "less worthy") and violence as a way of life in American society results in a greater likelihood of their victimization. Additionally, Katz (1979–1980) has suggested that ageism coupled with the (physically or mentally) impaired condition of an elderly person increases the likelihood of their being abused or maltreated.

Women predominate—numerically and proportionally—among the elderly. And because of the possibility of purse snatching; the likelihood of living alone, widowhood, rape or other forms of sexual abuse; and stereotypes pertaining to their inability to defend themselves, elderly women can be erroneous assumed to be more likely victims of crime and abuse. The fact that men, in general, are often offenders contributes to the popular view of crime and abuse being committed mainly against elderly women.

In fact, there has been very little attention paid to the victimization of elderly men. Yet, research has found that not only are many elderly men victims of crime and abuse, but they may be especially vulnerable to adversity at the hands of others.

FEAR

As had been indicated, research has found that fear of crime is more prevalent among the elderly than younger populations. Such findings generally have not differentiated between groups of elderly by racial or ethnic background, by age group, nor by gender.

Although the findings are somewhat dated, Powell (1980) surveyed the literature on crime against the elderly and reported on a study of the extent of experienced victimization and anticipated victimization (fear) of three samples of elderly populations (African-Americans, Mexican-Americans and whites) in Los Angeles. He reported that, with slight variations, the African-American sample (both males and females) were more fearful than the Mexican-American sample. The white sample was generally less fearful. There were differences between these three groups by gender and age group; and although females in all three groups generally were more fearful than the males, the differences were not great, or significant, and were influenced by family income and occupational status. Ragan (1977) also found differences in the belief that crime is one of the most serious problems and adversely affects one's ability in getting around on the part of elderly men and women from African-American, Mexican-American, and white populations.

Such findings are believed to underscore the fact that discussing the conditions of all elderly men, as opposed to all elderly women, glosses over important distinctions. Further, when discussing elderly men, specificity is required to better understand the social, psychological, and economic variables which are related to fear, crime, or victimization. And while Powell's and Ragan's reports date back to 1980, there is no reason to believe that the extent of fear, the distinctions between the three groups, or differences by gender have significantly changed. Indeed, given contemporary crime rates in large cities, higher rates of fear among the elderly might be projected.

In a study of the elderly in Baltimore County, Wan et al. (1982) found that a younger sample of males (aged 60 to 74) experienced the greatest level of fear of crime, while older females (75 years of age and older) experienced the lowest. Among the explanations given was that the younger sample of elderly men were in situations where crimes were more apt to occur (i.e., leaving home to go to work, going out socially) and that this population was more aware of the existence of crime as reported in the news. Here, too, it is suspected findings are currently valid.

Thus, there are conflicting findings on fear of crime between elderly men and women. Fear of crime can be a deterrent; those more fearful are less likely to become victims. Yet, those who are fearful still venture out of their dwellings—to be exposed to the possibility of crime. And this is especially true of elderly men, by virtue of their lifestyles and their employed status.

CRIME

It is contended that elderly men, despite being a numerical and proportional minority, are more than likely to be the victims of criminal activity against the elderly. "Except for rape and personal larceny with contact, older men were more likely to be victims of personal crimes than older women for all types of personal crimes" (Yin, 1985, p. 25). Wan et al.

(1982) found that elderly men have higher rates of victimization for the crimes of robbery and larceny. And Fattah and Sacco (1989) have written "It appears that males are more frequently victimized than females and that they are more likely to be victims of serious crime. Thus, men tend to outnumber women among victims of assault and robbery." (p. 171).

Liang and Sengstock (1983) also found that elderly men were more likely to be victims of crime. Yin (1985) indicated that typical older victims are unmarried men and those who frequent public places which attract younger groups. Also, elderly men who are victimized are those who go out during evening hours.

Bachman (1992) has identified certain groups of elderly who are especially vulnerable to being victims of crime: African-Americans, those separated or divorced, renters, urban dwellers, and males. The 1994 National Crime Victimization Survey (U.S. Department of Justice, 1994) indicated that for *violence*, there were 12 elderly African-American males, 10 elderly African-American females, six elderly white males, and three elderly white females for every victim per 1,000 persons (over 12 years of age). For *personal theft*, there were 18 elderly white females, 15 elderly white males, 13 elderly African-American males, and nine elderly African-American females for every victim per 1,000 persons (over 12 years of age). Such statistics suggest that crime victimization is influenced by age, race, gender, and form of criminal activity. Generalizations drawn from crime statistics, thus, are relatively questionable.

The U.S. Department of Justice (1994) survey also differentiated crime rates by age group. For *violent crimes*, the rate was 8.5 for those 50 to 64 and 4.0 for those 65 and over per 1,000 persons over 12 years of age; for *personal theft*, the rate was 38.3 for those 50 to 64 and 19.5 for those 65 and older per 1,000 persons over 12 years of age; and for *household crime*, the rate was 133.0 for those 50 to 64 and 78.5 for those 65 and older per 1,000 persons over 12 years of age. The conclusion to be reached is that, regardless of the type of crime, rates of victimization among the elderly are lower for older groups.

Wan, Odell, and Lewis (1982) suggest that elderly persons in better health and from higher social classes experience lower levels of victimization. Fattah and Sacco (1989) have concluded that those who suffer debilitating physical or mental conditions increase their dependency upon others (who might subject them to harm). Additionally, they indicate that those from racial and economic minority groups—especially if living in high-crime areas—have an increased risk of victimization.

Underscoring the need to differentiate between age groups of elderly men, Yin (1985) suggested that the likelihood of older men venturing out decreases as they get older. Supporting such a contention, Wan et al. (1985) reported that victims tended more often to be males between 60 and 74 years of age. Additionally, those elderly men who were at high risk of becoming victims had never married.

Among explanations for the findings (or belief) that elderly men are more likely to be victims of crime include their lifestyles and vocational or avocational activities (Fattah & Sacco, 1989; Hindelang, Gottredson, & Garofalo, 1988). This is to suggest that, due to their work or leisure-time activities, older men—more so than older women—are likely to be in public places (where crimes are likely to occur). So too are older men likely to go out at night where, therefore, they are exposed to greater risk.

Men tend to be found in places where they can be targets for criminal activities (i.e., bars, skid-rows, nightclubs). In addition, older men (erroneously believing themselves to be able to resist any threat to their person or their possessions) might place themselves in potentially dangerous situations. Inasmuch as research has found that elderly men are more likely to be homeless (Keigher, 1991), or otherwise found living in high crime-rate areas of a city (i.e., transient hotels, on skid row, halfway houses), there is an increased probability of their being a victim of crime.

Fattah and Sacco (1989) have discussed the risk of crime (exposure to criminal harm) as being related to age-segregated residences. Congregate living situations for the elderly (i.e, homes for the aged, public housing, single room occupancy hotels) can attract criminals who prey upon older persons (Kosberg, 1988). In addition, living with others or sharing a residence leads to a greater likelihood of older persons being victimized by a family member, significant other, or a coresident. The case could be made that elderly men, either living with a spouse or with another individual, might be especially vulnerable to not only victimization by strangers but also by those with whom they live.

Any effort to focus upon the special vulnerability of elderly men must include attention to the increasing number of elderly homosexuals in society. Despite an optimistic assumption regarding the increasing sensitivity to and acceptance of this subpopulation of elderly men, it is believed—nonetheless—that elderly gays may continue to be at high risk of violence directed to them by those suffering from homophobia (as well as by younger gays). Comstock (1991) has suggested that violence against gay men (and lesbians) must be seen as a another significant social problem in American society, along with violence against women, children, and ethnic and racial populations.

Rubenstein (1986) has written about older men who live alone. This group includes those who are short- or long-term widowers, the never-married, and those divorced. He suggests that feelings of loneliness, and seeking companionship or friendship, may place such older men in potentially harmful situations (and with persons having questionable motivations).

ABUSE

Pillemer and Finkelhor (1988), in their study of elder abuse in one urban area (using a limited definition of abuse), found there to be an equal number of abused elderly men and women. Given the preponderance of elderly women, they projected that the risk of being abused is twice as great for elderly men as for elderly women, and concluded: "Thus, men seem more vulnerable to elder abuse" (p. 55).

Tatara (1993) also explored the rate of abuse by gender, as recorded by state protective service agencies, and considered the ratio of elderly men to women. His survey led him to conclude there was a greater vulnerability to abuse for elderly men than for elderly women, given that the proportion of elderly male victims exceeded the proportion of elderly men.

Fattah and Sacco (1989) have referred to a community survey which found that rates of abuse for men were twice as high as the rates experienced by women. They suggested that the mistreatment of elderly females is more likely to show up on official statistics because women are more likely to experience serious injuries and are less likely to tolerate abuse than are elderly men.

There are several explanations for the vulnerability of elderly men. Butler et al. (1991) have stated: "Abuse by a spouse is the most prevalent form of abuse, followed by abuse from an adult child" (p. 207). Given a greater proportion of elderly men still married, the conclusion can be made that there will be a higher risk for elderly men to be abused (by their spouses).

Inasmuch as most elderly husbands are older than their wives, they are likely to be in poorer physical and mental health. This frailty places pressures upon their spousal caregivers, or on any caregiver, which can result in abusive behavior out of design or frustration. Additionally, the greater frailty of elderly husbands also results in their inability to protect themselves.

The increasing dependency of elderly husbands on others can lead to their being abused for several reasons. It may be that an abused elderly man had been either a child or spouse abuser earlier in his life. Tatara (1993) has referred to the possibility that as men are often older and more impaired than their spouses, they can be "paid back" for the abuse of their children or spouses. This is to suggest that elder abuse may represent a "turning of the tables" of a longstanding pattern of spouse abuse. A resentful, retaliatory wife may abuse her once-abusive husband, who is now infirm and vulnerable. Adult children may abuse an elderly father who abused them, or they may wish to "get even" for their father's harsh treatment of their mother at an earlier period in time (Kosberg & Nahmiash, 1995).

Elderly men are more likely to abuse alcohol, or other substances, and such problems can be associated with their being victims of abusive behavior (Kosberg & Nahmiash, 1995). They will be unable to make appropriate judgements about the care they are receiving and may be incapable of leaving the situation (i.e., their home, a residential setting, or a shelter). Their vulnerability is exacerbated by the existence of physical and/or mental health problems along with the drinking problem.

A general area of needed research pertains to physical, psychological, or economic abuse against the elderly perpetrated by both professional and non-professional formal caregivers within the home (i.e., home aides, visiting nurses) and in the community (i.e., in day care programs, within the offices of physicians or attorneys). Similar to private dwellings, abuse behind the closed doors of offices or otherwise not seen by members of the general community pose special challenges. Research on the extent of such abuse is necessary, as is a determination of the interrelationship between the characteristics of both abused elderly persons and those of the formal caregiving abusers. Such an exploration should determine the importance of gender (as well as many other important considerations). Finally, inasmuch as abuse is a "hidden probem," it will be important to determine whether or not the rural location of elderly men place them at special risk (as is true, of course, for their general vulnerability to victimization).

INSTITUTIONAL MALTREATMENT AND ABUSE

Over the decades, institutions for the elderly have been widely criticized for ineffective care and inhumane treatment. The preponderance of proprietary facilities has exacerbated the level of discontent, reflecting a belief that proprietary facilities cannot simultaneously provide a profit for owners and quality care for the residents (a belief not supported by empirical research).

There is very little reliable information on the victimization of the elderly within institutional settings (Pillemer, 1988), and certainly even less on the special vulnerability of elderly men within such settings. Authors of one study of elder abuse in institutions (Pillemer & Moore, 1989) admitted that their study probably suffered from an under-reporting of abuse. Additionally, there are differing definitions of abusive behavior within institutional settings. Usual definitions include the theft and misappropriation of possessions and funds, neglectful behavior, and physical maltreatment, among others. Yet, the maltreatment of impaired institutionalized populations might include more subtle considerations—those difficult to identify and measure: touch, facial expression, eye contact, posture, head movement, spatial position, and gesture by staff (Hoffman, Platt, & Barry, 1988).

One study of elder abuse, based upon Ombudsmen Office records in California (Watson, Cesario, Ziemba, & McGovern, 1993), found that more women were reported to be abused than men. This is "no surprise," for not only were there many more institutionalized elderly women than men, but it is suspected that the underreporting of victimized elderly men believed to exist in the community might well explain a similar phenomenon within institutional settings.

There are reasons for believing that elderly men may be at high risk for maltreatment within institutional settings. Current cohorts of elderly men possibly have been socialized during an era when independence and self-reliance were very important to their self-concept. Men were traditionally the breadwinners and took pride in their ability to influence the lives of family members. In certain subcultures, the dominant role of men in a marriage, in the family, and with regard to others is even greater and extends into their later years. Current cohorts of elderly women are likely to have been socialized to be more dependent on others. Thus, it can be concluded that placement within an institutional setting might be more psychologically disruptive for some elderly men than for elderly women.

It may be that this incongruity results in higher levels of unhappiness and depression for institutionalized elderly men. Although not referring to the importance of gender, Schulz (1976) suggested that some characteristics observed among the institutionalized aged (such as depression, helplessness, and accelerated physical decline) are, in part, attributable to a loss of control. There is no reason to believe that such relationships (potentially affecting institutionalized elderly men) have lessened over the past 20 years since the work by Schulz.

In a dated study (Turner, Tobin, & Lieberman, 1972), it was found that persons most likely to survive institutionalization were rated as being aggressive, demanding, active, and narcissistic. One might wondered whether these attributes were—or are—especially characteristic of institutionalized elderly men. But what are the consequences?

While older men might survive the institutionalization process, what can be said of the care given to them? Clearly, within institutional settings—as is true within private dwellings in the community—caregivers (be they family members, professionals, or agency staff) can act out against the nonconforming, noncooperating care recipient. Although it seems plausible to conclude that there is a relationship between the provocative nature of an institutionalized person (seeking independence and control) and the quality of their care (acts of omission and commission), empirical research is needed to determine if such speculation can be substantiated and if findings are especially likely for institutionalized elderly men.

Institutions for the elderly care for mainly female populations, in that elderly men are more likely to have a surviving spouse providing care within community-based settings. Nonetheless, elderly men are institutionalized and, in being in the minority, there is reason to wonder if elderly men are receiving qualitatively and quantitatively different care and attention.

In addition, there will be an increase in the number and proportion of Alzheimer's Disease (A.D.) patients within institutional settings (U.S. Congress, 1992). Care of such populations may pose additional caregiving problems for staff members resulting from the behavioral problems of these patients, and from administrative and family demands and expectations. Accordingly, there is a need to ensure that A.D. residents are not maltreated; this is a concern pertaining to all A.D. patients within long-term care facilities, but especially for elderly men, who are less likely to have family visitors to provide surveillance over their care (Joiner & Freudiger, 1993).

CONCLUSION

Kosberg (1990) has written about methods by which to assist elderly victims of abuse and crime, including adequate assessment and interventions. Admittedly, gender was not an issue for discussion. Yet, we know that elderly men are often self-assured, have erroneous assumptions regarding their physical abilities, and are especially likely to place themselves in harm's way. In addition, it is known that they often fail to admit to having been victimized and do not seek and use necessary community resources. Accordingly, efforts are needed which specifically provide education to elderly men for the prevention of crime and abuse, and which seek to work with victimized groups of elderly men (whether using individual or group interventions). Roles for the researchers and practitioners are obviously prodigious.

The purpose of this chapter is not to point out the special vulnerability of elderly men to crime and abuse by minimizing the importance of the problems for elderly women. Indeed, by suggesting the special problems of elderly men, it is hoped that there will be renewed attention to the causes of general victimization of all elderly persons. While there seem to be particular explanations for the crime and abuse of present cohorts of elderly men, in all likelihood, the distinctions—social, psychological, economic, etc.—will be dissipating as gender equity continues to make substantial gains in American society.

Accordingly, the specific factors cited for the propensity of victimization of elderly men (their lifestyles, living arrangements, relationships, etc.) may increasingly become true also for elderly women in the future. Clearly, such future possibilities for the victimization of all elderly persons—males and females—necessitate preventive planning to preclude their anticipated potential victimization.

The major intent of this chapter is to suggest that though they are a statistical minority among the elderly as a group, elderly men are especially vulnerable to crime and abuse, and the fearful anticipation of such. The scarcity of attention directed toward victimized elderly men might be understandable, given their minority status and the general lack of sympathy for them. Yet, findings of their particular susceptibility to being victimized, coupled with the underreporting of their problems, should compel all who favor equity in the treatment of victims in contemporary society to consider the prevention of, and interventions for, elderly men—no differently than for elderly women.

REFERENCES

Bachman, R. (1992). *Elderly victims.* Washington, DC: U.S. Department of Justice.

Butler, R. N., Lewis, M., & Sunderland, T. (1991). *Aging and mental health: Positive psychosocial and biomedical approaches* (4th ed.). New York: Macmillan.

Comstock, G. D. (1991). *Violence against lesbians and gay men.* New York: Columbia University.

Fattah, E. A., & Sacco, V. F. (1989). *Crime and victimization of the elderly.* New York: Springer-Verlag.

Hindelang, M., Gottfredson, M. R., & Garofalo, J. (1978). *Victims of personal crime: An empirical foundation for a theory of personal victimization.* Cambridge, MA: Ballinger.

Hoffman, S. B., Platt, C. A., & Barry, K. E. (1988). Comforting the confused: The importance of nonverbal communication in the care of people with Alzheimer's disease. *The American Journal of Alzheimer's Care and Related Disorders and Research, 3,* 25–30.

Joiner, C. M., & Freudiger, P. T. (1993). Male and female differences in nursing home adjustment and satisfaction. *Journal of Gerontological Social Work, 20,* 71–85.

Katz, K. D. (1979–80). Elder abuse. *Journal of Family Law, 18,* 695–722.

Keigher, S. M. (Ed.). (1991). *Housing risks and homelessness among the urban elderly.* New York: Haworth.

Kosberg, J. I. (1988). Preventing elder abuse: Identification of high risk factors prior to placement decision. *Gerontologist, 28,* 43–49.

Kosberg, J. I. (1990). Assistance to crime and abuse. In A. Monk (Ed.) Handbook of gerontological services (pp. 450–473). New York: Columbia University Press.

Kosberg, J. I., & Nahmiash, D. (1995). Characteristics of victims and perpetrators and milieus of abuse and neglect. In L. A. Baumhover & S. C. Beal (Eds.), *Abuse, neglect, and exploitation of older persons: Strategies for assessment and intervention* (pp. 29–47). Baltimore: Health Professions Press.

Liang, J., & Sengstock, M. C. (1983). Personal crimes against the elderly. In J. I. Kosberg (Ed.), *Abuse and maltreatment of the elderly: Causes and interventions* (pp. 40–67). Boston: John Wright–PSG.

Pillemer, K. (1988). Maltreatment of patients in nursing homes: Overview and research agenda. *Journal of Health and Social Behavior, 29,* 227–238.

Pillemer, K. A., & Finkelhor, D. (1988). The prevalence of elder abuse: A random sample survey. *The Gerontologist, 28,* 51–57.

Pillemer, K. A., & Moore, D. W. (1989). Abuse of patients in nursing homes: Findings from a survey of staff. *Gerontologist, 29,* 314–320.

Powell, D. E. (1980). The crimes against the elderly. *Journal of Gerontological Social Work, 3,* 27–39.

Ragan, P. K. (1977). Crimes against the elderly: Findings from interviews with Blacks, Mexican-Americans, and Whites. In M. A. Y. Rifai (Ed.), *Justice and older Americans* (pp. 25–36). Lexington, MA: Lexington Books.

Rubenstein, R. L. (1986). *Singular paths: Older men living alone.* New York: Columbia University.

Schulz, R. (1976). Effects of control and predictability on the physical and psychological well-being of the institutinalized aged. *Journal of Personality and Social Psychology, 33,* 563–573.

Tatara, T. (1993). Understanding the nature and scope of domestic elder abuse with the use of state aggregate data: Summaries of the key findings of a national survey of state APS and aging agencies. *Journal of Elder Abuse and Neglect, 5,* 35–59.

Turner, B. F., Tobin, S. S., & Lieberman, M. A. (1972). Personality traits as predictors of institutional adaptation among the aged. *Journal of Gerontology, 27,* 21–68.

U.S. Congress, Office of Technology Assessment (1992). *Special Care Units for people with Alzheimer's and other dementias: Consumer education, research, regulatory, and reimbursement issues.* Washington, DC: U.S. Government Printing Office.

U.S. Department of Justice (1994). *Elderly crime victims: National Crime Victimization Survey* (DOJ Publication No. NCJ–147186). Washington, DC: U.S. Government Printing Office.

Wan, T. T. H., Odell, B. G., & Lewis, D. T. (1982). *Promoting the well-being of the elderly: A community diagnosis,* New York: Haworth.

Watson, M. M., Cesario, T. C., Ziemba, S., & McGovern, P. (1993). Elder abuse in long-term care environments: A pilot study using information from long-term care ombudsman reports in one California county. *Journal of Elder Abuse & Neglect, 5,* 95–111.

Whitaker, C. J. (1987). *Elderly victims.* Washington, DC: U.S. Department of Justice.

Yin, P. (1985). *Victimization and the aged.* Springfield, IL: Charles C Thomas.

E. Formal and Informal Assistance

CHAPTER 14

Informal Caregiving by Older Men*

Lenard W. Kaye, D.S.W.

INTRODUCTION

This chapter considers the experiences of older men who have assumed the role of "informal caregiver," defined as an individual who takes on responsibility for the assistance needed by an impaired relative, friend, or neighbor. Given the demographics of male caregiving, such a discussion must, necessarily, emphasize primarily the efforts of husbands, and to a lesser degree sons, who fulfill this function for their dependent spouses and parents, respectively.

Traditionally, men who become engaged in the caregiving enterprise have usually been characterized as performing an extremely restricted range of concrete or instrumental tasks for disabled family members, including such activities as home and yard repair and maintenance, transportation, intervening to obtain community entitlements and benefits, and financial management. These same men have tended, it is further maintained, to avoid engagement in tasks that require personal, hands-on assistance (e.g., grooming, bathing, or dressing the care recipient) or that are otherwise likely to require emotional support or affec-

*The research on which this chapter is based was supported by a grant from the AARP Andrus Foundation.

tive expression. Yet, there may be circumstances under which men are willing to accept the obligation of care and undertake a range of intimate personal care functions from which they conceivably may derive identity and reward. These men, it is postulated, are driven by motives and experience challenges similar to those of female caregivers.

For the purposes of this discussion, older men who assume this level of intensity in their informal caregiving efforts will be categorized as "primary caregivers," defined as individuals who take on responsibility for the majority of assistance needed by an impaired person. At the same time that male primary caregivers experience the responsibilities of helping in ways similar to those of women engaged in the same tasks, it is suggested that there are unique dimensions to the older male caregiving experience that separate it from that of female caregivers.

This chapter will present the available evidence suggesting that, contrary to popular belief, older men—especially spouses—are heavily engaged in the caregiving enterprise. Their involvement can and does consume significant portions of their lives and requires substantial allotments of physical and emotional commitment. Indeed, in the research that reports on spousal caregiving, men are generally found to provide equal or greater proportions of care, compared to their female counterparts. Thus, marital status and age appear to play important parts in determining caring responsibility. As suggested by Fisher (1994), by revealing the importance of both age and marital status in the analysis of caregiving, it is believed that our understanding of filial care and the role of gender in caregiving is going to be necessarily altered.

Evidence will also be offered suggesting that older males engaged in primary informal caregiving tend to display a strong and enduring tendency to present a stoic, "stiff upper lip" orientation to their role and function in the caregiving experience. It is suggested that a consistent and concerted effort is frequently made by these primary male caregivers to "tough it out," resisting in various ways the assistance and support of both informal and formal sources of supplementary aid. As such, this discussion may challenge conventional wisdom which minimizes men's inclination and capacity to care for others. At the same time, the argument will be made for the impressive caregiving contributions, both in the instrumental and affective domain, of these same men, even in the face of their own failing health. Various demands of caregiving serve to highlight that older men may downplay the level of stress and strain associated with providing informal care. Nevertheless, there is a heavy burden placed on them in performing this role when they become engaged in helping a relative for extended periods of time who is suffering from the destructive consequences of Alzheimer's Disease, arthritis, cancer, heart disease, stroke, and the like.

THE SCOPE AND BREADTH
OF FAMILY CAREGIVING

The caregiving experience of family members and other informal supports has emerged as a phenomenon of significant interest to the scientific and lay community. Montgomery and Datwyler (1990) argue that the expansion of informal caregiving, which they categorize as service provided by unpaid workers, is due not only to the unprecedented growth in the aged population, but also to the preoccupation with acute care problems on the part of those formal providers of care who comprise the medical system. Informal supports (e.g., family, friends, and neighbors) have, in combination with ancillary health personnel (e.g., nurse's aides, homemakers, housekeepers, home health aides, and the like) filled the resultant service gap in care to the aged. These low-pay or no-pay providers represent a central and pervasive feature in the lives of most impaired elders. Indeed, only a minority of elders receive formal organizational services. Nor has the informal provision of aid undergone significant changes, even though families are growing smaller, significant geographic distance between family members is increasingly commonplace, and female participation in the labor force has undoubtedly increased (Morris & Morris, 1992).

While the elder caregiving experience has received considerable attention in recent years from the research community, male caring remains a phenomenon studied much more sparingly. Caregiver research samples have, as a rule, been dominated by a preponderance of female subjects. Resultant conventional wisdom has fixed on the premise that caregiving is a female-centered area of familial activity and, in particular, one dominated by the efforts of daughters. Some observers appear frustrated by the presumed gender bias in viewing the family caring experience, referring to the inequity of a system whereby women continue to carry the predominant share of family support tasks (Montgomery & Datwyler, 1990). For others, the dearth of knowledge of the caregiving experience of men has undoubtedly resulted in misunderstandings about the roles and motivations of male carers (Parker, 1993).

When males have been included in research samples, they are often undifferentiated in data analyses, thus obscuring possible intragroup differences in their experiences. Male research subjects have also tended to be adult children rather than husbands, despite reports that spouses are more likely to assume caregiving responsibilities. Dwyer and Coward (1991) point to other potential gender-related deficiencies in caregiving research: 1) the failure to account for the wide range of characteristics beyond gender that may be associated with the provision of care to an older person; 2) the focus of research on those children who are currently providing help, rather than on the total sibling network of potential providers of assistance; and 3) the fact that sons tend to help with different caregiving tasks than daughters.

Arber and Gilbert (1990), in surveying the British experience, conclude that men are indeed the "forgotten carers." They argue that men make a larger contribution to caring for incapacitated family members than is often recognized. They identify three widely endorsed, yet false, assumptions about male caregivers: 1) men are very unlikely to be primary carers of infirm elderly people; 2) elderly men receive more support from statutory and voluntary services than female caregivers; and 3) men who serve as caregivers are more likely to obtain supplemental assistance from other relatives.

The substantial role played by Americans generally, and men in particular, is highlighted in the Commonwealth Fund (1992) report, *The Nation's Great Overlooked Resource: The Contributions of Americans 55+.* This national survey, conducted by Louis Harris and Associates, Inc. of 2,999 Americans (1,069 men and 1,930 women) age 55 and over, documents that more than 70% of older Americans contribute to society, their families, and their communities through working, volunteering, and caring for sick and disabled persons. It confirms that, contrary to the stereotype, men play a larger role than expected as caregivers. In total, 28% of men and 29% of women 55 years and over are helping sick or disabled parents, spouses, other relatives, friends, and neighbors. Among married couples, 1.6 million men and 1.8 million women are caring for their sick or disabled spouses. Furthermore, 1.2 million men and 1.9 million women are caring for their sick or disabled parents, while 2.1 million men and 3.1 million women are caring for sick or disabled friends or neighbors. Taken together, these men and women are contributing in caregiving effort the equivalent of more than 20 million full-time

workers (Commonwealth Fund, 1992). Stone and Kemper (1989) estimate that there are as many as 13.3 million potential family caregivers in
the United States who have disabled spouses or parents 65 years of age
and older. Given estimates that between one-quarter and one-third of
elder caregivers are men, there were between 1.7 million and possibly as
many as 2.3 million men caring for elderly relatives in the United States
in 1989. Their numbers can be expected to have grown in the 1990s.
Given the propensity for married men to fulfill caregiving functions for
their incapacitated wives, it can be assumed that a substantial portion of
these men are aging themselves.

UNDERSTANDING THE NATURE
OF MALE CAREGIVING

Understanding the unique experience of male caregiving requires that
attention be directed toward the attitudes, expectations, and needs of
men acting as caregivers for their elderly relatives. Unfortunately, research has rarely addressed these dimensions of the experience in the
case of the older male caregiver. A comprehensive picture of the male
experience will only be arrived at if consideration is directed to multiple
dimensions of caregiving: 1) the distinctive characteristics and coping
strategies of men performing this role; 2) the factors that instigate the
allocation of elder caregiving responsibilities to men in families; 3) the
incentives and disincentives for successful male caregiving performance;
4) the unique interpersonal relationship dynamics that influence the
quality of caregiving interchanges between males and their dependent
relatives; and 5) the extent to which respite services, home health care
programs, caregiver support groups, and other community service interventions are able to respond to the needs of male family caregivers.

PROFILING THE MALE CAREGIVER

Men engaged as primary caregivers are, more likely than not, older
husbands caring for their incapacitated wives. Indeed, it is conceivable
that men constitute slightly more than half of spousal caregivers (Archer
& MacLean, 1993). The majority of such individuals are likely to be in
their 50s or older. The proportion of male caregivers that are men of

color or representative of minority groups is difficult to ascertain, given that the vast majority of surveys of male caregiving have failed to tap the experiences of ethnic and racial minorities. While primary spousal caregivers are more likely than not to be retired, a substantial minority (perhaps around 25%) combine the responsibilities of caregiving simultaneously with the demands of part-time and full-time employment. The majority of primary male caregivers live with the person to whom they are providing care and, more likely than not, have resided with that person for an extended period of time.

Contrary to popular belief, primary caregiving men have been found to perform a rather broad range of assistive tasks, from hand-holding to home repair. They are capable of carrying out social and emotional support tasks, instrumental- and case management-type tasks, and even "hands-on" personal care tasks (although research confirms that the latter tend to be performed least often). The rather commonplace performance of social and emotional support tasks by older male spousal caregivers (Kaye & Applegate, 1990), in particular, appears to challenge the traditional view of men as inexpressive and emotionally detached and may lend support to the notion that men in middle and later life become more focused on family relations, nurturance, and affective connectedness.

As has been suggested, care recipients of male caregivers appear most likely to be spouses, with lesser proportions of men caring for a parent or parent-in-law. Men appear even less likely to be caregivers for siblings or friends. Given the high proportion of men who are spousal caregivers, and the greater likelihood that women will be diagnosed with Alzheimer's Disease than men, it can be expected that substantial proportions of these helpers are assisting wives suffering from Alzheimer's Disease or a related disorder, who consequently exhibit varying degrees of mental dysfunction. The demands placed on the caregiver helping a victim of Alzheimer's Disease can be expected to be especially great.

CONTRIBUTIONS TO CARE
FROM FAMILY MEMBERS

Researchers have repeatedly documented uneven, if not rather limited, levels of assistance received by primary caregivers from other members comprising the family constellation. The dearth of assistance provided individuals who have assumed primary responsibility for support of a significant other has been observed for older male caregivers as well (Kaye & Applegate, 1990). It is not particularly uncommon for older male caregivers (spousal helpers, in particular) to report family assistance to occur rather seldom. In fact, substantial numbers of these caregivers (as many as a third or more) discover they are the sole providers of care. It is relatively unusual for more than two other individuals to bear some portion of the older male caregiver's responsibility.

The most common sources of supplementary family assistance for men engaged in caregiving appear to be the care recipients' spouses and children. Interestingly, Kaye and Applegate (1990) discovered that sons were cited more often than daughters as stepping in to provide secondary support for male caregivers. While this observation may be unexpected for those who subscribe to traditional views of female-dominated patterns of caregiving, it reinforces Barusch and Spaid's (1989) conclusion that caregivers tend to turn to children of the same gender for supplementary aid.

Increments in the frequency of supplementary family assistance appear to be associated with decrements in the care recipient's level of behavioral orientation and overall mental health. While relatives are involved on a more frequent basis during the course of a care recipient's emotional and mental decline, the absolute number of family members who engage in this supplemental help tends to decline over time. This rather disturbing pattern of supplementary aid was observed by Stoller (1985) who concluded that as elder caregiving stretches into chronicity, it becomes a drama cast with fewer and fewer committed family players.

NEEDING AND UTILIZING FORMAL COMMUNITY SERVICES

There continues to be conflicting findings in terms of the extent to which male caregivers utilize available community services to ease the burden associated with maintaining informal supports in the community. Earlier research and conventional wisdom have maintained that male caregivers receive comparatively high levels of outside assistance with their tasks.

On the other hand, if men who are caring for spouses or other males who are engaged in caregiving as primary helpers are separated out, community service utilization levels appear to decline. Furthermore, it does not appear particularly unusual for male caregivers to minimize the extent to which they make use of formal organizational services.

At the same time, male caregivers may express the belief that they are not necessarily receiving adequate support from the formal service system. Among those services that may be needed by these men are traditional in-home services (i.e., homemakers, home health aides) as well as congregate-organized adult day care. Such services can be seen to provide, at best, brief respite, rather than extended relief, from the responsibilities of family care. Motenko (1989) found that men preferred to carry on with their caregiving tasks with the assistance of only limited ancillary services, thus enabling only brief—rather than extended or permanent—respite. Perhaps like the men in Miller's research (1991), the men in Motenko's sample wished to remain in control, transferring customary roles of authority from the traditional workplace to the home setting. This possibility finds support from the Kaye and Applegate research (1990) which documented the tendency for caregiving men to assume the role of service monitor or manager during times of community service provision.

As observed by Kaye and Applegate (1990), receipt of services appears not to be significantly associated with the elder care recipients' perceived physical health or their degree of mental impairment. Put differently, persons who are judged to be severely impaired, physically and mentally, may be no more likely than less-incapacitated care recipients to receive outside agency services when male caregivers are engaged as primary helpers. In such instances, it would seem that these male caregivers, with limited assistance from other relatives, are picking up the slack and becoming increasingly burdened by the demands of long-term family care as the health of their care recipients deteriorate.

The Kaye and Applegate (1990) data do confirm the expected: the deteriorating status of care recipients is accompanied by increments in caregivers' views of the need for formal community service intervention. Positive correlations were observed between service need and the degree of care recipient physical illness and mental impairment. Furthermore, decrements in caregiver financial status were accompanied by increases in perceived need for outside assistance. It would therefore appear, according to these data, that even though male caregivers are able to testify to an increased need for help during the course of decline in care recipient health, they are not particularly likely to have those needs satisfied by community agency personnel. Interestingly, the Kaye and Applegate data confirm no significant differences in the extent to which services were used when comparing spousal to nonspousal caregivers, employed to unemployed caregivers, and primary to secondary caregivers. On the other hand, it is interesting to note that those men who lived with their care recipients reported significantly greater use of community services than those who did not. Indeed, the coresidence variable has been suggested to be a key measure in understanding patterns of informal care and use of formal community services (Tennstedt, Crawford, & McKinlay, 1993).

Additional analyses reported by Kaye and Applegate (1990) confirm that the age of the caregiver, his overall health, the gender and age of the care recipient, levels of supplemental family assistance, and whether or not the care recipient is thought to have Alzheimer's Disease are not associated with differing levels of community service consumption. Only when the perceptions of spousal and nonspousal caregivers are compared do significant differences surface. Specifically, spousal caregivers believe there to be significantly lower levels of need for agency assistance than do their nonspousal counterparts. This finding parallels that of other research which suggests that when husbands are primary caregivers, the likelihood of supplementary assistance is reduced (Tennstedt, McKinlay, & Sullivan, 1989).

Other characteristics of male caregivers and their elder care recipients are not found to vary in relation to community service usage, save for the recipients' perceived capacity to perform activities of daily living (ADLs) (Kaye and Applegate, 1990). Elder recipient ADL limitations are found to be significantly greater for those male caregivers who indicate they are receiving community services. However, male caregiver financial status, life satisfaction levels, age, overall health, overall mental health, and functional status do not significantly vary when comparing those receiving and not receiving community services. Furthermore, care recipient age, overall health, and overall mental health do not vary when comparing those who are receiving and are not receiving formal outside assistance. Thus, an older person's functional capacity (as measured by ADL limitations), rather than physical and mental health, would seem to be a more strategic variable in understanding the utilization of agency services by older male caregivers and their incapacitated elders.

THE CHALLENGE OF OLDER MALE CAREGIVING

Older male caregivers are challenged by the helping experience. It is not unusual for older men who are primary carers, as opposed to secondary carers, to report significantly lower levels of life satisfaction (Kaye & Applegate, 1994). Primary carers also tend to be significantly older than secondary carers, and are likely to rate their overall health, overall mental health, and functional health lower. Similarly, these men can be expected not to register particularly high assessments of their own emotional health. Nor is it unusual for these men to indicate that their health limits the care that they are able to provide to their impaired relatives. Increasing amounts of time devoted to caregiving by men is associated with declining financial well-being, overall health, and overall mental health, and increases in age. It would appear that those men who can less easily assume the role of primary caregiver are nevertheless more likely to assume the responsibility and at the same time derive less satisfaction from the experience.

As has been highlighted throughout this chapter, intense caregiving is commonly a spousal experience, especially for men. Furthermore, husbands who become caregivers appear to be at greater risk than their female counterparts, as well as other categories of men. Those caregivers who are spouses and who reside with the care recipient are likely, in particular, to be at-risk. They tend to be older, have more health problems, survive on lower incomes, perform more caregiving tasks, care for more disabled persons, report more stress-related symptoms, and generally are more adversely affected by providing care than nonspousal caregivers (Barusch & Spaid, 1989). Whether the marital relationship has historically been rewarding or not, the disruptions and discontinuities caused by illness can create alterations in the marital relationship and resultant distress for husbands (Motenko, 1989).

Spousal caregivers may be vulnerable, in particular, to emotional stress. Spousal caregivers have been found to be more depressed, have higher negative affect, more likely to use psychotropic drugs, have more symptoms of psychological distress, and suffer from more physical health problems than the general population (Pruchno & Potashnik, 1989). It is understandable that O'Bryant, Straw, and Meddaugh (1990) describe spousal caregiving as an encapsulating experience which serves to shape and intensify the special nature of that experience.

While both male and female caregivers are stressed, some factors appear to mitigate the expression, if not intensity, of burden for men. Gender remains an important predictor of caregiver burden when other sociodemographic variables are taken into consideration. Men, it has been suggested, may feel a less strong sense of responsibility and commitment to the caregiving role than women—as expressed in lesser effort, emotional involvement, and personal concern for the care receiver (Kramer & Kipnis, 1995). Interpreted somewhat differently, the orientation of older male caregivers has been characterized as one of "rationality with feeling;" an "industrial" approach that is quite task-oriented and systematic, if not stoic, at the same time that significant measures of intimacy are expressed (Kaye & Applegate, 1994). In the case of spousal primary caregivers, both men and women appear to express an exceedingly strong sense of responsibility and commitment to the caregiving role. Older men, as opposed to younger men, may be more disposed to commiting themselves to the responsibilities of long-term caregiving. For these individuals, the characterization of their experiences as comprising a caregiving "career" does not appear to be overstated.

THE POTENTIAL CONSEQUENCES OF MALE CAREGIVER STOICISM

Primary male caregivers—especially spousal male caregivers—do not, it has been argued, present themselves as frequent beneficiaries of informal or formal supplemental care. In particular, they appear to be restrained in their utilization of community services, even as their own health and functional status may be on the decline. Whether motivated by male stoicism, a desire to retain control, or the gratification realized from sustaining a meaningful relationship, primary male caregivers can be observed to go it alone with minimal help received from others. Nor do they appear inclined, necessarily, to escape or flee from the responsibilities of family care.

This pattern would suggest that those engaged in policymaking and program planning affecting male caregivers generally—and, in particular, primary, older male spousal caregivers—should emphasize forms of assistance that support and sustain these men, rather than replacing or substituting for their caregiving roles and responsibilities. It would also seem that a substantial part of the effort of programmers will need to be focused on convincing these men to partake of available community services in the first place. One should not assume that primary male caregivers (whether they be husbands or sons) aim to escape from the responsibility of care at the first opportunity. Rather, a more compelling urge for these men may be to resist, over the long-term, critical assistance—even as their own personal resources are dwindling.

One question remaining to be asked concerns itself with these men's service utilization patterns. Does the limited degree of service usage evidenced by these men reflect comparatively low levels of needed assistance, a resistance to asking for help, or—rather—lack of caregiver knowledge and/or relative unavailability of particular home-delivered interventions in a given geographic community? While community services would appear to be an important buffer against stress, limited information remains available as to the adequacy and appropriateness of both formal and informal support services required by elderly male caregivers, in particular, and spouses. It is clear, however, that men who are new to the caregiving role could benefit from training offered by community programs in the development of specific caregiving skills.

A CLINICAL PERSPECTIVE ON MALE CAREGIVING

From a clinical perspective, the potential consequences for primary caregiving men of maintaining a stoic, "stiff upper lip" mentality throughout the course of caregiving are worrisome. It is very hard to be a caregiver for extended periods of time. For older men who are, themselves, increasingly subject to the physical and emotional decrements associated with aging, "toughing it out" can mean the inevitable buildup of potentially unhealthy and, ultimately, disruptive levels of frustration, hostility, guilt, and fatigue. The responsibilities of caregiving for a family member with a chronic and severely disabling condition, such as Alzheimer's Disease, can overwhelm the man and alter the balance of his relationship with the care recipient. When help, assistance, and affection become ultimately unidirectional, moving only from the caregiver to the care recipient, the level of stress experienced by the former can be expected to rise, especially as caregiving endures over time and the status of the care recipient deteriorates. It is conceivable that some proportion of these caregivers will ultimately come to express substantial measures of resentment and anger which can be expected to impact negatively on their caregiving behavior. At the least, it may result in the premature burnout of caring men such that they choose to terminate the experience significantly sooner than would otherwise have been expected. Either way, the consequences for the incapacitated elder receiving care are serious.

The causes of caregiver stress for men can potentially be examined from several different perspectives. First, stress may be disaggregated into categories according to the source. Some stresses may derive from patient characteristics, some from caregiver characteristics, and some from the external environment. Furthermore, stresses may be classified as primary or secondary. Finally, caregiver stress may be measured objectively or subjectively by means of self-reports.

Of course, a stoic posture can have negative consequences for the health of these caregivers as well. The assumption of an inordinate amount of caregiving responsibility without supplementary aid or temporary respite may accelerate their own physical and emotional decline. In turn, their physical and emotional capacity to care for another person may be reduced significantly.

Spousal caregivers, representing the majority of men engaged in the caregiving function, are aging themselves and vulnerable. They are at considerable risk for a host of emotional and physical health problems. In fact, they may be in little better health than their care recipients. For those men who downplay their incapacities and the burden associated with caregiving, at the same time that they resist accepting assistance from relatives and community agencies, the caregiving experience may be a particularly disabling one with potentially negative consequences (Pruchno & Potashnik, 1989).

Caregivers serving Alzheimer's Disease victims are more likely to be men than women. These caregiving men appear to be at particular risk of illness, which in turn undermines their capacity to persevere in the caregiving role. Working with Alzheimer's Disease and related disorder patients is a predictor of increased caregiver strain (Bass, McKee, Deimling, & Mukherje, 1994) as it serves to highlight the ultimate mortality of both care recipient and care provider. The special demands placed on caregivers of Alzheimer's Disease patients are likely to be especially great for spousal caregivers as compared to adult children. At the same time, men who care for Alzheimer's Disease victims may represent an especially nurturant group of family-oriented males. O'Bryant et al. (1990) rightly conclude that providing care to an Alzheimer's Disease victim may be the ultimate test of spousal commitment, because of the gradual process of mental and physical decline prior to the patient's death.

For caregivers who are determined to "go it alone," caregiving can be isolating and lonely. The work of caregiving necessarily replaces time that otherwise might have been spent with others. More that 95% of the men in the Kaye and Applegate sample (1990) had been caregivers for more than 1 year, while almost two-thirds had done so for 3 years or longer. More than one-half of the sample were providing in excess of 60 hours of care each week, with an additional 24% reporting weekly caregiving involvement levels between 21 and 60 hours. Furthermore, it is likely that primary caregivers, both male and female, will perceive at varying points in the caregiving experience a lack of reciprocity, or acknowledgment by the care recipient, in terms of the emotional support offered by such individuals. That is, primary caregivers may feel that they are providing for someone else without equivalent expressions of affective return. The relative lack of perceived reciprocity between the male caregiver and care recipient, in the area of mutual support, concern, and affection, can be expected to further test the resiliency of the caregiving experience for these men.

The fear that making formal services available to informal supports would weaken the "glue" that connects caregiver to care recipient has never been borne out (Morris & Morris, 1992). Such a concern may actually be moot in terms of spousal caregivers, given their extremely limited use of community services. Pruchno and Potashnik (1989) have also reported that caregiving spouses use medical services at rates which are similar to or lower than those reported by the general population. While caregiving spouses may prefer to do the tasks themselves, continuing as long as possible in the role with minimal use of community resources, increased service utilization by caregiving men may serve to extend the life of the caregiving bond rather than weaken it, as it buttresses caregiver and care recipient against the inevitable wear and tear of the demands of long-term caregiving.

SUPPORT GROUPS AND RESPITE
FOR CARING MEN

Caregiver support groups may represent a major untapped programmatic resource for men engaged in elder care. In particular, groups providing social support may help buffer the male caregiver from the negative effects of stress on mental health. Men are capable of being regular and active participants in these groups. Moreover, once engaged, they express considerable satisfaction with the rewards derived from group association, and are grateful for the opportunity to receive social support and share their experiences with other men (and women) like themselves (Kaye & Applegate, 1993).

Unfortunately, it is rare for support group facilitators to make special efforts to reach out to male caregivers. Specialized outreach and recruitment directed at men appears crucial if they are to be helped to overcome their inclination to resist participation. It is likely that support groups, in order to appeal initially to men, will need to be strategically marketed, stressing the availability of expert advice and the provision of concrete information. Caregiving spouses, in particular, are likely to benefit from straightforward help in learning to perform the caregiving role and developing caregiving routines at home (Mui & Morrow-Howell, 1993). Once engaged, however, it is suggested that men can be expected to benefit as much as women from the emotional return realized from mutual sharing in the group setting and ventilation of common problems and challenges associated with caregiving.

While caregiver support groups are deemed a useful formal intervention for men engaged in caregiving, it should be anticipated that certain subgroups of men will exhibit greater resistance than others in terms of attending group sessions. Hispanic male caregivers and other minority ethnic groups can be expected, in particular, to find caregiver support groups and other mainstream interventions to be less responsive to their needs (Monahan, Greene, & Coleman, 1992). Such individuals will require extra outreach on the part of support group facilitators to encourage their attendance.

Temporary, short-term respite appears highly desirable as well for older primary male caregivers. A national survey carried out by the Office of Technology Assessment (1987) confirmed that 96% of caregivers caring for elders with dementia need respite. Unfortunately, only about 2% of caregivers receive any kind of supportive community services of this type. When offered, caregiver respite services can work to reduce caregiver burden (Skelly, McAdoo, & Ostergard, 1993). Like support group programs, the challenge for respite services appears to be one of transmitting their programmatic message in a way that encourages men to make use of the intervention rather than rejecting it out of hand, because it is perceived to serve as evidence of failure to fulfill their caregiving responsibilities.

RECOMMENDATIONS FOR FUTURE RESEARCH, POLICY, AND PROGRAMMING

The research on male caregivers, as alluded to earlier in this chapter, has reflected a variety of flaws and limitations. As a rule, male caregiver research samples have not been particularly large or geographically diverse. When they are, they unfortunately tend to represent self-selected groups of subjects studied at single points in time. Cross-sectional designs make inferring causal relationships between caregiving and various impacts suspect, given the dynamic nature of helping behaviors and relationships.

Furthermore, most of the caregiver research, including that which focuses on men, cannot claim substantial diversity in terms of the socio-economic status, racial/ethnic background, and sexual preference of the subjects. Samples are remarkably homogeneous, reflecting—more often that not—a cohort of urban or suburban white, relatively well-educated, heterosexual, middle-class men. Studies that examine the comparative experiences of caregivers and care recipients differing in terms of geographic location, ethnicity, race, class, and sexual orientation are long overdue. At the same time, there may be certain advantages derived from studying caregivers in smaller, more homogeneous subgroups. Indeed, the value of much caregiving research has been reduced because samples have been so diverse, especially in terms of relationship status, making it impossible to distinguish between variables.

The selection effects associated with drawing samples from the membership rosters of particular community programs, services, and housing residences may also limit the generalizability of findings. One has no way of knowing whether or not those men who utilize particular community interventions are typical of the vast majority of male caregivers who choose not to be affiliated with such programs and organizations. Certainly, random samples drawn from the larger population of unaffiliated male caregivers would maximize representativeness and allow for greater assurance when drawing conclusions or making generalizations. As such, further research is needed in order to insure a more thorough understanding of the male caregiving experience. Analyses need to reflect a more comparative perspective both in terms of considerations of different subgroups of male caregivers as well as male and female caregiving experiences. Until those analyses have been performed, perspectives such as those put forward in this chapter must, unfortunately, await full confirmation.

Ultimately, research, policy, and programming addressing the needs of caregivers may need to be reassessed given likely bias toward (1) understanding family obligation based on the practice of white, majority-culture families; (2) the assumption that men have marginal capacity to care with commitment and ability that derives both from a sense of affection and duty; and (3) the enduring belief in a "gender boundary" for intimate care (Fisher, 1994). Following the lead of British analysts of the caregiving experience, rather than being primarily determined by gender, the obligation to care for an incapacitated elder may actually be influenced more strongly by marital relationship and long-term coresidence than by gender. Older men, especially spouses, are capable of expressing both a sense of personal obligation and feelings of affection when confronted with caregiving responsibilities, and have done so through responsible long-term engagement in a variety of helping tasks. Taken together, these realities will need to wield greater influence on the mindset of policymakers, program developers, and researchers if the circumstances of caregivers are to be fully understood and responded to responsibly.

REFERENCES

Arber, S., & Gilbert, N. (1990). Men: The forgotten carers. *Sociology, 23,* 111–118.

Archer, C. K., & MacLean, M. J. (1993). Husbands and sons as caregivers of chronically ill elderly women. *Journal of Gerontological Social Work, 21,* 5–23.

Barusch, A. S., & Spaid, W. M. (1989). Gender differences in caregiving: Why do wives report greater burden? *The Gerontologist, 29,* 667–676.

Bass, D. M., McKee, J. M., Deimling, G, & Mukherje, S. (1994). The influence of a diagnosed mental impairment on family caregiver strain. *Journal of Gerontology: Social Sciences, 49,* S146–S155.

Commonwealth Fund. (1992). *The nation's great overlooked resource: The contributions of Americans 55+.* New York, NY: Author.

Dwyer, J. W., & Coward, R. T. (1991). A multivariate comparison of the involvement of adult sons versus daughters in the care of impaired parents. *Journal of Gerontology: Social Sciences, 46,* S259–S269.

Fisher, M. (1994). Man-made care: Community care and older male carers. *British Journal of Social Work, 24,* 659–680.

Kaye, L. W., & Applegate, J. S. (1990). *Men as caregivers to the elderly: Understanding and aiding unrecognized family support.* Lexington, MA: Lexington Books.

Kaye, L. W., & Applegate, J. S. (1993). Family support groups for male caregivers: Benefits of participation. *Journal of Gerontological Social Work, 20,* 167–185.

Kaye, L. W., & Applegate, J. S. (1994). Older men and the family caregiving orientation. In E. L. Thompson, Jr. (Ed.), *Older men's lives* (pp. 218–236). Thousand Oaks, CA: Sage.

Kramer, B. J., & Kipnis, S. (1995). Eldercare and work-role conflict: Toward an understanding of gender differences in caregiver burden. *The Gerontologist, 35,* 340–348.

Miller, B. (1991). Elderly married couples, gender, and caregiver strain. *Advances in Medical Sociology, 2,* 245–266.

Monahan, D. J., Greene, V. L., & Coleman, P. D. (1992). Caregiver support groups: Factors affecting use of services. *Social Work, 37,* 254–260.

Montgomery, R. J. V., & Datwyler, M. M. (1990). Women & men in the caregiving role. *Generations, 14,* 34–38.

Morris, J. N., & Morris, S. A. (1992). Aging in place: The role of formal human services. *Generations, 16,* 41–48.

Motenko, A. K. (1989). The frustrations, gratifications, and well-being of dementia caregivers. *The Gerontologist, 29,* 166–172.

Mui, A. C., & Morrow-Howell, N. (1993). Sources of emotional strain among the oldest caregivers: Differential experiences of siblings and spouses. *Research on Aging, 15,* 50–69.

O'Bryant, S. L., Straw, L. B., & Meddaugh, D. I. (1990). Contributions of the care-giving role to women's development. *Sex Roles, 23,* 645–658.

Office of Technology Assessment. (1987). *Losing a million minds: Confronting the tragedy of Alzheimer's and other dementias* (OTA–BA–323). Washington, DC: U.S. Government Printing Office.

Parker, G. (1993). *With this body: Caring and disability in marriage.* Buckingham, England: Open University Press.

Pruchno, R. A., & Potashnik, S. L. (1989). Caregiving spouses: Physical and mental health in perspective. *Journal of the American Geriatrics Society, 37,* 697–705.

Skelly, M. C., McAdoo, C. M., & Ostergard, S. M. (1993). Caregiver burden at McGuire Veterans Administration Medical Center. *Journal of Gerontological Social Work, 19,* 3–14.

Stoller, E. P. (1985). Elder-caregiver relationship in shared households. *Research on Aging, 7,* 175–193.

Stone, R. I., & Kemper, P. (1989). Spouses and children of disabled elders: How large a constituency for long-term care reform? *The Milbank Quarterly, 67,* 485–504.

Tennstedt, S., Crawford, S., & McKinlay, J. B. (1993). Determining the pattern of community care: Is coresidence more important than caregiver relationship. *Journal of Gerontology: Social Sciences, 48,* S74–S83.

Tennstedt, S., McKinlay, J. B., & Sullivan, L. M. (1989). Informal care for frail elders: The role of secondary caregivers. *The Gerontologist, 29,* 677–683.

CHAPTER 15

Community Programs and Services

Sheldon S. Tobin, Ph.D.

Community programs and services are intrinsic to the focus of many of the previous chapters. Retirement communities provide programs for their residents. Rural Americans use programs and services. Community mental health centers are ubiquitous. Services are available to the physically ill, substance abusers, those elderly persons physically or mentally abused and their perpetrators, and for assistance to family caregivers. There is, indeed, a numerous array of programs and services on the American landscape; some are in the public sector while others are in the private sector, some are for-profit, and other are not-for-profit, and some are sectarian in nature.

Whereas classifying these disparate, nonarticulating programs and services for the aging and their families is a challenge, one approach is to use two trichotomies: first, community-based, homebased, and congregate residential programs; and second, services for minimally, moderately, and severely impaired individuals (Tobin & Toseland, 1990).

For minimally impaired elderly persons, community-based programs include senior centers, congregate dining programs, information and referral services, and counseling. In turn, homebased services include transportation, home repair services, and telephone reassurance. Congregate residential programs encompass retirement communities and various kinds of senior housing arrangements.

For moderately impaired people, community-based services encompass multipurpose senior centers, community mental health centers, outpatient health services, and case management systems. Homebased services are comprised of foster family care, homemaker services, meals-on-wheels, and case management for family caregivers and their elderly impaired members. Congregate residential care includes group homes, sheltered residential facilities, board and care homes, and out-of-home respite care.

For severely impaired persons, there are community-based programs such as medical day care, psychiatric day care, and Alzheimer's family groups. Homebased services include home health care and protective services. Congregate residential services encompass acute hospitals, mental hospitals, nursing homes, and hospice care facilities.

FAMILY LIFE AND USE OF PROGRAMS AND SERVICES

Given this array of programs and services, can any generalizations be made regarding gender differences in use? It is, indeed, possible, because the normative pattern of family life changes with age. When aging couples are minimally impaired, they will use programs and services together. Then, because husbands usually become severely impaired before their wives, home care for husbands by elderly wives is the norm. Later, when women become widows, they will use the diversity of available programs for minimally impaired elderly persons if their health is adequate to permit them to do so. If moderately or severely impaired, care responsibilities for widowed women fall heavily upon their adult children, usually daughters and daughters-in-law, who may rely upon available services for the homebound.

This scenario of normative aging in the later part of life provides a blueprint for differential use of community programs and services by men and women. When both elderly spouses are minimally impaired, they will use the programs and services available to them as a couple. Together they will attend senior centers, dining programs, and attend counseling sessions (if there is marital discord). If neither drives, they will use discounted public transportation or special transportation for elderly persons. They may choose to relocate to senior housing or to move to a retirement community in a warmer climate.

When their aging husbands become ill, wives will seek community-based services (such as day care programs) to assist in caring, and also services brought into the home, including homemaker and home health services. If she becomes too burdened from caring, she may seek in-home or out-of-home respite care.

After her husband's death, she will enter the world of survivors—the world of widows—and may go alone to a senior center or to a congregate dining program. She will maintain her house, either by herself or with help from her children. As her health fails, she will depend more upon her children, and may move in with a daughter or daughter-in-law who may quit work to care or rely heavily on aides coming into the home. Later, she may enter a nursing home.

Which of the many available services will be used depends on many factors. The very religious may organize their service use around church and synagogue, and sectarian offerings also include counseling agencies and nursing homes. Nearness of children and the willingness of children to be of assistance will determine the extent of reliance on formal services. And, of course, more affluent senior citizens can afford luxurious retirement housing and continuing care communities, as well many kinds of in-home helpers.

Yet it is apparent that the normative scenario provides for only a general understanding of gender differences in how available programs and services are used. Moreover, the scenario elucidates why there is a chapter on women in Monk's (1990) comprehensive *Handbook of Gerontological Services,* but not a chapter on men. This chapter (Simon, 1990) is entitled "Services to widows and elderly women" and the author states: "In contrast with American elderly men, three-fourths of whom are married and live with their wives, three-fifths of elderly women have no spouse" (p. 327). Elderly women who become widows are likely to be impoverished (Minkler & Stone, 1985) and to need a great many community programs and services. But these facts should not imply that elderly men have no need for such community resources.

DIFFERENTIAL UTILIZATION

The scenario explains why the ratio of women to men for the moderately, as well as severely, impaired is quite high. Indeed, reports have revealed that three women for every man use family service agencies

(Kosberg & Garcia, 1988), community mental health centers (Mosher-Ashley, 1993), community-based supportive health services, as evidenced by participation in the federally funded National Long-Term Care Demonstration (better known as the "Channeling Demonstration") (Rabiner, 1992), and meal programs for the poor in senior service centers (Kirk & Rittner, 1993). This consistently high ratio of three women for every man across disparate kinds of services seems to reflect demographic differences of increasing percentages of women to men with advanced ages, added to by their status as widows who are more likely to be living alone with less income.

Kirk and Rittner (1993), for example, show that men and women who used daytime meal programs for the elderly poor in South Florida were remarkably similar. Although in the sample of 1,083 participants, of which over 90% were over 75 years of age, three-fourths (77.4%) were women; a very large majority of each gender were unattached (84.5% of the men and 91.5% of the women) and lived alone (70.2% of the men and 72% of the women). In turn, more than 9 of 10 lived in either an apartment or hotel which was rented on a weekly or monthly basis. Quality of life self-assessments differed somewhat: men reported higher levels of social interaction, and—whereas loneliness was ubiquitous, as was an overall poor quality of life—men reported being somewhat less lonely and having a somewhat better quality of life. Therefore, in this rare study, because of the focus on contrasting male and female participants in a service program, demographic variables revealed gender similarities with differences only in self-assessments of quality of life.

The Rabiner (1992) analysis of data from the Channeling Demonstration also revealed that, whereas the ratio again was three to one favoring the participation of women (74% women) in the sample that averaged nearly 80 years of age, gender *per se* had no effect on the extent of utilization. In the Channeling Demonstration, being African-American (which possibly was a proxy for socioeconomic status) and severe incapacities in the Activities of Daily Living were most associated with utilization. Men, however, reported being more satisfied with services than women, a finding congruent with that of Kirk and Rittner (1993).

Extant data suggest that both men and women with similar demographic characteristics, and apparently with the same needs, use available community services. However, use by so many more women than men could suggest an underutilization by men, particularly because of the conventional wisdom that younger men use mental and physical health services less than women. There is no evidence, however, that among elderly persons, men underutilize available services. Rather, it is more likely that they have a lesser need for these services because they are less likely to be widowed and, thereby, feel isolated and pauperized.

ATTITUDES TOWARD USAGE

Different attitudes by gender toward use of family service agencies, community mental health centers, community-based social and health services, and meal programs for the poor elderly, therefore, are not in evidence. This is not so for adult day care, which also is used more by women than by men. Kaye and Kirwin (1990), for example, found that female family caregivers (e.g., wives and daughters) were more likely than men (e.g., husbands and sons) to use adult day care as an "alternative to institutionalization;" that is, as an alternative to nursing home placement. In turn, Cohen-Mansfield, Besansky, Watson, and Bernhard (1994) found, among family members who chose not to use adult day care, females (mostly wives, but also daughters) either denied they needed help or believed it was their responsibility to provide the care.

Differences in caregivers' approaches to care by gender are congruent with how men (particularly husbands) focus on instrumental concerns, whereas women (particularly wives) focus on affective concerns. An illustration of how this difference in instrumental and affective aspects of care affects use of service can be found in a study on accessing adult day care (Force, 1993). In the study, husbands, wives, and daughters were compared. As expected, comparisons among 20 individuals in each group revealed that daughters were less ambivalent than spouses about using adult day care. Husbands in contrast to wives, however, were more concerned about the opinion of others, preferred to care at home, and valued their ability to provide care. Still, when home care became too overburdening, male spouses sought adult day care.

When queried on the timing of use, differences between husbands and wives emerged. Wives discussed their wish to delay the use of day care until care at home became physically draining and emotionally exhausting. Husbands, however, generally felt that as long as they were able to provide transportation for their wives, that they would have no need for day care. The availability of service-provided transportation was of negligible importance.

To be explicit, husband's maintenance of driving provided self-assurance that their caregiving was manageable. Husbands often said that "As long as I can drive, we are okay." Their instrumental, managerial approach to care was also evident in their greater use of home care services. Therefore, if husbands drive, their objective care burden is felt as less excessive, and they are less likely to use out-of-home day services in caring for their spouses. Wives, in turn, experiencing more affective burden, are likely to use day programs sooner for their husbands. Stated another way, a counterpart of the differences between elderly husbands and wives (in their attitudes toward spouse-caring) is their attitude toward use of out-of-home services, used later in the process of spouse-caring by husbands than by wives.

SENIOR CENTERS

Miner, Logan, and Spitze (1991) used the 1984 Supplement on Aging of the National Health Interview Survey to extend the analysis of Krout, Cutler and Coward (1990) regarding predictors of the frequency of attendance at senior centers. Although women attend senior centers more than men, gender was unrelated to the extent of attendance. When attendance was trichotomized into rarely, sometimes, or frequently attended, about one-fourth of both men and women attended rarely, close to one-third attended sometimes, and a little less than one-half attended frequently. Related to frequency of attendance were increasing age, less-educated, more social interaction, more volunteering, being white, and eating meals at the center. The predictor variables are a confusing set because "less educated" and "eating meals" reflects a service function needed more by those with lower income, whereas "more social interaction" and "more volunteering" reflect a social function welcomed by higher-income participants.

Although men and women apparently use senior centers for similar reasons, a finer-grained portrait reveals some differences. Volunteering, for example, is not only more a woman's activity, but whereas female volunteers give social and altruistic reasons for volunteering, male volunteers are likely to give only altruistic reasons (Morrow-Howell & Mui, 1989).

Then, too, interaction in senior centers may reveal differential gender behavior because of the shortage of available men as companions. Anecdotal reports of interaction in senior centers, in retirement communities, and in senior housing are often revealing of how widows compete for the too few widowers, particularly to be companions at meals. An 88-year-old widow in upscale senior housing said, "I am nice to everybody here but I have a special friend, Ben, who eats dinner with me. He lost his wife after a long illness." Similar comments can be heard in nursing homes among widows who are not severely demented.

THERAPEUTIC ENCOUNTERS

Throughout the settings of programs and services, as well as for individuals at different levels of impairment, there are therapeutic encounters that enhance functioning of elderly persons and their families. These encounters range from advice-giving to counseling to psychotherapy. Advice-giving, which is sometimes referred to as consultation, consists of providing information about, and discussing, alternative courses of action that can be followed. Counseling goes further by helping patients and clients to understand their current behaviors. In turn, psychotherapy seeks this understanding, often referred to as insight, by assisting patients and clients to explore in-depth relationships between current behaviors and their causes in early socialization; that is, the uncovering of unconscious feelings and motives.

All three kinds of therapeutic encounters appear in the gerontological literature. The focus of advice-giving and counseling, however, has largely been on families that include aging persons (Smith, Tobin, Robertson-Tchabo, & Power, 1994). Still, it is rare to find any discussions of gender differences for the three kinds of encounters. Whereas therapists, when treating elderly persons, are likely to experience evoked feelings of dependency, deterioration, and death, as well as concerns related to care of their own parents, there is no evidence that elderly men evoke these common countertransference issues more than do woman. Yet, beyond the idiosyncracies of each therapist and elderly individual in treatment, gender will influence countertransferences.

Instructive is the Poggi and Berland (1985) experience. When these two male child psychoanalysts convened a newcomers' group of elderly women in senior housing, they felt infantilized when the women referred to them as "boys." They were unable to perceive the women as gender-specific women until they (the two authors) discussed their feelings with each other and together noted their avoidance of reaffirming the women's identities by focusing on the women's deficits and needs for concrete assistance. The desexualizing would not have occurred if the group consisted of men or if the cotherapists were women, because there would not be the need to desexualize the maternal figures. Possibly, however, when women treat elderly men, there is a corresponding need to desexualize paternal figures.

Although there are both anecdotal and study reports of successful outcomes to treatment of elderly men and women, little has been written contrasting outcomes for men and women. An exception is the study of Lazarus and Groves (1987). Eight patients, four men and four women, were treated by different, experienced, psychodynamically oriented therapists for 15 weekly sessions of 50 minutes each. Significant gender differences were found in treatment effects for the group. Men showed less symptomatic improvement and psychodynamic change than women, and their improvements occurred later in the therapy. Also, they did not maintain the degree of symptomatic improvement as well as the women at 6-month followup. These differences in outcome were explained by Lazarus and Groves:

> In contrast to the women patients, the men were far less active psychologically, or physically, in trying to resolve their focal conflicts. Instead they tended to remain enmeshed in the provocative interpersonal relationship or situation that precipitated their entry into psychotherapy. The therapist was used by the men as a substitute for nurturant, supportive, and calming objects currently not available in their intrapsychic or external worlds (pp. 287–288).

The women, however, needed their therapists "to reaffirm their competency and to gain permission to carry out some assertive instrumental plan. They became free to recognize, discharge, and even enjoy the masculine, aggressive aspects of their personalities which had been suppressed" (p. 286). These interpretations used to explain differences in outcomes by gender are congruent with Gutmann's (1987) formulation for developmental androgynous changes following the parental imperative.

The Lazarus and Groves study (1987) of brief psychodynamic therapy contrasts with the anecdotal reports of psychoanalysis with older patients. In their review of these reports, Brody and Semel (1993) found that men were reported to be amenable to psychoanalysis. Of course, successful psychoanalysis necessitates selected patients with sufficient ego strength to explore their innermost feelings and motives. They state: "It is evident in this brief review of several articles on the late life treatment of aging men that work issues were mentioned in the vast majority of those cases" (p. 110). This is certainly neither unanticipated nor surprising.

OTHER STUDIES

Cohen, Teresi, Holmes, and Roth (1988) studied the survival strategies of homeless men, many of whom are elderly. Shelter data suggest that one of four homeless males is 60 years of age or over, but this may be an underestimate, because many elderly men leave shelters because of fears of muggings and institutionalization.

Skid row inhabitants who live in "flop houses" and on the street can be considered an ignored population. Few have much income, and about one-half receive public assistance. Sicker than their aged peers, they rely for survival primarily on informal social supports from other homeless persons. Formal community programs which can exist in neighborhoods, however, assist in their survival. For example, soup kitchens under the auspice of religious organizations afford homeless men a warm meal and a warm place to stay. However, because the men often have to attend worship services to obtain warm meals, they may resist using such community resources.

Men also receive assistance from other religious organizations. Taylor and Chatters (1986) contrasted older African-American men and women receiving assistance from their churches. They found, as others have, that women attended church more frequently, were more likely to be church members, and expressed a higher degree of intrinsic religiosity than men. In this instance, the finding was among African-American elderly men and women. Yet, seredipitously and surprisingly, the level of assistance men and women received from church members did not differ. Social relationships and obligations, as well as social integration into their church, predicted assistance levels to individuals with gender having no effect on assistance.

Taylor and Chatters (1985) found that the assistance received is more of the informal type: three-fourths of 581 respondents reported receiving socioemotional support, and less than one of five (18.9%) reported receiving instrumental support. Yet, because churches and synagogues are formal organizations, they should be included in discussions of formal community programs, albeit congregations may function more as extended families than as impartial service providers. Palmore (1980), in commenting on their importance, wrote:

> Churches and synagogues deserve special consideration because they are the single most pervasive community institution to which the elderly belong. All the other community institutions considered together, including senior citizen centers, clubs for elders, unions, etc., do not involve as many elders as do churches and synagogues (p. 236).

CONCLUSION

The use of soup kitchens by homeless men, and assistance given by church members to African-American elderly men, are rare exceptions to the abundant literature on aging women. Streib and Binstock (1990) observed this discrepancy when discussing gender-oriented research:

> The contemporary growth of scholarship on women and aging seems to have received impetus from two major factors. One is the differential mortality patterns of men and women. . . . Gender scholarship on the social aspects of aging also appears to have evolved as part of the more general emergence of feminine studies in the social sciences (p. 3).

Congruent with this observation is the content of the popular general text *Social Gerontology*, written by Hooyman and Kiyak (1993). In the book, the only insertion for "men" in the index, for example, is "male climacterium," whereas under "women" there are 29 references including African-American, baby boomers, chronic disease, friendship, health status, mental health, sexuality, support systems, and volunteer work, among others. Only by more focused research on use of programs and services by men, on the attitudes of men toward programs and services, and on the outcomes of these programs and services for men can the neglect be rectified.

REFERENCES

Brody, C. M., & Semel, V. G. (1993). *Strategies for therapy with the elderly*. New York: Springer, 1986.

Cohen, C. I., Teresi, J., Holmes, A., & Roth, E. (1988). Survival strategies of older homeless men. *The Gerontologist, 28*, 58–65.

Cohen-Mansfield, J., Besansky, J., Watson, V., & Bernhard, L. J. (1994). Underutilization of adult day care: An exploratory study. *Journal of Gerontological Social Work, 22*, 21–39.

Force, L. T. (1993). *Spouses and children in accessing adult day care: Differences in attitudes and behaviors among daughters, husbands and wives.* Unpublished doctoral dissertation, University of Albany of the State University of New York.

Gutmann, D. (1987). *Reclaimed powers: Toward a psychology of men and women in later life*. New York: Basic Books.

Hooyman, N. R., & Kiyak H. A., (1993). *Social gerontology: A multidisciplinary perspective* (3rd ed.). Boston, MA: Allyn and Bacon.

Kaye, L. W., & Kirwin, P. M. (1990). Adult day care services for the elderly and their families: Lessons from the Pennsylvania experience. *Journal of Gerontological Social Work, 17*, 167–183.

Kirk, A., & Rittner, B. (1993). Old and poor: Comparison of female and male meal program participants. *Journal of Gerontological Social Work, 19*, 207–222.

Kosberg, J. I., & Garcia, J. L. (1987). The problems of older clients seen in a family service agency. *Journal of Gerontological Social Work, 11*, 141–153.

Krout, J. A., Cutler, S. I., & Coward, R. T. (1990). Correlates of senior center participation: A national analysis. *The Gerontologist, 30*, 72–79.

Lazarus, L. W., & Groves, L. (1987). Brief psychotherapy with the elderly: A study of process and outcome. In J. Sadavoy & M. Leszcz (Eds.), *Treating the elderly with psychotherapy* (pp. 265–293). Madison, CT: International Universities Press.

Miner, S., Logan, J. R., & Spitze, G. (1993). Predicting the frequency of senior center attendance. *The Gerontologist, 33*, 650–657.

Minkler, M., & Stone, R. (1985). The feminization of poverty and older women. *The Gerontologist, 25*, 351–357.

Monk, A. (Ed.). (1990). *Handbook of gerontological services* (2nd ed.). New York: Columbia University Press.

Morrow-Howell, N., & Mui, A. (1989). Elderly volunteers: Reasons for initiating and terminating service. *Journal of Gerontological Social Work, 13,* 21–34.

Mosher-Ashley, P. (1993). Referral patterns of elderly clients to a community mental health center. *Journal of Gerontological Social Work, 20,* 5–23.

Palmore, E. (1980). The social factors in aging. In E. Busse & D. Blazer (Eds.), *Handbook of geriatric psychiatry* (pp. 222–248). New York: Van Nostrand Reinhold.

Poggi, R. G., & Berland, D. I. (1985). The therapists' reactions to the elderly. *The Gerontologist, 25,* 508–513.

Rabiner, D. J. (1992). The relationship between program participation, use of formal in-home care, and satisfaction with care in an elderly population. *The Gerontologist, 32,* 805-812.

Simon, B. L. (1990). Services to widows and elderly women. In A. Monk (Ed.), *Handbook of gerontological services* (2nd ed.) (pp. 326–341). New York: Columbia University Press.

Smith, G. C., Tobin, S. S., Robertson-Tchabo, E. A., & Power, P. W. (Eds.). (1984). *Strengthening aging families; Diversity in practice and policy.* Thousand Oaks, CA: Sage.

Streib, G. F., & Binstock, R. H. (1990). Aging and the social sciences: Changes in the field. In R. H. Binstock & L. K. George (Eds.), *Handbook of aging and the social sciences* (3rd ed.). San Diego, CA: Academic Press.

Taylor, R. J., & Chatters, L. M. (1986). Church-based informal support among elderly blacks. *The Gerontologist, 41,* 637–643.

Tobin, S. S., & Toseland, R. W. (1990). Models of services for the elderly. In A. Monk (Ed.), *Handbook of gerontological services* (2nd ed.). New York: Columbia University Press.

CHAPTER 16

Support Groups for Older Men: Building on Strengths and Facilitating Relationships

Amanda Smith Barusch, D.S.W. * & Terry Peak, Ph.D.

INTRODUCTION

Participating in a support group does not match widespread notions of acceptable masculine activity. But careful examination suggests that this intervention modality may be surprisingly compatible both with men's experiences and their needs. Lacking the social support enjoyed by most women, older men are at a higher risk for alcohol abuse, suicide, and acute illness. Support groups that involve older men may effectively substitute for the support women derive from family and friends. As a result, support groups can serve a preventive function—protecting men from the effects of isolation and providing an opportunity for them to learn new ways of building emotionally satisfying relationships.

Yet, older men are less likely than older women to participate in, and more likely than older women to drop out of, most support groups offered by human service organizations (Yalom, 1985). These support groups are predominantly female. Most human service professionals and group leaders are women, as are most clients and group participants. The relative absence of older men from a setting dominated by women is hardly surprising. Although group structures and processes are not

---

* Authors are listed alphabetically.

designed to exclude men, their feminine bias can preclude the effective involvement of older men. This chapter is designed to identify those distinctive attributes of masculinity, and of older men, that have implications for support groups. Specific strategies are also offered for the effective recruiting and inclusion of older men in groups of various kinds.

MASCULINITY

The phrase "masculine mystique" has been used to describe the behaviors and attributes associated with traditional male socialization (Silverberg, 1986; Sternbach, 1990). Under this rubric, masculinity involves valuing independence over cooperation, cognition over emotion, and action over feelings. The traditional (stereotypic) male is strong and in control of both his emotions and his immediate environment.

Any discussion of "masculine," as a trait, risks stereotyping and overgeneralization. Clearly, an individual man (just like an individual woman) has both masculine and feminine traits. In this chapter, prototypic male traits are used primarily for illustrative purposes (recognizing, of course, the variations of masculinity that exist both within and among men).

Men become masculine in response to, and in interaction with, what they perceive to be the integral parts of the societal definition of masculinity. That definition is affected by both societal pressures—the social construction of masculinity (Kimmel & Messner, 1989)—and personal needs (that may change over time). While girls learn to establish intimate, confiding relationships with friends, peer contacts between boys are largely characterized by competition. Their involvement in team sports teaches them to play by the rules, and to play to win. The on-the-job experiences of males also train them not to share emotions, but to engage in parallel activities designed to accomplish clear and measurable goals. Some have argued that in their later years, men experience the freedom to explore more nurturing or feminine activities.

Concerns with gender equity, and a blurring of gender roles, are leading men and women away from the traditional socialization patterns. However, most older men still embrace these views of masculinity and, perhaps as a result, enjoy less emotional and social support than do their female counterparts.

THE USE OF SOCIAL SUPPORT

Cantor and Litwak offer contrasting descriptions of older people's use of social support. Cantor (1979) suggests a "hierarchical-compensatory model" that emphasizes the nature of the relationship between helper and help recipient. In Cantor's view, older adults seek assistance from individuals in their social networks in a clear order of preference, regardless of the specific task involved, beginning first with kin (spouse, then adult children), followed by friends and neighbors. The unmarried also turn to kin first—their children—followed by other relatives, then friends and neighbors. Litwak (1985) suggests a task-specific model, in which older adults select helpers according to their suitability for the needed task. In this view, an older adult who needs immediate help with a specific task would turn to neighbors, while one who needed long-term support or assistance of an intimate nature would approach family members.

Regardless of the process by which older adults seek assistance, social support is clearly associated with health benefits. Schwarzer and Leppin (1989), in their meta-analysis of 55 studies on the general topic of social support and health, concluded that "ill health is more pronounced for those who lack support" (p. 11). In their major review article on this topic, House, Landis, and Umberson (1988) stated that the absence of social relationships may constitute a risk factor for health. Cohen and Syme (1985), in *Social Support and Health*, write that one value of social support is in promoting positive self-change by altering behavior and emotions. Modifying a person's social support environment may be the most cost-effective method for coping with chronic stressors and health problems.

Men and women differ in both the structure of their support networks and the processes by which they seek assistance. Older men are more likely than older women to be married and, hence, to have a spouse able to provide assistance. Older women compensate for the lack of a spouse through rich patterns of mutual assistance with friends and neighbors. Throughout their adult years, most married women maintain exchanges of assistance with friends and neighbors that are more active and intense than similar exchange patterns among married men. Lifelong tendencies to reach outside the marital relationship for social support prepare older women for active participation in support groups.

SUPPORT GROUPS IN THE UNITED STATES

Most support groups in the United States consist of voluntary associations formed for mutual benefit. The first documented support group was established by the Jewish Blind Society in 1819. It was followed 100 years later by the "Not Forgotten Association of Wounded War/Veterans" in 1920, and the "National Deaf and Blind Helpers League" in 1928 (Goldstein, 1990). Alcoholics Anonymous was founded in 1947 in Great Britain, and rapidly became one of the most well-known self-help organizations in the U.S. The National Alliance for the Mentally Ill was established in the U.S. in 1979, and has been a major force in policy development for the chronically mentally ill.

During the 1980s, the availability of support groups increased dramatically, so much so that an estimated 15 million people participated each week (Leerhsen, Lewis, Pomper, Davenport, & Nelson, 1990). Indeed, the importance of the self-help movement was recognized by former Surgeon General C. Everett Koop, who established a nationwide clearinghouse for information on mutual support groups. This active support from the Surgeon General helped to promote the growing acceptance of self-help groups as a treatment modality (Riessman & Gartner, 1987). The self-help movement has been seen as a way to empower individuals and to democratize everyday life.

Support groups are also viewed as an inexpensive, yet effective, method of providing support that can, in a wide variety of situations, lessen the stress and anxiety caused by difficult circumstances. Support groups have been formed to address a tremendous array of problems. Targets of support group intervention can range from individuals who are themselves suffering with a chronic ailment or problem to those who are involved in caregiving and support. Support groups have been formed for people who have cancer as well as for people who are related to someone with cancer, for people who are recovering from an addiction as well as those for people related to someone who is in either recovery or denial, for couples who are infertile, for parents who are interested in home schooling, for parents of a child who is gay or lesbian, for mothers of twins, for women who believe strongly in breastfeeding, and for those who want to lose weight, as well as for those with an eating disorder.

Given their diversity, it is difficult to speculate on the demographics of support groups. In 1989, Toseland and Rossiter observed: "Most participants in caregiver groups are white, middle-class persons" (p. 447). This probably holds true for most support groups offered through human service organizations. Groups are also more likely to be available in urban, rather than rural, settings. It is unclear to what extent, if any, the phenomenal growth of self-help and support groups has increased their availability to ethnic-minority and low-income populations.

Support groups can prevent the burden of a problem from overwhelming a person's resources. Support groups typically offer information about services available in the community, as well as understanding that is generally derived from personal experience with the problem. A frequent topic of discussion is how to obtain assistance from family members and friends—to build an effective individual support network. General sharing of feelings is another common group activity. In fact, for participants, the freedom to discuss and share feelings among nonjudgmental peers may be the most utilized component of support groups (Peak, 1993).

Cohen and Syme (1985) refer to three issues that help determine whether a support group will have a positive impact on its participants. One important issue is reciprocity. The opportunity to assume both roles, that of giver and receiver, can increase the perceived equity of a social transaction and, hence, the effectiveness of a support group. Reciprocity is particularly important for involvement of older men, who may feel more comfortable receiving help after they have given some. A second issue is the match between the type of support offered and the type of problem. A support group can provide its participants with support, education, and concern in a nonjudgmental environment to sustain and/or improve their well-being. A third issue has to do with timing. Support groups may be more effective at some times than at others. For example, a group that reaches people in the early stages of a chronic illness may be more effective than one offered in middle or later stages. Further, the reliable long-term provision of social support may increase feelings of well-being.

The support offered by a group may increase participants' sense of well-being. Weiss (1974) identified six dimensions of social support: attachment, social integration, opportunity for nurturance, reassurance of worth, a sense of reliable alliance, and the obtaining of guidance. He suggested that support groups offer assistance along each dimension, and that all six are necessary for individuals to feel they are adequately supported. Support group members give and receive help and information. Support group interactions help to instill hope in group participants. Members learn they are not alone with their problems and, as a result, are able to normalize their problems through the group interaction.

SUPPORT GROUP EFFECTIVENESS

If support groups were not overwhelmingly perceived as helpful, their numbers would not continue to grow. Popular evidence aside, there have been other, more rigorous, attempts to document the effectiveness of this model. Unfortunately, methodological limitations reduce the capacity of most research to demonstrate the effectiveness of support groups. For example, as Haley (1989) points out, a typical problem in conducting research on support group effectiveness is difficulty recruiting a pool of participants of sufficient number for various statistical tests. A related issue is the general lack of random assignment of participants to treatment conditions. Another problem has been the length of time that groups meet. Support groups that have been the focus of research efforts are short-term in nature, typically meeting for 8 weeks or less. An effect would have to be very powerful to be significantly evident after 8 weeks.

Despite these limitations, some evidence does suggest that support groups are effective. Evaluations have revealed moderate effectiveness on outcome measures, such as caregiver burden (Barusch & Spaid, 1991) and health (Spiegel, 1995). With a few exceptions, most evaluation studies have not explicitly examined cost savings as an outcome measure but, in cost-conscious times, this is beginning to change. For example, a recent study that looked at the cost-effectiveness of a support group for caregivers of frail elderly veterans found that participants had significantly lower health care costs than did members of a control group (Peak, Toseland, & Banks, 1995).

Perhaps the greatest testimony to the effectiveness of support groups is their widespread popularity. Participants consistently report high levels of satisfaction with their groups, even when evaluations show little or no improvement on global measures of well-being (Barusch, 1991; Gallagher, Lovett, & Zeiss, 1989; Toseland & Rossiter, 1989; Zarit & Teri, 1991). Their satisfaction is critical. Participants are probably the most important constituency supporting development and continuation of support groups.

Later Life Challenges

Late life presents some men with nontraditional challenges, such as caregiving and widowerhood, for which their socialization and life experiences may have left them ill-prepared. Others may find that normative changes, such as retirement, challenge their lifelong coping patterns. Failure to accommodate to these changes may leave older men at risk for problems related to social isolation, such as substance abuse and suicide.

Support groups designed to accommodate the needs and interests of older men can help them cope with these challenges. Caregiver support and bereavement groups differ slightly from those designed to address substance abuse problems. While utilizing the same positive self-help group components, caregiver support and bereavement groups act in a preventive capacity by reducing the likelihood that participants will experience the isolation associated with late-onset alcoholism. Clearly, groups designed to support people through these challenges can also serve an important suicide-prevention function.

Caregiving

As the number of elderly in need of care expands, and the size of families shrinks, older men are increasingly finding themselves in the role of family caregivers. As Kaye and Applegate (1990) noted, men respond differently to caregiving than women. Men consistently report lower levels of burden associated with caregiving, perhaps because their experiences are substantially different (Barusch & Spaid, 1989). Men who assume the caregiving role are usually older than women. Despite the physical limitations often associated with advanced age, older caregivers may experience less role strain. Caregiving men also receive more instrumental assistance with caregiving tasks than do women. While female caregivers generally have more sources of emotional support, men typically receive more help with tasks such as home nursing and housework. Gender differences have also been reported in the type of care provided by men (Barusch & Spaid, 1989). While women are more involved in personal care, men charged with caregiving typically find personal care extremely difficult and delegate it whenever possible.

Kay and Applegate (1990) suggest that men who are successful caregivers increasingly assume functions traditionally associated with the feminine role. Indeed, in their study of caregivers, they found men reporting that they derived the greatest degree of satisfaction from the provision of emotional and social support. Caregiving may provide men the opportunity to reconceptualize their understanding of masculinity.

Caregiver support groups can provide men a forum for accomplishing this task, even as they provide opportunities for exchange of information and problem solving around the daily challenges of caring for a disabled loved one. Perhaps more importantly, as one caregiver newsletter put it "They are living proof that you are truly not alone" (Northwest Caregiver, Winter/Spring 1996, p. 6).

Widowhood

Bly (1986) has said "Grief is the doorway to a man's feelings." Although the vast majority of widowed people in the United States are female, a significant proportion (estimated at 17% by the National Widowed Persons Service in 1988) is male (Brabant, Forsyth, & Melancon, 1992). When Israeli Prime Minister Menachem Begin resigned soon after his wife's death, many suggested his high level of distress was typical of male widowers—that men experience greater emotional distress upon bereavement than do women. In fact, there is little conclusive evidence that widowers have more depression, anxiety, or mental illness than widows; yet, men do have a higher risk of mortality during the first year of their bereavement than women (Jacobs & Ostfeld, 1977).

There is evidence that widowed women ask for, and receive, more social support throughout their bereavement process than do men. This may be because men do not know how to ask for help in dealing with intense personal feelings of loss. Most men rely on their spouses for intimate emotional support and are ill-prepared to reach out to others. As mentioned above, women maintain a wider network of confiding relationships that may include other family members, friends, and neighbors. The loss of a spouse may be equally devastating for men and women, but women have the social support networks and the help-seeking skills to cope with bereavement, whereas many older men lack both the networks and the skills. Widowhood also presents both men and women the challenge of assuming the tasks usually performed by a spouse. For older men this might involve learning to prepare meals and maintain a household.

Support groups for the widowed can provide a setting for learning these tasks. In mixed-gender groups, male participants might be called upon to teach women about the chores usually performed by husbands. In a reciprocal exchange, female participants might offer guidance on tasks often done by wives. Bereavement groups also help normalize the grieving process, allowing participants to understand that they are not alone in feeling like they are sometimes "going crazy." By providing supportive relationships, these groups constitute an important—even life-saving—resource for older men who have lost their wives.

Substance Abuse

Data from a national survey on drug abuse suggest that men abuse alcohol more then women at every age, by a ratio of at least four to one (Robbins, 1991). But the frequency of intoxication among men aged 65 and over is significantly higher than that of younger men. Isolation is often cited as a factor in the alcohol problems of older men. Indeed, older men who are married, or cohabiting, report being drunk significantly less than those who are widowed, never married, divorced, or separated. Role loss may also contribute to alcohol use and abuse among older men. Although employment status is not related to alcohol use among women, older men who are retired or work full-time drink significantly less than those who are unemployed or work in part-time jobs. Given the cross-sectional character of most representative surveys, it is difficult to ascertain whether isolation and role loss *cause* older men to drink or whether older men become isolated and unable to hold a full-time job as the *result* of alcohol abuse.

Late-onset alcoholism may account for one-third of adult alcoholism. Men who begin to have problems with drinking in their later years often do so upon loss of their spouses. While some have suggested this behavior reflects the absent spouse's role in regulating drinking, it may also be that older men use alcohol to numb their grief.

The success of Alcoholics Anonymous (AA) is testimony to the benefits of structured support groups for those coping with substance abuse. Most AA participants begin under some kind of mandate: court order, pressure from friends or family, from an employer or physician, or as an after-effect of treatment. Yet, continued participation in AA is testimony to the success of the treatment modality for this type of problem.

All the components of self-help—self-determination, mutuality, altruism, the small group format, personal, informal and direct interaction, and, most important, the promise of control over one's life—act in combination to strengthen the recovery process. For participants, the shared, common experience appears to be particularly helpful.

Suicide

Men over the age of 60 have the highest suicide mortality of any group in the United States. The overall 1988 rate of suicide in the U.S. was 12.4 per 100,000 population, compared to 21.0 per 100,000 elderly and 41.9 per 100,000 older men (McIntosh, 1992). Marriage, work, and finances seem to reduce the risk of suicide for older men. Married people, in general, have the lowest rates of suicide, followed by the never-married. Divorced and widowed adults have the highest risk of suicide. Consequently, bereaved men have been identified as a group with a particularly high risk of suicide. Similarly, men who are unemployed or retired are at higher risk than their working colleagues. Suicide among older men is also more common among lower-income than among middle- and upper-income men (Canetto, 1992).

Canetto (1992) offers an explanation of suicide rates for men that draws upon an understanding of male socialization and coping behavior, and suggests that socialization increases men's risk for suicide by reducing their flexibility. In Canetto's view, women are socialized to adapt to the needs of others and to the changing demands of their immediate environments. In contrast, men are taught to control their environments—to "shape the world" according to their needs. When faced with uncontrollable changes associated with age, men have a limited reper- toire of coping responses and are at greater risk of suicide.

With respect to suicide prevention, Canetto (1992) argues that "a balance of work and relationship commitments may be the best protec- tion against suicidal despair" (p. 94). In this view, the benefit of working lies in the relationship experiences and responsibilities. Similarly, rela- tionships increase the number of people adversely affected by a suicide. Support groups can reduce men's risk of suicide by expanding both their relationships and their responsibilities.

JOINING A SUPPORT GROUP

Participation in a support group has a cost. Apart from the obvious costs of transportation and time, participants also sacrifice their personal ob- jectives and preferences to the priorities of the group. Because control is part of the "masculine mystique," this loss of control may seem more costly to men than to women. Support groups may also carry a stigma for many older adults. While "baby boomers" may readily acknowledge an occasional need for help with personal and emotional problems, the current cohort of elderly is more reluctant to publicly acknowledge its need for help. Participation in a support group, particularly in a rural community, may constitute a public declaration of personal failure. Thus, inducements to join a group must be sufficient to compensate the older man for such potential costs.

Participants' motives for joining support groups vary tremendously. For some, despite the necessity to subsume some personal preferences to the group's will, membership is perceived as a way to be in control. There is an attractive antibureaucratic reliance on self (and similar others) inherent in support group participation that contributes to this sense of control. Another beneficial feature is the opportunity to explore universal aspects of the problem that unites all members. Because every- one in the group shares a certain amount of experience with the prob- lem, everyone is somewhat of an expert. Some group participants attend to compare their own situations with others, while others seek informa- tion or help with problem solving. Some look to support groups for emotional support and consolation; those overwhelmed by feelings of isolation are able to find companionship and relief from loneliness in the support group format (Bauman, Gervey, & Sigel, 1992; Levy & Derby, 1992). Whatever other benefits may accrue from group membership, the underlying principles of self-determination and empowerment (Madera, 1987) are the most universally redeeming qualities of support group participation.

While men are not typically members of support groups, they do serve as active participants and leaders in a wide range of voluntary associations. Groups designed to advance economic or political agendas are often controlled, staffed, and dominated by men. These include political action committees, Chambers of Commerce, investment clubs, and service organizations (such as the Elks, Kiwanis, and Rotary Clubs). Social and emotional support may not constitute inducements for men to join a group, whereas they may be more willing to enroll in task-focused groups.

RECRUITING OLDER MEN INTO SUPPORT GROUPS

Poorly designed recruiting activities can subtly discourage men from participation in support groups. Use of public service announcements and advertisements that present only women convey the message that a support group will not readily accommodate men. Similarly, sponsorship or location within a women's resource center, YWCA, or other women's organization might discourage men from participation. Scheduling a group during working hours clearly precludes participation by older men still in the labor force.

Efforts to recruit older men should be guided by an understanding of things men seek from a support group. Although they consistently report having less emotional support from family members and friends than do women, men typically do not seek emotional support from self-help groups. They tend to resist groups organized for therapeutic purposes (Van Zandt, Van Zandt, & Wang, 1994). The reasons men give for joining groups more commonly reflect their need for specific information and assistance with problem solving or their interest in comparing their situation with others. Thus, groups that offer educational activities and expert speakers may be attractive to men. Titles of group sessions, such as "Caregiver Seminar" or "Coping with Alzheimer's Disease," convey an educational focus that can be attractive to many men.

Sometimes men find the opportunity to *give* help more attractive than the chance to *receive* help. Davies, Priddy, and Tinkleberg (1986) reported that male caregivers of Alzheimer's patients resisted group therapy: "The concept of a small therapeutic group aroused a sense of skepticism in many of the male caregivers" (p. 386). Instead of offering emotional support or personal growth, Davies et al. recommended that men be given the opportunity to pilot a new intervention for male caregivers. The opportunity to participate in the development and evaluation of an intervention had much greater appeal for men. Clearly, for this group of older men, the opportunity to participate in the task of developing an intervention was more attractive than the chance to receive therapy.

Broad-based recruiting tools, such as public service announcements and newspaper advertisements, should present males as both participants and leaders in support groups. Individualized recruiting efforts should focus on each man's personal goals and interests, emphasizing the extent to which they are congruent with the group's mission and procedures. Some men may find the opportunity to serve as an "expert" an inducement to attend at least one session. As an introductory experience, a potential participant might be invited to present specific information to the group.

STRATEGIES FOR EFFECTIVE INVOLVEMENT OF OLDER MEN

The key to effective involvement of older men in support groups is designing an experience that builds on their strengths and is compatible with their relationship styles. Traditional male strengths include the capacity to "play by the rules" and to accomplish discrete, objective goals. Group formats that are well structured and that emphasize task achievement build on this strength. In contrast, process-oriented groups with less-structured formats may be uncomfortable for older men.

In relationships, the prototypical male emphasizes control, and avoids expressions of emotion. Here again, a process focus may create discomfort. Men are often uncomfortable with spontaneous outbursts of emotion. Predictable or ritualized expressions of emotion are less threatening. Thus, group rituals (such as an introductory handshake or a closing hug) offer safe expressions of affection for older men. Similarly, men in bereavement groups may find ritualized expressions of grief very satisfying.

There is some dispute over the relative merits of co-educational and gender-segregated support groups. Most older men had looked to women (their mothers and wives) for nurturance, and in co-educational groups men may look to women participants for emotional support. This tendency may represent an additional burden for support group women, who may be reluctant to reject the nurturing role. In an all-male support group, men must look to other men for emotional support. While some could argue that this represents a learning opportunity, it may also dampen the exchange of feelings. Pragmatically, most groups are organized not around gender, but around the problem situation. Although a few problems (such as prostate cancer) are exclusively male in nature, most involve men and women to various degrees. Leaders of support groups must be aware of the dynamics of gender, and be ready to intervene if the emotional needs of men increase the burdens of women participants.

Noting that, "Men are a hard to serve population group," Sternbach (1990, p. 23) described a therapeutic group for men. Called the "Men's Seminar," this ongoing group provides a supportive structure that encourages personal growth of men. The group process is very structured, with each participant required to "take a turn" talking without interruption. This benefits both speaker and listeners. The speaker enjoys the rare opportunity to explore his thoughts and feelings without judgement or distraction. The listeners have a chance to practice the art of "deep listening," a skill more often associated with women than men.

As evidence that men's desire for control may conflict with their preference for structure, Sternbach (1990) referred to the fact that men invariably question the structure of their group—a common experience for facilitators. When this happens, the leader acknowledges their concerns and suggests that the group structure be treated as an experiment and that they try it for a while, then reevaluate and revise the rules as necessary. Satisfied with this solution, participants generally agree to continue.

CONCLUSION

Men bring distinctive strengths and vulnerabilities to later life. They typically enter old age married and rely on a spouse for emotional support. Often, men are task-centered, prepared to achieve measurable goals. They look to their wives for nurturance and emotional intimacy, and lack an extended network of friends and confidants. Most older men predecease their wives. Those who do not are at higher risk of mortality and substance abuse. Older men, in general, are at higher risk for suicide than are older women. Many of these vulnerabilities have been linked to a lack of social and emotional support.

Groups tailored to recruit and involve older men can provide necessary, even life-saving, support. But older men are reluctant to join support groups, and have higher dropout rates than older women. It has been suggested that the dominant approach to group support has evolved within a feminine environment (human services), is implemented by women (human service professionals), and addresses primarily feminine concerns (emotional support). Older men may find this environment alien to their histories and personal styles.

Yet, the differences between older men and older women pale compared to their similarities. With a little consideration and accommodation, support groups can respond to the needs and relationship styles of older men. Inclusion of a male perspective will enrich the experience of all support group participants, even as it reinforces and expands the capabilities of older men.

REFERENCES

Barusch, A. S. (1991). *Elder care: Family training and support.* Newbury Park: Sage.

Barusch, A. S., & Spaid, W. M. (1989). Gender differences in caregiving: Why do wives report greater burden? *The Gerontologist, 29,* 667–676.

Barusch, A. S., & Spaid, W. M. (1991). Reducing caregiver burden through short-term training: Evaluation findings from a caregiver support group. *Journal of Gerontological Social Work, 17,* 7–33.

Bauman, L. J., Gervey, R., & Sigel, K. (1992). Factors associated with cancer patients' participation in support groups. *Journal of Psychosocial Oncology, 10,* 1–20.

Bly, R. (1986, April/May). Men's initiation rites. *Utne Reader.*

Brabant, S., Forsyth, C. J., & Melancon, C. (1992). Grieving men: Thoughts, feelings, and behaviors following deaths of wives. *The Hospice Journal, 8,* 33–47.

Canetto, S. S. (1992). Gender and suicide in the elderly. *Suicide and Life-Threatening Behavior, 22,* 80–97.

Cantor, M. H. (1979). Neighbors and friends: An overlooked resource in the informal support system. *Research on Aging, 1,* 434–463.

Cohen, S., & Syme, S. (1985). Issues in the study and application of social support. In S. Cohen & S. Syme (Eds.), *Social Support and Health* (pp. 3–22). Orlando, FL: Academic Press.

Davies, H., Priddy, J. M., & Tinkleberg, J. R. (1986). Support groups for male caregivers of Alzheimer's patients. *Clinical Gerontologist, 5,* 385–395.

Gallagher, D., Lovett, S., & Zeiss, A. (1989). Interventions with caregivers of frail elderly persons. In M. Ory & K. Bond (Eds.), *Aging and health care: Social science and policy perspectives* (pp. 167–190). New York: Routledge.

Goldstein, M. Z. (1990). The role of mutual support groups and family therapy for caregivers of demented elderly. *Journal of Geriatric Psychiatry, 23,* 117–128.

Haley, W. (1989). Group intervention for dementia family caregivers: A longitudinal perspective. *The Gerontologist, 29,* 478–480.

House, J., Landis, K., & Umberson, D. (1988). Social relationships and health. *Science, 241,* 540–545.

Jacobs, S., & Ostfeld, A. (1977). An epidemiological review of the mortality of bereavement. *Psychosomatic Medicine, 39,* 344–357.

Kaye, L., & Applegate, J. (1990). *Men as caregivers to the elderly.* Lexington, MA: Lexington Books.

Kimmel, M., & Messner, M. (1989). *Men's lives.* New York, NY: Macmillan.

Leerhsen, C., Lewis, S. D., Pomper, S., Davenport, L., & Nelson, M. (1990, February 5). Unite and conquer. *Newsweek,* 50–55.

Levy, L. H., & Derby, J. F. (1992). Bereavement support groups: Who joins; who does not; and why. *American Journal of Community Psychology, 20,* 649–662.

Litwak, E. (1985). *Helping the elderly: The complementary roles of informal networks and formal helping systems.* New York: Guilford.

Madera, E. (1987). Supporting self-help: A clearinghouse perspective. *Social Policy, 18,* 28–29.

McIntosh, J. L. (1992). Epidemiology of suicide in the elderly. *Suicide and Life-Threatening Behavior, 22,* 15–35.

Peak, T. (1993). Impact of a social support program for spouse-caregivers on the health costs and utilization of frail, elderly veterans. *Dissertation Abstracts International, 54,* 4, October, 1544-A.

Peak, T., Toseland, R., & Banks, S. (1995). The impact of a spouse-caregiver support group on care recipient health care costs. *Journal of Aging and Health, 7,* 427–449.

Peters, G. R., Hoyt, D. R., Babchuk, N., Kaiser, M., & Iijima, Y. (1987). Primary-group support systems of the aged. *Research on Aging, 9,* 392–416.

Riessman, R., & Gartner, A. (1987). The surgeon-general and the self-help ethos. *Social Policy,* 23–25.

Robbins, C. A. (1991). Social roles and alcohol abuse among older men and women. *Family and Community Health, 13,* 37–48.

Schwarzer, R., & Leppin, A. (1989). Social support and health: A meta-analysis. *Psychology and Health, 3,* 1–15.

Silverberg, R. A. (1986). *Psychotherapy with men: Transcending the masculine mystique.* Springfield, IL: Charles C Thomas.

Spiegel, D. (1995). How do you feel about cancer now? Survival and psychosocial support. *Public Health Reports, 110,* 298–300.

Sternbach, J. (1990). The men's seminar: An educational and support group for men. *Social Work with Groups, 13,* 23–39.

Toseland, R., & Rossiter, C. (1989). Group interventions to support family caregivers: A review and analysis. *The Gerontologist, 29,* 438–448.

Van Zandt, P. L., Van Zandt, S. L., & Wang, A. (1994). The role of support groups in adjusting to visual impairment in old age. *Journal of Visual Impairment and Blindness, 88,* 244–252.

Weiss, R. (1974). The provisions of social relationships. In Z. Rubin (Ed.), *Doing unto others* (pp. 17–26). Englewood Cliffs, NJ: Prentice-Hall.

Yalom, I. (1985). *The theory and practice of group psychotherapy* (3rd ed.). New York: Basic Books.

Zarit, S., & Teri, L. (1991). Interventions and services for family caregivers. In K. Warner Schaie (Ed.), *Annual review of gerontology and geriatrics*: Vol. III (pp. 287–310). New York: Springer.

CHAPTER *17*

The Institutionalization of Elderly Men*

Theodore H. Koff, Ed.D.

"Throughout recorded history, few fears have cut as deeply into the soul of man as the fear of growing old" (Moss & Halamandaris, 1977, p. 9). In addition, the fear of growing old has been accompanied for many by adverse experiences, such as aging with illness and severe disability, loss of loved ones (especially spouse and children), and institutionalization resulting from lack of resources to be cared for properly and to receive needed care in one's own home. For the oldest of the men in society, the prospect of living in a nursing home has become both a last refuge and a source of great anxiety.

For many, living in a nursing home may represent a short period of rehabilitation before returning home, a postponement of the pleasures of home, and a brief interlude in the trajectory of aging and disability. However, for many others, a transfer to a nursing home, rather than continuing to receive care in a hospital, may give rise to an unspoken fear of the nursing home becoming a permanent residence.

Changes in hospital payment mechanisms, especially the diagnostic-related group (DRG) system, has resulted in shorter periods of hospitalization and increased use of nursing homes for short-term rehabilitative periods, a type of care previously provided by hospitals. Older men,

*Appreciation for assistance in the preparation of this manuscript is extended to Bob Barba, Jai Larman and Sandy McGinnis.

socialized when hospital and nursing home use was significantly different from today, need to be helped to understand the changes that have
taken place and the purpose of institutionalization, especially if their
misunderstanding of the purpose conflicts with the contemporary role of
the institution. Therefore, it is important that the expectations for nursing home care be explored with a prospective resident and family members to establish a framework in which the nursing home staff, and its
intended service goals, are mutually understood.

Short-term residence, although having some of the same negative
characteristics older men fear in extended-care settings, is not the focus
of this chapter. Rather, the chapter focuses upon older men for whom a
nursing home will be a final residence.

In this context, a nursing home is intended to be a replacement for the
older man's prior home and his long-term residence. The events leading
to institutionalization, and its actual occurrence, form a period of trauma
for the intended resident as well as family members and friends. This
period is filled with the losses described above, anxiety about the uncer-
tainties of institutional life, the likelihood of some level of personal
incompetence, and awareness of personal proximity to death. Certainly,
becoming a permanent nursing home resident is not a status to be
celebrated. It is naturally associated with fear and avoidance encouraged
by a history of negative community attitudes based on poor care, abuse,
medical neglect, and denial of the respect that society should give its
elderly, in general, and older men, in particular.

How can this interlude in the living experiences of older men be made
an opportunity for continued growth, expression of self and, especially,
maleness? Responsiveness to the unique needs of the older man living in
an institution is often neglected. He is bathed, fed, dressed, entertained,
medicated, and nursed like anyone else in the nursing home without
concern for his maleness. Is maleness no longer important?

The Department of Veterans Affairs (formerly known as the Veterans Administration) has developed a network of facilities known as
nursing homes or domiciliaries. Because these programs are available to
those who have veterans' status, they are for the most part institutions
serving older men. Currently, the Department operates 130 nursing care
facilities and 39 domiciliaries, with 99% of the facilities occupied by
older men (J. Kolbe, personal communication, December, 1995). Many
states, through their own Departments of Veterans Affairs, own and
operate institutions for veterans and primarily serve elderly men. Some

communities also support private, subsidized nonhealth care institutions solely for men who, because of prior histories of drug or alcohol addiction or irregularities in their lifestyles or behavior, are thought to be inappropriate company for women. Obviously, it was intended that female residents not be part of the social fabric of these organizations.

THE LONG RIDE FROM HOME

A significant factor in adjustment to a move to a nursing home, from wherever the person may previously have resided, is willingness to move to the more restrictive setting. People rarely anticipate relocation into a nursing home with excitement and anticipation of new opportunities. Forcible relocation, whether implemented by legal entities, family, or medical constraints, is obviously the least desirable approach. It also should be recognized that persons from cultures which emphasize family care of the elderly (specifically, parents cared for by their children) may have the greatest difficulty dealing with involuntary transfer into an institutional setting.

Ethnic Minorities

For example, the rate of nursing home admissions is much higher for whites than for ethnic minority groups, indicating that ethnic minority families have an aversion to delegating the care of their elders to nursing homes. If an older minority male is living in a nursing home, it may mean that the individual's condition has deteriorated beyond the capacity of the family to provide the required care. In this case, it is likely that the family is not capable of implementing the cultural expectation of caring for elderly relatives, or that the family has adopted community mores and accepted that it is not wrong to institutionalize one's elders.

Providers of nursing home care should be especially sensitive to issues of familial strife or cultural dissidence within an ethnic minority family. When a nursing home is located on an Indian reservation or in the midst of an enclave consisting of a highly concentrated community of Asians or Hispanics, ethnic minority nursing homes (in which cultural traditions are observed) may have evolved because families live in close proximity to the home, and staff generally are representative of the population served. However, if American Indians who live in remote areas require institutionalization, they may find they have to be placed in nursing homes in unfamiliar urban communities where families are less able to visit on a regular basis. The absence of noninstitutional supportive services on reservations also contributes to the inability of families to care for older family members at home.

Easing the Transition

Whenever possible, it is important to permit the elderly person and close family members to be actively involved in issues related to moving to a nursing home. Even if reconsideration or reversal of the decision to institutionalize is not possible, the person to be affected can participate in the selection of a facility, the room or roommate, furniture, and personal items and clothing to be moved. The transfer may be eased through making several visits to the facility in order to meet the staff and, perhaps, participating in a meal and learning about life in the institutional setting. It can be helpful to introduce some male residents with whom the prospective resident might associate, and some male staff members who will provide personal care, meals, and activities. Such hospitality will help make the person feel that there is something to be gained by moving into the nursing home.

"It's no heaven, but I guess it's the best you can do when you need so much help." In a sense, this message often heard from those who currently live in health care facilities is sad, but it also reflects acceptance of the need for more care than can be provided at home. Any transfer to a nursing home from a hospital or the person's home should be a carefully orchestrated process that is very sensitive to the adverse issues of relocation trauma (Tesch, Nehrke, & Whitbourne, 1989).

Some male nursing home residents fight and contest every aspect of institutional care. One old man who had recently been admitted to a nursing home summarized the way he felt about institutional care when he said, "I have wanted to die ever since I went in that home in Summerville. I have thought of takin' my life. . . . I don't know why I hated that place so bad. I had no one. I was by myself. There was no menfolks in there too . . . there was one other man that you could get in a conversation with. There wasn't but three of us there" (Gubrium, 1993, p. 31).

Think about how hearing this plea—that death would have been preferable to having been sent to a nursing home—would have affected family members, other residents in the nursing home and, of course, the personnel who cared for this individual and had to deal with it on a recurrent basis.

HOME, AT LAST

A nursing home, frequently the care center of last choice for older men, must be responsive to both the residents' and family members' feelings about severe dependency and near-death experiences. Family members may need assistance in resolving issues related to cultural expectations of children's responsibilities to their parents, as well as to the fear of the impending loss of a parent and the consequences of that loss for their own lives.

On the other hand, there are those who speak of this living in an institution as an opportunity: "The best thing that could have happened to me. Three meals a day, lots of friends, housekeeping, laundry, transportation, entertainment, and even a cocktail party every evening before dinner. I never had it so good."

Do these individuals represent residents in the same institutions at the same time? Or do they, in fact, represent different cohorts of older persons living at different institutional settings for different reasons at different times? For some persons, institutional living responds appropriately to their dependency needs and reflects an enhancement of their lifestyle. Such men, like these, seem to make a favorable adjustment to living in a nursing home.

The most restrictive institutional environments disable their residents by limiting personal autonomy, independence, and opportunities for the expression of individual interests and preferences. Goffman (1961), in his landmark essay on the mental asylum (which represents the most restrictive of institutions), wrote that observations of the institutional restrictions of the asylum can be applied to other institutional living arrangements, because all such facilities have so much in common. Every institution has some value to the individual or to the society in which the individual resides. But all institutions also have encompassing tendencies, the most restrictive of which prevent or provide "the barrier to social intercourse with the outside and to departure (from the institution) that is often built right into the physical plant" (Goffman, 1961, p. 5).

Nursing homes, among the most restrictive of the institutions that respond to the needs of older persons, provide an environment beset with social hazards. They require residents to eat, sleep, and play with the same people, under the same authority, with the same set of rules, day after day. This results in boredom, the absence of stimulation, and possible depression. These adverse affects are most pronounced for older men because it is likely that they have a high level of disability and/ or absence of a helping spouse (the primary reasons for institutionalization), are less able to leave the setting intermittently, or are unable to express their autonomy by confronting upsetting rules or services. This set of circumstances dictates that those who are in greatest need for responsiveness by the institution are, in fact, in the greatest jeopardy of suffering the ultimate threat of living in an institution—the loss of autonomy. Institutions caring for older men must be especially sensitive to this issue and find ways to minimize its effects.

AUTONOMY, PATERNALISM AND BENEFICENCE

The due-process and equal rights protection guaranteed by the 14th Amendment to the Constitution are often abridged in the policies and admission agreements of nursing homes and compromised, especially in the care of men in nursing homes and in the absence of sensitivity on the part of health care practitioners (Hofland, 1988). Health care in the nursing home setting includes the provision of nursing and medical care and encompasses all aspects of food service, recreation, and various therapies, along with integration of these elements with the respective roles and contributions of friends and family members. The health care ethic of "beneficence," which prescribes a greater balance of good over harm in the provision of care, also requires alternatives in opportunities and variation in the types of care, and rejection of some activities considered undesirable by some persons. In displays of paternalism by health care providers, such rights for older men are often ignored.

Institutionalized people who are chronically ill often evoke in caregivers a strong sense of protectiveness, stemming from a belief in their own superior competence to provide care and nurturance to those in need of help. The resulting paternalism, or interference with the liberty of action of an individual, may be justified exclusively for reasons pertaining to the welfare, good, happiness, needs, interests, or values of the person being coerced. The traditional paternalism of health care is further encouraged by fears that debilitated and ill patients will make mistakes if left to make their own decisions (Hofland, 1988).

The Omnibus Budget Reconciliation Act of 1987 (OBRA, 1987) reinforced the rights of residents in nursing homes who are recipients of federal funds (as well as the rights guaranteed by the 14th Amendment) to maintain autonomy and to be informed of those rights, especially with regard to the acceptance or rejection of services administered by the members of the staff providing care within the institution. For older men, respect for rights must also deal with issues related to the expression of continuing maleness, including sexuality, autonomy, and leadership roles if those have been experienced over the years.

Another critical issue related to beneficence and/or paternalism involves the relationship between a physician and an older man. Where this relationship is of long standing and/or there are strong personal feelings, individual wishes as well as rights will be highly regarded and protected. However, this type of close relationship between a physician and an older man may have come to an end, with the growth of physician practices controlled by managed care or health maintenance organizations. Physician training has been and continues to be focused primarily on acute care (even though the increasing growth of the older population requires a much greater understanding of the dynamics of chronic care). Physicians providing care in nursing homes will be increasingly dependent on "physician extenders" like nurse practitioners and physician's assistants. During limited personal encounters, they may not recognize that there may be significant differences between the way they practice when dealing with an older man in a nursing home and in their acute care practice. It is possible that the time constraints imposed by organized medical practice will diminish opportunities to show sensitivity to the needs for autonomy of the older man.

> In acute care, patients have relatively short stays and face many potential life-and-death decisions requiring rapid resolution. In long-term

care, by contrast, older adults live for years with chronic conditions and often slow deterioration of health. Small everyday decisions are the heart of long term care and the time frame for decisions and opportunities for advanced planning expand considerably (Hofland, 1988, pp. 3–4).

Medical professionals who are unsympathetic to the sick-role expectations of institutionalized older men, and who believe them to be incompetent, discourage independence and nurture dependency (Chowdhary, 1990). The adverse impact of current changes in medical care practice in nursing homes is no more clearly stated than in the words of a newly qualified young physician, assigned to a nursing home practice, when he advised the attending nurse by telephone to deny a request for a man to have dinner with his family outside of the home. If the man could leave the facility, the physician reasoned, there was no need for him to be in an institution. In this case, having the older man's autonomy reduced by the rejection of the request probably caused greater harm to him than did any of the chronic conditions leading him to enter the nursing home. Such acts of paternalism should not be accepted in the practice of nursing home care. Nor should there be a need to ask permission from a physician for an individual to express his autonomy.

SOME DEFINITIONS

Initially, this chapter introduced some critical issues related to nursing homes in general. An important next step is to define some of the various types of institutional settings that are available to, and generally occupied by, older men.

"Nursing home" has evolved as the generic name for institutional care that provides some level of assistance to its residents. The category includes facilities that offer board and care, personal care, adult care, adult congregate living, sheltered care, assisted living, intermediate care, nursing care, and continuing care (retirement communities). This list is not exhaustive but merely representative. In some situations, state licensure requirements define a nursing home, irrespective of what name a facility uses to describe its care. In other settings, the focus is directed less on medical care than on the personal care needs of residents.

If an organized hierarchy of institutions serving older men were to exist, the nursing home would represent the most restrictive environment serving the most debilitated population. It is in these settings that the greatest problems with autonomy and paternalism can exist, as this population is likely to be more dependent on others for care.

Nursing homes call themselves by names that are intended to alleviate the fears of nursing homes by older persons. These names may be euphemisms like Golden Years, Summerville, or Happy Acres, or they may bear the corporate name of a sponsor such as Manor Care, Life Care, or Beverly Manor.

Despite attempts to disguise the fact that they are, indeed, nursing care facilities, the real distinguishing institutional characteristic is the formal licensing of the facility and the expectation of services provided by facilities holding that license. While a license (or the absence of same) may establish the range of services that are available, it also governs the range of needs presented by applicants for services and a facility's ability to continue to serve residents (in light of changing health care requirements).

Data from the 1991 National Health Provider Inventory (National Center for Health Statistics, 1991) show that there were approximately 379,130 men in nursing homes and approximately 115,307 men in board and care homes, a total of approximately 494,437 men institutionalized in these two settings alone. Not included are the number of men who may reside in some other kind of residential setting. This data source also reports that men occupy 38.1% of the beds in nursing homes and 26.6% of the beds in board and care facilities. Clearly, older men are in the minority in either setting, and where their percentages are increased, as in nursing homes, they are likely to suffer more impairments and require more health care than the men in board and care homes. The following paragraphs, therefore, are an interpretation of issues and concerns that affect the half million plus older men who are institution-alized in health care settings, and the need of these men for responsive care.

With the average age of nursing home residents about 84, it can be anticipated that this institutional population will have deteriorated in both physical and mental impairments.

Older men are typically cared for at home by a wife and/or other members of the family, and are institutionalized only when their care needs exceed the capacity of family members (or there is no family member) to provide care. The presence of a spouse decreases the likeli-hood of institutionalization for older men (Burr, 1990). Men typically marry women younger than themselves and women typically live longer than men, resulting in the expectation that most older men who suffer significant impairment in their activities of daily living will be cared for in their own residence by their wives. However, in the absence of the wife, or when care requirements exceed the capacity of the spouse, then institutionalization needs to be considered.

Yet, there are differences between African-American and white men in institutional use. Race is an important demographic characteristic because elderly whites are more likely to be living in an institution than elderly nonwhites. Yet, African-American men of the same generation are generally in poorer health, have less education, and have considerably lower incomes (Burr, 1990). The probability of being in a nursing home increases as a factor of demographics, economics, and health. Thus, as African-American men achieve longer life spans, their poorer health and lower economic status will increase their incidence of institutionalization. Burr (1990) further suggests that with marital disruption continuing to be a social problem for them, more older African-American men will find themselves in institutions instead of relying on family for the provision of care at home.

IT IS A FEMALE WORLD

Understanding the demographics of older men and women is critical to appreciating several of the more important attributes of older men in nursing care institutions. One of these is that an older man typically arrives at a nursing care institution much older than his female counterpart. He probably is in much greater need of institutional care because he has been cared for at home for a long time. In contrast, a woman arrives at an earlier age and with less dependency needs, having received far less care at home. Her spouse may have been disabled and unable to provide her with the needed care for any extended period of time; or he died.

Second, most nursing homes are essentially female environments, because, in general, fewer men survive to old age; and those who do are most likely to be in a severely disabled condition and live in the institution for a shorter time. In addition, there is a preponderance of female workers in this area of the health care field; it is a common complaint of men that they miss the opportunity to be with, and have time to spend with, men in male-oriented activities. Obviously, the existence of activities for older men is not the same across facilities, and it is difficult to duplicate a male resident's social and cultural environment prior to his institutionalization. However, nursing care institutions, because they are staffed predominantly by women providing care for women residents, view the opportunity for male recreational and creative activities through the filter of a female orientation. Even though female recreational staff and female nursing staff may do all that they can to accommodate the needs of the male residents, any male-oriented activities generally evolve from the perspective of the female employees. As a consequence, these activities often miss the mark of what would respond best to the needs of male residents. Furthermore, to introduce so-called "male-oriented" activities without regard for the uniqueness of each male resident would be to commit the institutional crime of "batching" all male residents.

What is needed is sensitivity to the needs of male residents expressed by taking the necessary time to interact with male residents and determine what in their life experiences could be continued within the institutional setting. Preferably, the institution would have available a competent male member of the staff with whom the male residents could relate. An additional challenge is that men often are admitted to a nursing home because they have lost a caretaker (or spouse) and may be experiencing a sense of loneliness, isolation, and depression.

Some might envy older men living as a minority in a female-oriented environment; but although this circumstance appears to offer opportunities for socializing activities, there are limitations to this minority status. Some men have expressed concern for having to bathe, dress, or use the toilet in the presence of female staff. They may resent having to be seen nude in their dependent circumstance. Modesty, and perhaps prior association with the same spouse for many years, causes discomfort at having to expose themselves in front of an unrelated female. This problem calls for greater sensitivity by female staff members to male modesty, negating the myth of the "dirty old man" wanting to expose himself to female employees. The need for male staff caretakers within the nursing care facility is the obvious approach for minimizing this concern regarding modesty.

WHAT ABOUT SEX?

The issues of intimacy and sexual activity (or fantasy) are frequently raised by men in nursing care institutions. Bullard-Poe, Powell, and Mulligan (1994) conceptualized physical intimacy as sexual and non-sexual, and reported that their findings showed that older men in institutions gave highest priority to what they refer to as social intimacy over any form of sexual intimacy. Some men have reported that female residents and staff seemed uncomfortable when a man attempted to engage in social intimacy with female residents—without any attempt to seduce a woman into sexual activities.

Sexual interest among older men exists, and is active, yet "few interventions are being taken to facilitate the expression of sexuality among residents of long-term care facilities . . ." (Wallace, 1992, p. 308). Nursing homes generally deprive their residents of their sexual rights. "The aged in nursing homes must frequently live in celibacy. The physical setting of many nursing homes desexualizes the environment" (Kaas, 1978, p. 373).

There are several major inhibitors to sexual encounters in institutions. One of these is absence of privacy, since most rooms are shared by two persons of the same gender and no provision is made to lock the bedroom for privacy. One nursing care center established a privacy room for residents and discovered, to their disappointment, that it was not used. Part of the problem may have been the need to reserve the room, thereby announcing to staff an intention to use the room for intimate purposes. Obviously, monitoring intimacy in this formal way does not encourage spontaneity.

Another inhibitor is disapproval on the part of nursing home staff members (predominantly female), who may attempt to protect the "unaware female resident," or who frown upon sexual behavior for those severely disabled who are institutionalized. Expression of intimacy within an institution is curtailed as a result of social constraints imposed by the visibility of behaviors in the very open living environment of an institution. What may happen in one corner of the institution is immediately known by all—staff and residents, and soon by the families of the residents—who may object to the behavior.

Intimacy for an older man who is interested and capable of sexuality is typically submerged, and may find expression in even less acceptable activities. Yet, the findings of Bullard-Poe et al. (1994), as related to institutionalized men, suggest that when "intimate interactions are increased, quality of life will improve even for the institutionalized elder" (p. 235).

WHO IS IN CONTROL?

One of the more difficult adjustments older men have to make in the institutional environment is having to relinquish control. Following the major adjustments that had to be made on entering an institution, even greater concessions to loss of control must be made. It becomes necessary to give up control over when meals are served, when to sleep and be awake, when to bathe, what to eat, whom to befriend, and whom to trust. If a man has earlier been in control, or perceived himself to be in control, of major issues of family, marriage, household, employment, leisure time, and religious beliefs and observations, he finds that all of these must be compromised in institutional living.

Older men who are in poor health may find themselves particularly isolated and deeply affected by the consequences of role loss (Ferraro & Barresi, 1982). Especially significant is diminishing control over continuing family relationships and friendships, particularly those that have been sustained over an extended period. "What can I contribute to this relationship to make it important for my family and friends to continue their social intimacy with me?" is a question frequently asked by older men (in words to that effect).

A significant adverse consequence of loss of control for older men may be depression. It is known that the incidence of depression among institutionalized older men is even greater than among older men living in the community. While it would be an error to attribute lack of control as the major cause of depression for a large group of institutionalized males, it appears that when giving up control over life's events represents a major change in an individual's lifestyle, it is a significant contributor to depression.

RESPONDING EFFECTIVELY TO COMPLEX NEEDS

When an older man has had to endure the complexity of losses that may have initially required him to enter an institution, he subsequently has to endure additional losses while living there. Multiple losses could include loss of spouse, health, functional capacities, income, role, status and—especially—autonomy, or the expression of self. The severity of the losses experienced by any individual depends upon that person's lifelong pattern of dealing with losses and the availability of supportive social contacts.

It might appear that little can be done by an institution to ameliorate the losses experienced prior to admission to a nursing home. In fact, the facility can either exacerbate or minimize the impact of these losses. An environment can and does have an impact on any individual. Whether the impact is positive or negative may be a product of the limits imposed by the institution, the extent of the disability or functional capacity of the individual, and the sensitivity of the institution for maintaining the autonomy and overall quality of life for its residents.

Obviously, an institution that provides a comfortable life style for rich and capable individuals is far less likely to impose upon its residents' autonomy. In relatively costly life care or retirement communities, the residents may be responsible for the facility's management. They select the management firm, control the budget and expenditures, and may even control who may be admitted into their midst. Within reason, they control their own choice of menus, hours of eating, time for play, and the nature of their recreational activities.

Such autonomy is not a reality in the conventional nursing home to which residents are admitted, because disabling health problems prevent their continued living in their own homes. In these facilities, autonomy may be compromised by acts of paternalism by care providers, who presume that residents need others to act on their behalf.

Quality of life in an institution seems to depend most on the sensitivity of all of the participants in the institutional setting to the unique needs of each resident. Provision of appropriate care should, wherever possible, respect the need of any individual to retain individual autonomy. In particular, the needs of the male residents need to be seen through the eyes of a male.

Issues related to ethics, personal values, freedom, and paternalism are part of the complex of chronic care (Koff, 1988). The providers of services need to be guided by the ethical standards of the organization, as reinforced by continuing education and the modeling of ethical behavior by the organization's leadership. Chronically ill older persons can be unwittingly exposed to the indignities of paternalism, abuse, or other unethical behavior because of the desire to respond to the needs of those who are severely dependent. Maintenance of the dignity of the person requires careful attention to, and review of, the patterns of care to make certain they reflect the ethical standards expected of providers of chronic care.

REFERENCES

Bullard-Poe, L., Powell, C., & Mulligan, T. (1994). The importance of intimacy to men living in a nursing home. *Archives of Sexual Behavior, 23*, 231–237.

Burr, J. (1990). Race/sex comparisons of elderly living arrangements. *Research on Aging, 12*, 507–530.

Chowdhary, U. (1990). Notion of control and self-esteem of institutionalized older men. *Preceptual and Motor Skills, 70*, 731–738.

Ferraro, K., & Barresi, C. (1982). The impact of widowhood on the social relations of older persons. *Research on Aging, 4*, 227–247.

Goffman, E. (1961). *Asylums*. Garden City, NY: Anchor.

Gubrium, J. (1993). *Speaking of life: Horizons of meaning for nursing home residents*. New York: Aldine DeGruyter.

Hofland, B. (1988). Autonomy in long term care: Background issues and a programmatic response. *The Gerontologist, 28*(Suppl.), 3–9.

Kaas, M. (1978). Sexual expression of the elderly in nursing homes. *The Gerontologist, 18*, 372–378.

Koff, T. (1988). *New approaches to health care for an aging population*. San Francisco: Jossey-Bass.

Moss, F., & Halamandaris, V. (1977). *Too old, too sick, too bad: Nursing homes in America*. Germantown, MD: Aspen.

National Center for Health Statistics. (1991). *National Health Provider Inventory* (unpublished tables). Atlanta: U.S. Department of Health, Public Health Service, Centers for Disease Control and Prevention/National Center for Health Statistics.

Tesch, S., Nehrke, M., & Whitbourne, S. (1989). Social relationships, psychosocial adaptation, and intrainstitutional relocation of elderly men. *The Gerontologist, 29*, 517–523.

Wallace, M. (1992). Management of sexual relationships among elderly residents of long-term care facilities. *Geriatric Nursing*, 308–311.

F.   Conclusion

CHAPTER 18

The Status of Older Men: Current Perspectives and Future Projections

Jordan I. Kosberg, Ph.D. & Lenard W. Kaye, D.S.W.

STEREOTYPIC GENERALIZATIONS

Thompson's chapter, "Older Men as Invisible Men in Contemporary Society," in his edited book, *Older Men's Lives* (1994) cogently discusses the reasons why elderly men have not been the focus of professional research and practice, or public concern, and—thus—are invisible. Their marginality, in part, results from the fact that elderly men exist in smaller numbers and proportion in relationship to elderly women.

But among other explanations for the failure to focus upon the needs of elderly men is the view that older men enjoy a better quality of life than do elderly women. Yet, an alternate (and paradoxical) explanation for the failure to be concerned about providing nonmedical resources, in particular, to elderly men is the belief that they are primarily highly impaired and need only health care. Finally, Thompson suggests that the masculinities of individual elderly men have been "marginalized," rendering them a homogenized (and faceless) group.

To the generalizations of elderly men being privileged and powerful, or—alternatively—impaired and dependent, can be added the deprecating humor which portrays them as "dirty old men" or bumbling incompetents. It is wondered whether a film entitled "Grumpy Old Women" would have been produced and tolerated by the general public, as has

"Grumpy Old Men" and its sequel. The practice of making fun of elderly men has long existed in the mass media, and it is demeaning.

Any effort to broadly describe elderly men (or any group of elderly, for that matter) is to engage in a gross over-generalization which is inaccurate and unfair, and glosses over differences between subgroups of the elderly differentiated by age and a myriad of other socio-demographic characteristics. Moreover, any effort to describe elderly men must be done comparatively, in relation to a comparison group.

THE NEED FOR A COMPARATIVE APPROACH

As suggested by the chapters within this book, discussions of elderly men should have a comparative frame of reference upon which conclusions are drawn. The major comparison group, no doubt, would be elderly women; yet, comparisons of elderly men to younger men also have importance.

In a similar vein, comparative studies may include a sample of elderly men as their own control. This is to suggest a view of the changes which impact men as they age, and the adversities which affect the quality of their lives as they pass through the various stages of the life continuum.

If men are alleged to enjoy more benefits in life, they also have more to lose during the aging process. As suggested by Barer (1994), while it can be true that men—even older ones—might face fewer decrements, enjoy more independence, and exercise more control over their environments, their well-being may be in greater jeopardy as a result of such unanticipated events as widowerhood, caregiving, and relocation. It is realized that this notion of possible greater relative deprivation suffered by men will not result in sympathetic responses from all persons.

The utility of the comparative theme is made more complex, of course, by the diversity of elderly men. In discussing the losses faced by elderly men, and the likelihood of their using informal assistance and formal services, Wan and Odell (1983) give importance to prior levels of participation, the kin network size, and social class considerations as being more important than the relative role losses experienced alone or role losses experienced with resulting negative life changes. Thus, neither notions of relative deprivation nor past history (in seeking assistance) will suffice in arriving at conclusions about whether or not men face special disadvantages in their old age.

In fact, there are no simple reasons for believing that elderly men, *in toto*, can and should be referred to in sweeping generalities. Certainly the chapters in this book suggest that elderly men, as a group, appear more dissimilar than alike, and chapter authors also suggest the strong interrelationships between idiosyncratic characteristics (i.e., personalities, sexual orientations, and values) of elderly men and the problems that they face. Additionally, authors in this book have addressed the importance of such social and cultural variables as socioeconomic class, racial and ethnic background, urban-rural location, religion, and marital status, among others.

In conclusion, it can be assumed that elderly men, as a group, may be more heterogeneous than homogeneous. And might it be that there are more similarities between elderly men and women than there are differences?

The following represents an overview of the issues which have emerged from the chapters with regard to both commonalities and differences in the characteristics and problems of elderly men. This overview is not meant to be exhaustive, but suggestive of the need for further research which will both highlight the characteristics and the needs of elderly men, and will offer possible policy and programmatic guidelines for improving efforts to better meet their needs.

CHAPTER SUMMARIES

While elderly men might be considered to be "better off" than older women, in fact, this is true primarily for heterosexual, married, middle-class, white, elderly men. Consistently, throughout the book, there were suggestions that race, ethnicity, and social class must be factored into any discussion regarding the inherent challenges and opportunities of later life for men.

Certainly, more privileged (and mainly white) groups of elderly men can expect to experience the continuation of a variety of benefits associated with the more affluent in American society with regard to greater longevity, more employment opportunities, superior housing and retirement alternatives, and lower rates of victimization and incarceration.

However, those elderly men from lower socioeconomic classes and/or racial and ethnic minority groups can often anticipate a different set of benefits, including lower suicide rates, lower levels of economic loss resulting from retirement and unemployment, and more likely to be eligible for certain types of means criteria-driven programs and services.

Other key variables which preclude generalizations of elderly men pertain to sexual orientation, marital status, and geographic (urban/suburban/rural) location. Clearly, homosexual partnerships and friendships, and the supportive nature of the gay community, provide the elderly gay man with an effective alternative to more traditional forms of family support and care. Yet, discrimination may result in some programs not adequately serving a gay population. Furthermore, gays may choose not to seek assistance from resources serving straight elderly men and/or elderly women.

While elderly men in urban areas might be particularly vulnerable to inner-city crime, life for elderly men within rural communities has probably been romanticized, in that they may neither have family or other informal support systems in geographical proximity, nor readily accessible formal service systems. Again, efforts to discuss elderly men, and to compare them to elderly women, must be tempered by qualifications and specificity regarding similarities and differences in group characteristics when gender is being considered.

But, it is undeniable that older men do face the greater propensity for certain adversities than do older women, and ignoring or minimizing such situations is unfortunate. Elderly men, of course, suffer from male-related health conditions (i.e., heart disease, prostate cancer), and in addition are more likely to commit suicide, to be involved in car and job-related accidents, and to live out their old age within prisons. Elderly men are more likely to become victims of crime or abuse. They are more likely to abuse alcohol—explained (in part) by their male socialization and loss of self-image. And the very fact that men are less long-lived compared to women, may be the ultimate measure of how difficult the aging experience is for them (Rubinstein, 1996).

APPLIED IMPLICATIONS

From an applied perspective, there are special challenges in meeting the needs of elderly men. As caregivers, older men may not be well prepared for their responsibilities. They may be more likely to remain stoically burdened, isolated, and lonely. And they may be less likely to become involved in support groups or access caregiver respite services. As has been discussed, support groups generally do not meet the needs of lower-class, racial, and ethnic minority group members of any age, and they continue to be underutilized by elderly men.

At a more subtle, but not necessarily a less important, level, elderly men are more likely to find themselves in the minority within retirement communities, institutional settings, and as participants in community-based services and programs. Resulting—in part—from negative attitudes toward help-seeking behavior, they may be precluded from participating in support groups and community services, even when such interventions are available to meet their needs. The fact that such resources are often female-dominated can be expected to add to the reluctance on the part of elderly men to participate.

Community services for the elderly have been discussed as being either couple-oriented or dominated by female participants. Elderly men have been found to be underutilizers of community resources, not necessarily motivated to assume roles as volunteers, and less likely to use therapeutic interventions that are of a clinical nature. Institutional care may, in particular, represent a challenge to the male's desire for control and independence, given the likelihood that—once institutionalized—elderly men can expect to find themselves in a "world" dominated by female residents and female members of the staff.

Perhaps in this period of economic conservativism in expenditures for community services, any thoughts regarding the need for greater specificity in the populations targeted for community resources will be viewed as naive and wasteful. Yet, the question must be asked whether or not community resources for the elderly should be configured in a manner which reflects greater sensitivity to the potential benefits of separate programs, services, groups, and facilities for men and women. Implicit in such a consideration is the awareness of the unique nuances of specific activities that are likely to be successful in reaching out and attracting elderly men and ultimately meeting the needs of this population. For example, in a study of an outpatient treatment program for alcohol-and pharmacological-abusing elderly, Kosberg and Dobson (1994) found that older men were uncomfortable verbalizing their problems in proximity to female program participants, and that the older women were uncomfortable being in physical proximity to substance-abusing men.

Also implicit in such a question regarding separateness in service provision is whether or not it is gender—rather than such considerations as religion, education, ethnicity, race, or social class—which is related to resource acceptance and consumption. In the Kosberg and Dobson (1994) study, the ability to speak the dominant language, to be expressive and articulate, and hold dominant values were all influential in acceptance of, and continuation in, the treatment program.

While it is unlikely that there will be social settings constructed on a large-scale basis especially for unmarried heterosexual elderly men (i.e., retirement communities, institutions), there is a good possibility that such separate facilities will exist for gay elderly men. Indeed, inasmuch as social and health services exist specifically for elderly gay men (whether or not related to AIDS), it is more than likely that housing options will also increasingly become available for such elderly males.

FUTURE PROJECTIONS

Chapters in this book have primarily focused upon current cohorts of elderly men and women. Thus, it is important to anticipate likely changes in the future in the differences and similarities between elderly men and women. While occurring too slowly for some, gender equity is increasingly evidenced. With it, the narrowing of distinctions between the economic, social, and psychological profiles of the sexes can be anticipated.

Women have been "emancipated" from the home and from traditional female-oriented jobs. Men, too, have been "emancipated" from their gender dominance at home and on the job. Men have also been released from their traditional macho self-images, probably resulting from either the consequences of the feminist movement in the United States or from the acculturation of immigrating individuals who had embraced antiquated and traditional gender-related norms of behavior.

The increased blurring of gender distinctions challenges the projections of futurists. Indeed, in considering the characteristics of elderly men in the future in relationship to present cohorts, there are several questions in need of answers. First of all, how extreme and extensive will be the blurring of the distinctions between men and women, generally, and between older men and women, in particular?

One might ask whether there will be greater economic and employment equity resulting in the reduction of economic privileges for men and an increase in economic privileges for women. While such equity is to be applauded, might such "improved" conditions for women be associated with an increase in the incidence of certain types of problems generally associated with the male gender: suicide, job-site accidents, substance abuse, victimization, and adverse consequences of retirement and relative deprivation? One can also speculate upon possible benefits to men resulting from a reduction in the macho ideal and involvement in the "rat race," and a sharing with women of both family and economic responsibility.

Additionally, one might inquire as to whether there will be a lessening of distinctions on the basis of race and ethnicity. Always a powerful influence, the socioeconomic status of elderly men may become more important than their racial or ethnic or religious backgrounds. And, again, what will the relationship be between backgrounds, status, and gender in the incidence of problems and solutions to such problems?

Where will the elderly men of the future dwell? Will there be a migration from rural to urban areas, where there exists more affordable housing and community resources? Or, will there be a migration from urban areas, where crime and overcrowding may exist, to surrounding suburban areas?

With the current trend for longer, and permanent, prison sentences and, therefore, the likelihood of a growing elderly prison population, will elderly prisoners live out their lives integrated with younger prison populations, segregated into separate wards and facilities, or discharged back into the community? Will retirement communities continue to exist for white middle-class and better educated elderly persons, or will such housing options be available and utilized by a more representative sample of all elderly persons?

WHO SHALL SPEAK FOR ELDERLY MEN?

A great deal has been learned about the current cohort of elderly men. Less is known about future cohorts of elderly men and the society within which they will coexist with elderly women and younger persons of both sexes. It has been pointed out, at the beginning of this chapter, that elderly men have been perceived to be an invisible group; yet—at once—powerful, privileged, impaired, and incompetent. Who shall take the lead in correcting biased and stereotypic generalizations about elderly men? Will men assume responsibility for taking the lead themselves?

Certainly, there appear to be examples of opportunities for increasing the self-awareness and self-identity of men in contemporary American society. Beginning with *The Seasons of a Man's Life* (Levinson, 1978), the study of men from four occupational groups, there have been a number of books focusing upon men and masculine issues. A few examples are *Iron John: A Book About Men* by Bly (1992); *Being A Man: A Guide to the New Masculinity* by Fanning and McKay (1993); *The Male Stress Syndrome* by Witkin (1986); *The Seven Seasons of a Man's Life* by Morley (1995); *The Worth of a Man* by Dravecky (1996); and *Double Bind: Escaping the Contradictory Demands of Manhood* by Cooper (1996).

Although focusing upon men, aside from the Levinson book, only in Bly's book is there reference made to elderly men, and then the discussion pertains to changes in the role of older men resulting in their presently being "distrusted." The other texts fail to focus upon the elderly and—in fact—are either self-help books (Fanning & McKay, 1993; Witkin, 1986) or have a decidedly Christian orientation (Cooper, 1996; Dravecky, 1996; Morley, 1995).

Even in Levinson's "classic" study (1978) of the developmental perspectives on adulthood in a sample of 40 men, the age range is from the late teens until the latter 40s. There is minimal attention to men in their later middle-age and old-age years. Thus, the literature has neither adequately addressed the needs of elderly men, nor advocated for increased concern and attention for this group of men.

There have been several relatively recent events which have focused upon men in contemporary American society. While many persons, African-American and others, might question the motivations of its convener, Reverend Louis Farrakhan, the recent Million Man March in Washington, D. C. has been widely applauded for attempting to confirm the importance and role of African-American men. And, there is evidence to suggest that such assemblies may now be organized at the regional and local levels.

Promise Keepers, a fast growing Christian-oriented men's movement in North America, seeks to reconfirm the responsibility of men as loving, sensitive, and faithful husbands and fathers. In addition to large rallies, members meet in small groups where they hold each other accountable for spiritual, moral, ethical, and sexual purity, and for building strong marriages through the expression of love, protection, and Biblical values. Not addressed by these efforts nor specifically included for discussion, however, are the needs and concerns of elderly men in contemporary society.

Such groups and such assemblies can be perceived to represent a defensive response to widespread criticisms of men as irresponsible, absent, and unfaithful. While true of some men, such negative views of contemporary man are simplistic and are unfair to those who are very much committed to being loyal, lawful, and moral persons. Again, it is difficult to detect if any of these efforts at reconfirming the role of men in the family have any particular concerns regarding the role and importance of elderly men.

DIVERSE GROUPS OF ADVOCATES

In a general way, there are several different collectivities advocating for men, in general, and potentially for elderly men, in particular.

The first group are those who may be said to advocate for the feminization of males so to embrace some of the attributes which are characteristic of females. It has been suggested that men need to be more "female-like," sensitive, caring, sympathetic, etc. It is believed that this perspective envisions men being in a defensive and apologetic stance, and encourages them to assume supportive and secondary roles to women. These advocates seek to compensate women (and society) for the powerful and domineering role of men earlier in the history of American society.

It is suspected that older men, socialized during earlier times, might not be particularly inclined to support goals and objectives that may be perceived as promoting the demasculination of contemporary men. Indeed, with some justification, some elderly men (and younger men) might believe that these male advocates seek to empower women and, as a result, place men (not women) in dependent roles.

Another group of advocates for men's issues may be considered to be a response to the efforts (and success) of the feminist movement. Many of these men are motivated by the perceived injustices having been perpetrated against contemporary men in the workplace and in the home. Special considerations given to females in hiring and promotion and from the judicial system's actions against men (as husbands, former husbands, and fathers) are developments not well received by some men. Possible collective actions by men in this "camp" include challenges to court decisions regarding placement of children with mothers, alimony payments, visitation rights with children, and preferential treatment given by government to female owners of businesses and preferential hiring and promotion of female employees.

On the one hand, men who take issue with these developments can be viewed to be conservative reactionaries or traditionalists. However, others are responding to injustices they see resulting from the militancy of the women's movement and/or resulting from traditional gender-specific roles which are, in fact, changing in contemporary society. For example, there has been increasing attention given to the possibility of men as single parents. Indeed, it has been suggested that homes where single fathers care for children younger than 18 years of age are the fastest-growing family group in America, and that the group of more than 9 million single fathers found in the 1990 census is expected to increase (J. Getlin, *Miami Times*, 1996).

The publication of recent books on the topic of single fathers include *Dance Real Slow* (Jaffe, 1995); *Another Way Home* (Thorndike, 1996); *The Magic Summer: A Season with my Son* (Grant, 1995); *Single Fatherhood* (Gregg, 1995); and *Family Man* (Coltrane, 1996). There is a widely held belief that increasingly men are not only raising children, but being economically dependent upon women, and choosing to be "househusbands." Thus, court decisions and public policies which routinely favor women as opposed to men must be re-evaluated.

Thus, it is believed that concern about the needs and problems of men in contemporary society is growing, but it is still unclear whether or not such a movement will touch upon the needs of elderly men. It is unknown whether or not the concerns regarding this cadre of men will continue longitudinally as they age, or whether their concerns around the issue of male fatherhood will blossom into other areas of male concern, including those facing elderly men.

It is suspected that although some elderly men might have been penalized as a result of inequitable divorce decrees or had raised children singlehandedly, past court actions were most likely expected and accepted during times when the role of wife and mother was dependent (socially, psychologically, and economically) upon the man. And the man, seen as the powerful one in the family, was always seen to be the guilty and/or responsible one.

A third collective of male advocates concerns itself with the status of homosexual men. Generally, this group has not coalesced as well as it might with other men's groups, and cannot be viewed, as yet, to be a major player in efforts to ensure the rights of all men. Interestingly, though, if there are any effective efforts to improve and safeguard the lives of elderly men, it is those aimed at elderly gay men, and change is being advocated by a cross-section of the gay community. Clearly, in the "elderly man's movement," the gay community is in the vanguard.

A final collective of men that can be identified is the emergence of male advocates who neither embrace the notion of women's nor men's rights, but rather affirm the notion of gender equity. This group has linkages with both groups, and seeks to ensure that a blind preoccupation with gender does not impair notions of justice, equity, and fairness. While such notions might have given the impetus and direction to the women's movement, more contemporary efforts are needed to ensure that gross and negative overgeneralizations do not inappropriately stain the image of contemporary man. This concern for "fair play" applies to the view and treatment of elderly men in contemporary society.

Although it remains to be seen whether or not these four general orientations toward men can coalesce with one another, it is doubtful. In the future it will it be disclosed whether or not the needs and rights of elderly men will be better represented in scientific research, in the community resources available to the elderly, and in the concerns and policies of the citizenry. While attention toward, and the study of, men in contemporary society is minute compared to women, it is suspected that the future will disclose increased attention. Whether or not the contemporary efforts focusing upon younger groups of men will expand to include attention to older men, whether those currently engaged in advocacy of younger men will first become concerned about the rights of elderly men as they enter old age, or whether those concerned about elderly men will provide the impetus for action remains to be seen in the coming years.

CONCLUSION

Whether seen in stereotypic fashion through humor, the media, or in popular opinion, the view of elderly men is in need of more realistic and equitable treatment. Such a perspective is needed not only out of a sense of fairness to older men, but—as discussed throughout this book—in recognition that elderly men have problems which need to be identified, understood, and responded to by effective programs and services.

Who will be the advocates for this group—gerontologists, representatives of the elderly, representatives from the men's movement, concerned citizens, or human service workers? What seems clear is that there is currently the need for attention to the special needs of elderly men and the special challenges to meet their needs. Only to the extent that support can surface from multiple sectors of the professional and lay community will advocacy efforts likely become more meaningful and effective.

And as newer cohorts of elderly men emerge, so too will their needs and challenges undergo change. Thus, not only must there be assurance that elderly men will no longer remain an invisible group, but that their changing profiles will continuously be monitored.

This chapter, this book, is not about emphasizing the needs of elderly men at the expense of the needs of elderly women. That would be as unfortunate as continuing to disregard the needs of elderly men. Indeed, feminist gerontologist, Dr. Nancy Hooyman (1996), in debating the case that aging is more problematic for women than men, comes to the conclusion that " . . . , our energies as practitioners and researchers should be focused on identifying ways to improve the lives of both women and men who fall below the poverty line, face loneliness and physical and mental health problems, and are denied access to adequate health and long-term care" (p. 135). Yet, it is believed, such as balanced concern for elderly men and elderly women necessitates a balanced degree of concern and regard for the elderly men equal to that of elderly women.

What is called for is a rejection of over-generalizations which portray all elderly men as well-off, powerful, and content (or all elderly women as impoverished, dependent, and depressed). Such conclusions are doomed to be incorrect, unfair, and will preclude the level of specificity needed for effective programmatic interventions. Elderly men, as a group, are more dissimilar than they are alike. Yet, they do have special needs which demand special consideration by those in the helping professions and from those entrusted to enact effective policies and procedures which focus upon the needs of all citizens — males and females.

REFERENCES

Barer, B. M. (1994). Men and women aging differently. *The International Journal of Aging and Human Development, 38*, 29–40.

Bly, R. (1992). *Iron John: A book about men.* New York: Vintage Books.

Coltrane, S. (1996). *Family man.* Oxford: Oxford University Press.

Cooper, L. (1996). *Double bind: Escaping the contradictory demands of manhood.* Grand Rapids, NY: Zondervan.

Dravecky, D. (1996). *The worth of a man.* Grand Rapids, NY: Zondervan.

Fanning, P., & McKay, M. (1993). *Being a man: A guide to the new masculinity.* Oakland, CA: New Harbinger.

Gent, P. (1995). *The last magic summer: A season with my son.* New York: Morrow.

Getlin, J. (1995). *Authors explore the lives of suddenly single dads. The Miami Times*, March 27, pp. C1, C3.

Grant, A. (1995). The magic summer: A search with my son. Fairfield, NJ. Morrow Press.

Gregg, C. (1995). *Single fatherhood.* New York: National Book Network.

Hooyman, N. R. (1996). Is aging more problematic for women than men? Yes. (pp. 125–135). In A. E. Scharlach & L. W. Kaye, (Eds.), Controversial issues in aging. Needham Heights, MA: Allyn & Bacon.

Jaffe, M. G. (1995). *Dance real slow.* New York: Farrar, Straus, & Giroux.

Kosberg, J. I., & Dobson, F. (1993). *Group treatment for older substance abusers: Issues related to the homogeneity and heterogeneity of group composition.* Unpublished paper presented at the 22nd Annual Scientific and Educational Meeting of the Canadian Association of Gerontology (October), Montreal, Quebec.

Levinson, D. J. (1978). *The seasons of a man's life.* New York: Ballantine.

Morley, P. M. (1995). *The seven seasons of a man's life.* Nashville, TN: Thomas Nelson.

Rubinstein, R. L. (1996). Is aging more problematic for women than men? No. (pp. 125–135). In A. E. Scharlach & L. W. Kaye, (Eds.), *Controversial issues in aging.* Needham Heights, MA: Allyn & Bacon.

Thompson, E. H., Jr. (1994). Older men as invisible men in contemporary society. In E. H. Thompson, Jr. (Ed.), *Older men's lives* (pp. 1–21). Thousand Oaks, CA: Sage.

Thorndike, J. (1996). *Another way home.* New York: Crown.

Wan, T. T. H., & Ode, B. G. (1983). Major role losses and social participation of older males. *Research on Aging, 5*, 173–196.

Witkin, G. A. (1986). *The male stress syndrome.* New York: Newmarket.

Index

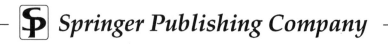 *Springer Publishing Company*

Fatherhood and Families in Cultural Context

Frederick W. Bozett, RN, DNS
Shirley M.H. Hanson, RN, PhD, Editors

Defining "culture" in its broadest sense, this multidisciplinary volume synthesizes contemporary research and theories about males as parents—and the multiple cultural factors influencing their socialization and enactment of the family role. Foreword by Michael E. Lamb.

Contents

Springer Series: Focus on Men
1991 290pp 0-8261-6570-2 hardcover

536 Broadway, New York, NY 10012-3955 • (212) 431-4370 • Fax (212) 941-7842

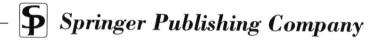

Gender Issues Across The Life Cycle

Barbara Rubin Wainrib, EdD, Editor

This diverse and fascinating volume goes beyond simply helping to sharpen the existing models of male and female adult development. It probes the implications of those developmental and social shifts for clinicians struggling with day-to-day gender issues arising within the clinical context. The result is a richly conceived and well-executed exploration of issues that are basic to us all—as people and as practitioners.

> Gender
> Issues
> Across the
> Life Cycle
>
> *Barbara Rubin Wainrib*
> Editor
>
> 🅢 *Springer Publishing Company*

Partial Contents:

Who's Who and What's What: The Effects of Gender on Development in Adolescence, *W.J. Cosse* • Clinical Issues in the Treatment of Adolescent Girls, *A. Rubenstein* • The Worst of Both Worlds: Dilemmas of Contemporary Young Women, *N. McWilliams* • Gender Issues of the Young Adult Male, *M. Goodman* • The New Father Roles, *R.F. Levant* • The Thirty-Something Woman: To Career or Not to Career, *F. Denmark* • Thirty-Plus and Not Married, *F. Kaslow* • Motherhood in the Age of Reproductive Technology, *S. Mikesell* • Helping Men at Midlife: Can the Blind Ever See? *A.L. Kovacs* • Motherhood and Women's Gender Role Journeys: A Metaphor for Healing, Transition, and Transformation, *J.M. O'Neil and J. Eagan*

Behavioral Science Book Service Selection
1992   224pp   0-8261-7680-1   hardcover

536 Broadway, New York, NY 10012-3955 • (212) 431-4370 • Fax (212) 941-7842

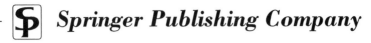

Springer Publishing Company

Men Healing Shame
An Anthology

Roy U. Schenk & **John Everingham,** Editors
Featuring **Robert Bly** and **Gershen Kaufman**

In this pioneering work, the editors and contributors identify the underlying (previously hidden) social and cultural causes of shame in men's lives, as well as its effects, and then discuss theoretical models and methods of treatment to help men process their shame. This volume also considers the possible impact of the women's movement on men's feelings of shame and is inspired by the current men's movement in psychology. This volume will be of interest to psychologists and professionals who counsel men.

Springer Series: Focus on Men
1995   352pp   0-8261-8800-1   hardcover

536 Broadway, New York, NY 10012-3955 • (212) 431-4370 • Fax (212) 941-7842

Springer Publishing Company

Becoming A Father
Contemporary Social, Emotional, and Clinical Perspectives

Jerrold L. Shapiro, PhD, **Michael J. Diamond,** PhD, and **Martin Greenberg,** MD, Editors

Foreword: **T. Berry Brazelton**

One of the most important events in men's lives is becoming a father. This transition has life long psychological, social, and emotional effects. In this volume, the editors and contributors explore both the dramatic increase in the involvement of fathers in pregnancy, childbirth, and early parenting, as well as the implications of fatherhood from a sociocultural, psychodynamic, and personal perspective.

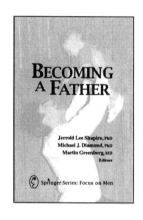

Partial Contents:

I. The Social Perspective. The Changing Role of Fathers, *M. Lamb* • The Paternal Presence, *K. Pruett* • Bringing in Fathers: The Reconstruction of Mothering, *D. Ehrensaft* • The Mother's Role in Promoting Fathering Behavior, *P. Jordan* • When Men Are Pregnant, *J. Shapiro* • Support for Fathers: A Model For Hospital-Based Parenting Programs, *P. Shecket* • Fatherhood, Numbness, and Emotional Self-Awareness, *R. Levant* • Teaching Responsible Fathering, *C. Ballard & M. Greenberg* • Teen Fathers: The Search for the Father, *M. Greenberg & H. Brown*

II. Personal Perspective. Three Tries To Get It Right, *L. Peltz* • Essay for Father's Day, *L. Kutner* • The New Father and The Old: Understanding the Relational Struggle of Fathers, *S. Osherson* • The Father Wound: Implications for Expectant Fathers, *J. Pleck* • Engrossment Revisited, *A. Bader*

III. The Clinical Perspective. Shifting Patterns of Fathering in the First Year of Life, *J. Hyman* • Becoming a Father, *M. Diamond* • Some Reflections on Adaptive Grandiosity in Fatherhood, *P. Wolson* • A Delicate Balance, *W. Pollack* • During the Transition to Fatherhood, *B. Sachs*

Springer Series: Focus on Men
1995 408pp 0-8261-8400-6 hardcover

536 Broadway, New York, NY 10012-3955 • (212) 431-4370 • Fax (212) 941-7842